Biorefineries –
Industrial Processes and
Products

Edited by
Birgit Kamm,
Patrick R. Gruber,
and Michael Kamm

Related Titles

Elvers, B. (Ed.)

Handbook of Fuels
Energy Sources for Transportation

2006
ISBN 3-527-30740-0

Olah, G. A., Goeppert, A., Prakash, G. K. S.

Beyond Oil and Gas: The Methanol Economy

2006
ISBN 3-527-31275-7

Shahidi, F. (Ed.)

Bailey's Industrial Oil and Fat Products
6 Volume Set

2005
ISBN 0-471-38460-7

Ocic, O.

Oil Refineries in the 21st Century
Energy Efficient, Cost Effective, Environmentally Benign

2005
ISBN 3-527-31194-7

Biorefineries – Industrial Processes and Products

Status Quo and Future Directions

Volume 1

Edited by
Birgit Kamm, Patrick R. Gruber, and Michael Kamm

WILEY-VCH

WILEY-VCH Verlag GmbH & Co. KGaA

The Editors

Dr. Birgit Kamm
Research Institute
Bioactive Polymer Systems
biopos e.V.
Kantstr. 55
14513 Teltow
Germany

Dr. Patrick R. Gruber
President and CEO
Outlast Technologies Inc.
5480 Valmont Road
Boulder, CO 80301
USA

Michael Kamm
Biorefinery.de GmbH
Stiftstr. 2
14471 Potsdam
Germany

1st Edition 2006
    1st Reprint 2006

Library of Congress Card No.: applied for

British Library Cataloguing-in-Publication Data:
A catalogue record for this book is available from the British Library.

**Bibliographic information published by
Die Deutsche Bibliothek**
Die Deutsche Bibliothek lists this publication in the Deutsche Nationalbibliografie; detailed bibliographic data is available in the Internet at <http://dnb.ddb.de>

© 2006 WILEY-VCH Verlag GmbH & Co. KGaA, Weinheim, Germany

Typesetting K+V Fotosatz GmbH, Beerfelden
Printing Betz-Druck GmbH, Darmstadt
Binding Litges & Dopf Buchbinderei GmbH, Heppenheim

Printed in the Federal Republic of Germany
Printed on acid-free paper

ISBN-13: 978-3-527-31027-2
ISBN-10: 3-527-31027-4

Contents

Volume 1

Biorefineries – Industrial Processes and Products. Status Quo and Future Directions. Vol. 1
Edited by Birgit Kamm, Patrick R. Gruber, Michael Kamm
Copyright © 2006 WILEY-VCH Verlag GmbH & Co. KGaA, Weinheim
ISBN: 3-527-31027-4

Volume 2

Editor's Preface

In the year 2003 when the idea for this set of books "Biorefineries, Biobased Industrial Processes, and Products" arose, the topic of biorefineries as means of processing industrial material and efficient utilization of renewable products had been primarily a side issue beyond the borders of the United States of America. This situation has changed dramatically over the last two years. Today in almost every developed and emerging nation much work is being conducted on biorefinery systems, driven by the rising cost of oil and the desire of to move away from petrochemical-based systems.

In these books we do not claim to describe and discuss everything that belongs or even might belong to the topic of biorefineries – that would be impossible. There are many types of biorefinery, and the state of the technology is changing very rapidly as new and focused effort is directed toward making biorefineries a commercial reality. It is a very exciting time for those interested in biorefineries – technologies for bio-conversion have advanced to a state in which they are becoming practical on a large scale, economics are leaning more favourably to the direction of renewable feedstocks, and chemical process knowledge is being applied to biobased systems.

As the editors of the first comprehensive biorefinery book we saw it as our duty to provide, first of all, a general framework for the subject – addressing the main issues associated with biorefineries, the principles and basics of biorefinery systems, the basic technology, industrial products which fall within the scope of biorefineries, and, finally, technology and products that will fall within the scope of biorefineries in the future.

To provide a reliable description of the state of biorefinery research and development and of industrial implementations, strategies, and future developments we asked eighty-five experts from universities, research and development institutes, and industry and commerce to present their views, their results, their implementations, and their ideas on the topic. The results of their contributions are thirty-three articles organized into seven sections. Our very special thanks go to all the authors.

We are especially indebted to Dr. Hubert Pelc from Wiley-VCH publishing, who worked with us on the concept and then, later, on the development and implementation of the book. Thanks go also to Dr. Bettina Bems from Wiley-

Biorefineries – Industrial Processes and Products. Status Quo and Future Directions. Vol. 1
Edited by Birgit Kamm, Patrick R. Gruber, Michael Kamm
Copyright © 2006 WILEY-VCH Verlag GmbH & Co. KGaA, Weinheim
ISBN: 3-527-31027-4

VCH publishing, who managed with admirable professionalism and very much patience, and to the three editors and eighty-five authors from three different continents. We are also indebted to Hans-Jochen Schmitt, also of Wiley-VCH publishing, who had the not always easy task of arranging the manuscripts in a form ready for publication.

Maybe in 2030, when a biobased economy utilizing biorefinery technology has become a fundamental part of national and globally connected economies, someone will wonder what had been thought and written about the subject of biorefineries at the beginning of the 21st century. Hopefully this book will be highly representative. Until then we hope it will contribute to the promotion of international biorefinery developments.

Teltow-Seehof (Germany)   Birgit Kamm
Boulder, CO (USA)   Patrick R. Gruber
Potsdam (Germany)   Michael Kamm

November 2005

Foreword

One-hundred-and-fifty years after the beginning of coal-based chemistry and 50 years after the beginning of petroleum-based chemistry industrial chemistry is now entering a new era. In the twenty-first century utilization of renewable raw materials will gain importance in the chemical conversion of substances in industry. Partial or even complete re-adjustment of whole economies to renewable raw materials will require completely new approaches in research, development, and production. Chemical and biological sciences will play a leading role in the building of future industries. New synergies between biological, physical, chemical, and technical sciences must be elaborated and established and special requirements will be placed on raw material and on product-line efficiency and sustainability. The necessary change from chemistry based on a fossil raw material to biology-based modern science and technology is an intellectual challenge for both researchers and engineers. Chemists should support this change and collaborate closely with their colleagues in adjoining disciplines, for example biotechnology, agriculture, forestry, and the material sciences.

The German Chemical Society will help direct this necessary development by supporting within its structure new kinds of organization for chemists to work on this subject in universities, research institutes, and industry.

This two-volume book is based on the approach developed by biorefinery-systems – transfer of the logic and efficiency of today's petrochemical product lines and product family trees into manipulation of biomass. Raw biomass materials are mechanically separated into substances for chemical conversion into other products by different methods, which may be biotechnological, thermochemical, and thermal. Review of biomass processes and products developed in the past but widely forgotten in the petroleum age will be as important as the presentation of new methods, processes, and products that still require an enormous amount of research and development today.

Henning Hopf
President of the German Chemical Society
Frankfurt (Germany)

November 2005

Biorefineries – Industrial Processes and Products. Status Quo and Future Directions. Vol. 1
Edited by Birgit Kamm, Patrick R. Gruber, Michael Kamm
Copyright © 2006 WILEY-VCH Verlag GmbH & Co. KGaA, Weinheim
ISBN: 3-527-31027-4

Foreword

On October 5, 2005, the Nobel Prize Committee made an interesting and important statement with regard to the prize in chemistry. It said, "This represents a great step forward for 'green chemistry', reducing potentially hazardous waste through smarter production. [This research] is an example of how important basic science has been applied for the benefit of man, society and the environment." By making this statement, the Nobel committee recognized what a new generation of scientists has known for quite some time, that by working at the most fundamental level – the molecular level – we are able to design our products, processes, and systems in ways that are sustainable.

There is general recognition that the current system by which we produce the goods and services needed by society is not sustainable. This unsustainability takes many forms. It would be legitimate to note that in our current system of production we rely largely on finite feedstocks extracted from the Earth that are being depleted at a rate that cannot be sustained indefinitely. It is equally legitimate to recognize that our current production efficiency results in more than 90% of the material used in the production process ending up as waste, i.e. less than 10% of the material ends up in the desired product. Yet another condition of unsustainability is in our current energy use; this not only relies largely on finite energy sources but also results in degradation of the environment that cannot be continued as the growing population and demands of the developing world emerge over the course of the twenty-first century. Finally, the products and processes we have designed since the industrial revolution have accomplished their goals without full consideration of their impact and consequence on humans and the biosphere, with many examples of toxic and hazardous substances being distributed throughout the globe and into our bodies.

If we are to change this unsustainable path, it will need the direct and committed engagement of our best scientists and engineers to design the future differently from the past. We will need to proceed with a broader perspective such that when we design for efficiency, effectiveness, and performance, we now must recognize that these terms include sustainability – a minimized impact on humans and the environment.

An essential part of meeting the challenge of designing for sustainability will be based on the nature of the materials we use as starting materials and feedstocks. Any sustainable future must ensure that the materials on which we base

Biorefineries – Industrial Processes and Products. Status Quo and Future Directions. Vol. 1
Edited by Birgit Kamm, Patrick R. Gruber, Michael Kamm
Copyright © 2006 WILEY-VCH Verlag GmbH & Co. KGaA, Weinheim
ISBN: 3-527-31027-4

our economic infrastructure are renewable rather than depleting. The rate of renewability is also important because certainly one could argue that petroleum is renewable if you have a few million years to wait. Serious analysis would, however, necessitate that the rate of renewability is connected to the rate of use. There are options for how to approach this technological challenge, for example using waste products from one process as a feedstock for another, that are well thought through in industrial ecology models. There is, however, recognition that an essential part of a sustainable future will be based on appropriate and innovative uses of our biologically-based feedstocks.

This book addresses the essential questions and challenges of moving toward a sustainable society in which bio-based feedstocks, processes, and products are fundamental pillars of the economy. The authors discuss not only the important scientific and technical issues surrounding this transition but also the necessary topics of economics, infrastructure, and policy. It is only by means of this type of holistic approach that movement toward genuine sustainability will be able to occur where the societal, economic, and environmental needs are met for the current generation while preserving the ability of future generations to meet their needs.

While it will be clear to the reader that the topics presented in this book are important, it is at least as important that the reader understand that these topics – and the transition to a sustainable path that they address – are urgent. At this point in history it is necessary that all who are capable of advancing the transition to a more sustainable society, engage in doing so with the level of energy, innovation, and creativity that is required to meet the challenge.

Paul T. Anastas
Director of the Green Chemistry Institute
Washington, D.C.

November, 2005

List of Contributors (Volume 1 and 2)

José A. M. Agnelli
Universidade Federal de São Carlos
Departamento de Engenharia
de Materiais
Rodovia Washington Luis (SP-310)
São Carlos, São Paulo
Brazil

Margrethe Andersen
AgroFerm A/S
Limfjordsvej 4
6715 Esbjerg N
Denmark

Rolf Bachmann
McKinsey and Company Inc
Zurich Office
Alpenstrasse 3
8065 Zürich
Switzerland

Ursula Biermann
Fachbereich Chemie
Carl von Ossietzky Universität
Oldenburg
Postfach 2603
26111 Oldenburg
Germany

Robert C. Brown
Center for Sustainable Environmental
Technologies
Iowa State University
286 Metals Development Building
Ames, IO 50011
USA

Gösta Brunow
Department of Chemistry
University of Helsinki
A. I. Virtasen aukio 1
00014 Helsinki
Finland

Stefan Buchholz
Degussa AG
Creavis
Projecthouse ProFerm
Rodenbacher Chaussee 4
63403 Hanau-Wolfgang
Germany

Rainer Busch
Dow Deutschland GmbH & Co. OHG
Industriestrasse 1
77836 Rheinmünster
Germany

Biorefineries – Industrial Processes and Products. Status Quo and Future Directions. Vol. 1
Edited by Birgit Kamm, Patrick R. Gruber, Michael Kamm
Copyright © 2006 WILEY-VCH Verlag GmbH & Co. KGaA, Weinheim
ISBN: 3-527-31027-4

Grant M. Campbell
Satake Centre for Grain Process
Engineering
School of Chemical Engineering and
Analytical Science
The University of Manchester
Sackville Street
Manchester M60 1QD
UK

Joel R. Cherry
Novozymes Biotech Inc
1445 Drew Ave
Davis, CA 95616
USA

Gopal Chotani
Genencor International
925 Page Mill Road
Palo Alto, CA 94304
USA

L. Davis Clements
Renewable Products Development
Laboratories
3114 NE 45th Ave.
Portland, OR 97213
USA

Bruce E. Dale
Department of Chemical Engineering
and Materials Science
Michigan State University
East Lansing, MI 48824
USA

Bill Dean
Genencor International
925 Page Mill Road
Palo Alto, CA 94304
USA

Tim Dodge
Genencor International
925 Page Mill Road
Palo Alto, CA 94304
USA

Donald L. Van Dyne
Agricultural Economics
University of Missouri – Columbia
214c Mumford Hall
Columbia, MO 65211
USA

Wolter Elbersen
Agrotechnology and Food Innovations
B.V.
P.O. Box 17
6700 AA Wageningen
The Netherlands

Steve Fitzpatrick
Biofine
245 Winter Street
Waltham, MA 02154
USA

Paul Fowler
The BioComposites Centre
University of Wales
Bangor
Gwynedd LL57 2UW
UK

Wolfgang Friedt
Institut für Pflanzenbau
und Pflanzenzüchtung 1
Justus-Liebig-Universität Giessen
Heinrich-Buff-Ring 26–32
35392 Giessen
Germany

John Frye
Pacific Northwest National Laboratory
P.O. Box 999/K2-12
Richland, WA 99352
USA

Patrick R. Gruber
President and CEO
Outlast Technologies Incorporated
5480 Valmont Road
Suite 200
Boulder, CO 80301
USA

Dietmar R. Grüll
Südzucker Aktiengesellschaft
Mannheim/Ochsenfurt
Wormser Strasse 11
67283 Obrigheim/Pfalz
Germany

Daniel J. Hayes
Department of Chemical
& Environmental Sciences
University of Limerick
Limerick
Ireland

Michael H. B. Hayes
Department of Chemical
& Environmental Sciences
University of Limerick
Limerick
Ireland

David E. Henton
Nature Works LLC
(former Cargill Dow LLC)
15305 Minnetonka Blvd
Minnetonka, MN 55345
USA

James R. Hettenhaus
CEA Inc
3211 Trefoil Drive
Charlotte, NC 28226
USA

Karlheinz Hill
Cognis Deutschland GmbH & Co. KG
Paul-Thomas-Straße 56
40599 Düsseldorf
Germany

Thomas Hirth
Fraunhofer-Institut
Chemische Technologie
Joseph-von-Fraunhoferstraße 7
76327 Pfinztal
Germany

John Holladay
Pacific Northwest National Laboratory
P.O. Box 999/K2-12
Richland, WA 99352
USA

Franz Jetzinger
Zuckerforschung Tulln
Gesellschaft mbH
Josef-Reither-Strasse 21–23
3430 Tulln
Austria

Donald L. Johnson
Biobased Industrial Products
Consulting
29 Cape Fear Drive
Hertford, NC 27944
USA

Ed de Jong
Agrotechnology and
Food Innovations B.V.
P.O. Box 17
6700 AA Wageningen
The Netherlands

Birgit Kamm
Research Institute Bioactive Polymer
Systems (biopos e.V.)
Research Centre Teltow-Seehof
Kantstraße 55
14513 Teltow
Germany

Michael Kamm
Biorefinery.de GmbH
Stiftstraße 2
14471 Potsdam
Germany
and
Laboratories Teltow
Kantstraße 55
14513 Teltow
Germany

Raphael Katzen
9220 Bonita Beach Road
Suite 2000
Bonita Springs, FL 34135
USA

Ralf Kelle
Degussa AG
R & D Feed Additives
Kantstrasse 2
33790 Halle/Westfalen
Germany

Pauli Kiel
Biotest Aps
Gl. Skolevej 47
6731 Tjæreborg
Denmark

Seungdo Kim
Department of Chemical Engineering
and Materials Science
Michigan State University
East Lansing, MI 48824
USA

Apostolis A. Koutinas
Satake Centre for Grain Process
Engineering
School of Chemical Engineering and
Analytical Science
The University of Manchester
Sackville Street
Manchester M60 1QD
UK

Martin Kozich
Zuckerforschung Tulln
Gesellschaft mbH
Josef-Reither-Strasse 21–23
3430 Tulln
Austria

George A. Kraus
Department of Chemistry
Iowa State University
1605 Gilman Hall
Ames, IA 50011-3111
USA

Thomas C. Kripp
Wella AG
Abt. FON
Berliner Allee 65
64274 Darmstadt
Germany

Stefan Kromus
BioRefSYS-BioRefinery Systems
Innovationszentrum Ländlicher Raum
Auersbach 130
8330 Feldbach
Austria

Siegmund Lang
Institut für Biochemie
und Biotechnologie
Technische Universität
zu Braunschweig
Spielmannstraße 7
38106 Braunschweig
Germany

Frieder W. Lichtenthaler
Institute of Organic Chemistry
Darmstadt University of Technology
Petersenstraße 22
64287 Darmstadt
Germany

Wilfried Lühs
Institut für Pflanzenbau
und Pflanzenzüchtung 1
Justus-Liebig-Universität Giessen
Heinrich-Buff-Ring 26–32
35392 Giessen
Germany

Guido Machmüller
FB 9 – Organische Chemie
Bergische Universität
GH Wuppertal
Gaußstraße 20
42097 Wuppertal
Germany

Paulo E. Mantelatto
Centro de Tecnologia Canavieira
(formerly Centro de Tecnologia
Copersucar)
Fazenda Santo Antonio
CP 162
13400-970 Piracicaba
Brazil

Achim Marx
Degussa AG
Creavis
Projecthouse ProFerm
Rodenbacher Chaussee 4
63403 Hanau-Wolfgang
Germany

Jürgen O. Metzger
Fachbereich Chemie
Carl von Ossietzky Universität
Oldenburg
Postfach 2603
26111 Oldenburg
Germany

Michael Narodoslawsky
Graz University of Technology
Institute of Resource Efficient and
Sustainable Systems (RNS)
Inffeldgasse 21 B
8010 Graz
Austria

Jefter Nascimento
PHB Industrial SA
Fazenda da Pedra
s/n – C. Postal 02
CEP 14150 Servana
São Paulo
Brazil

Glenn E. Nedwin
Novozymes Biotech Inc
1445 Drew Ave
Davis, CA 95616
USA

Ulf Prüße
Federal Agricultural Research Centre
(FAL)
Institute of Technology and
Biosystems Engineering
Bundesallee 50
38116 Braunschweig
Germany

E. Kendall Pye
Lignol Innovations Corp.
3650 Westbrook Mall
Vancouver, BC
V6S 2L2
Canada

René van Ree Rea
Energy research Centre
of the Netherlands (ECN) –
Biomass Department
P.O. Box 1
1755 ZG Petten
The Netherlands

Julia Richter
Institut für Chemie
Universität Potsdam
Karl-Liebknecht-Str. 24–25
14476 Golm
Germany

Jens Riese
McKinsey and Company Inc
Munich Office
Prinzregentenstraße 22
80538 München
Germany

Julian R. H. Ross
University of Limerick
Department of Chemical
& Environmental Sciences
Limerick
Ireland

Carlos Eduardo Vaz Rossell
Centro de Tecnologia Canavieira
(formerly Centro de Tecnologia
Copersucar)
Fazenda Santo Antonio
CP 162
13400-970 Piracicaba
Brazil

Mark Rüsch gen. Klaas
Department Technology
University of Applied Sciences
Neubrandenburg
Brodaer Straße 2
17033 Neubrandenburg
Germany

Hans J. Schäfer
Organisch-Chemisches Institut
Universität Münster
Corrensstraße 40
48149 Münster
Germany

Daniel J. Schell
National Bioenergy Center
National Renewable Energy
Laboratory
1617 Cole Blvd.
Golden, CO 80401-3393
USA

Matthias Schmidt
Biorefinery.de GmbH
Stiftstraße 2
14471 Potsdam
Germany

Manfred P. Schneider
FB 9 – Organische Chemie
Bergische Universität
GH Wuppertal
Gaußstraße 20
42097 Wuppertal
Germany

Margit Schulze
FB Angewandte Naturwissenschaften
FH Bonn-Rhein-Sieg
Grantham-Allee 20
53754 Sankt Augustin
Germany

Mathias O. Senge
SFI Tetrapyrrole Laboratory
School of Chemistry
Trinity College Dublin
Dublin 2
Ireland

Jack Starr
Cargill Dow LLC
15305 Minnetonka Blvd
Minnetonka, MN 55345
USA

Sarah A. Teter
Novozymes Biotech Inc
1445 Drew Ave
Davis, CA 95616
USA

Johan Thoen
Dow Europe GmbH
Bachtobelstrasse 3
8810 Horgen
Switzerland

Mette Hedegaard Thomsen
Risø National Laboratory
Biosystems Department
Frederiksbovgvej 399
4000 Roskilde
Denmark

Jeffrey S. Tolan
Iogen Corporation
8 Colonnade Road
Ottawa
Ontario K2E 7M6
Canada

Robert van Tuil
Agrotechnology and Food Innovations
B.V.
P.O. Box 17
6700 AA Wageningen
The Netherlands

Dan W. Urry
BioTechnology Institute
University of Minnesota
Twin Cities Campus
1479 Gortner Avenue
Suite 240
St. Paul, MN 55108-6106
USA
and
Bioelastics Inc.
2423 Vestavia Drive
Vestavia Hills, AL 35216-1333
USA

Fernando Valle
Genencor International
925 Page Mill Road
Palo Alto, CA 94304
USA

Klaus-Dieter Vorlop
Federal Agricultural Research Centre
(FAL)
Institute of Technology and
Biosystems Engineering
Bundesallee 50
38116 Braunschweig
Germany

Rouhang Wang
Satake Centre for Grain Process
Engineering
School of Chemical Engineering and
Analytical Science
The University of Manchester
Sackville Street
Manchester M60 1QD
UK

Marnik M. Wastyn
Zuckerforschung Tulln
Gesellschaft mbH
Josef-Reither-Strasse 21–23
3430 Tulln
Austria

Colin Webb
Satake Centre for Grain Process
Engineering
School of Chemical Engineering and
Analytical Science
The University of Manchester
Sackville Street
Manchester M60 1QD
UK

Volker F. Wendisch
Institute of Biotechnology 1
Research Center Juelich
52425 Juelich
Germany

Todd Werpy
Pacific Northwest National Laboratory
P.O. Box 999/K2-12
Richland, WA 99352
USA

Thomas Willke
Federal Agricultural Research Centre
(FAL)
Institute of Technology and
Biosystems Engineering
Bundesallee 50
38116 Braunschweig
Germany

Robert Wittenberger
Zuckerforschung Tulln
Gesellschaft mbH
Josef-Reither-Strasse 21–23
3430 Tulln
Austria

Feng Xu
Novozymes Biotech Inc
1445 Drew Ave
Davis, CA 95616
USA

Part I
Background and Outline – Principles and Fundamentals

Biorefineries – Industrial Processes and Products. Status Quo and Future Directions. Vol. 1
Edited by Birgit Kamm, Patrick R. Gruber, Michael Kamm
Copyright © 2006 WILEY-VCH Verlag GmbH & Co. KGaA, Weinheim
ISBN: 3-527-31027-4

1
Biorefinery Systems – An Overview

Birgit Kamm, Michael Kamm, Patrick R. Gruber, and Stefan Kromus

1.1
Introduction

The preservation and management of our diverse resources are fundamental political tasks to foster sustainable development in the 21st century. Sustainable economic growth requires safe and sustainable resources for industrial production, a long-term and confident investment and finance system, ecological safety, and sustainable life and work perspectives for the public. Fossil resources are not regarded as sustainable, however, and their availability is more than questionable in the long-term. Because of the increasing price of fossil resources, moreover, the feasibility of their utilization is declining.

It is, therefore, essential to establish solutions which reduce the rapid consumption of fossil resources, which are not renewable (petroleum, natural gas, coal, minerals). A forward looking approach is the stepwise conversion of large parts of the global economy into a sustainable biobased economy with bioenergy, biofuels, and biobased products as its main pillars (Fig. 1.1).

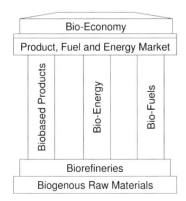

Fig. 1.1 3-Pillar model of a future biobased economy.

Biorefineries – Industrial Processes and Products. Status Quo and Future Directions. Vol. 1
Edited by Birgit Kamm, Patrick R. Gruber, Michael Kamm
Copyright © 2006 WILEY-VCH Verlag GmbH & Co. KGaA, Weinheim
ISBN: 3-527-31027-4

Whereas for energy production a variety of alternative raw materials (wind, sun, water, biomass, nuclear fission and fusion) can be established, industry based on conversion of sustainable material, for example the chemical industry, industrial biotechnology, and also the fuel generation, depends on biomass, in particular mainly on plant biomass.

Some change from the today's production of goods and services from fossil to biological raw materials will be essential. The rearrangement of whole economies to implement biological raw materials as a source with increased value requires completely new approaches in research and development. On the one hand, biological and chemical sciences will play a leading role in the generation of future industries in the 21st century. On the other hand, new synergies of biological, physical, chemical, and technical sciences must be elaborated and established. This will be combined with new traffic technology, media- and information technology, and economic and social sciences. Special requirements will be placed on both the substantial converting industry and research and development with regard to raw material and product line efficiency and sustainability.

The development of substance-converting basic product systems and poly-product systems, for example biorefineries, will be the "key for the access to an integrated production of food, feed, chemicals, materials, goods, and fuels of the future" [1].

1.2
Historical Outline

1.2.1
Historical Technological Outline and Industrial Resources

Today's biorefinery technologies are based (1) on the utilization of the whole plant or complex biomass and (2) on integration of traditional and modern processes for utilization of biological raw materials. In the 19th and the beginning of the 20th century large-scale utilization of renewable resources was focused on pulp and paper production from wood, saccharification of wood, nitration of cellulose for guncotton and viscose silk, production of soluble cellulose for fibers, fat curing, and the production of furfural for Nylon. Furthermore, the technology of sugar refining, starch production, and oil milling, the separation of proteins as feed, and the extraction of chlorophyll for industrial use with alfalfa as raw material were of great historical importance. But also processes like wet grinding of crops and biotechnological processes like the production of ethanol, acetic acid, lactic acid, and citric acid used to be fundamental in the 19th and 20th century.

1.2.2
The Beginning – A Digest

1.2.2.1 **Sugar Production**
The history of industrial conversion of renewable resources is longer than 200 years. Utilization of sugar cane has been known in Asia since 6000 BC and imports of cane sugar from oversea plantations have been established since the 15th century. The German scientist A.S. Marggraf was a key initiator of the modern sugar industry. In 1748 he published his research on the isolation of crystalline sugar from different roots and beet [2, 3]. Marggraf's student, F.C. Achard, was the first to establish a sugar refinery based on sugar beet, in Cunern/Schlesien, Poland, in 1801.

1.2.2.2 **Starch Hydrolysis**
In 1811, the German pharmacist G.S.C. Kirchhoff found that when potato starch was cooked in dilute acid the starch was converted into "grape sugar" (i.e. *d*-glucose or dextrose) [4]. This was not only a very important scientific result but also the starting point of the starch industry. In 1806 the French emperor Napoleon Bonaparte introduced an economic continental blockade which considerably limited overseas trade in cane sugar. Thus, starch hydrolysis became of interest for the economy. The first starch sugar plant was established in Weimar, Germany, in 1812, because of a recommendation of J.W. Döbereiner to grand duke Carl August von Sachsen-Weimar. Successful development of the sugar beet industry, however, initially obstructed further development of the starch industry [5]. In 1835, the Swedish Professor J.J. Berzelius developed enzymatic hydrolyses of starch into sugar and introduced the term "catalysis".

1.2.2.3 **Wood Saccharification**
In 1819 the French plant chemist H. Braconnot discovered that sugar (glucose) is formed by treatment of wood with concentrated sulfuric acid. 1855, G.F. Melsens reported that this conversion can be carried out with dilute acid also. Acid hydrolysis can be divided into two general approaches, based on (1) concentrated acid hydrolysis at low temperature and (2) dilute acid hydrolysis at high temperature. Historically, the first commercial processes, named wood saccharification, were developed in 1901 by A. Classen (Ger. Patent 130980), employing sulfuric acid, and in 1909 by M. Ewen and G. Tomlinson (US Patent 938208), working with dilute sulfuric acid. Several plants were in operation until the end of World War I. Yields of these processes were usually low, in the range 75–130 liter per ton wood dry matter only [6, 7]. Technologically viable processes were, however, developed in the years between World War I and World War II. The German chemist Friedrich Bergius was one of the developers. The sugar fractions generated by wood hydrolyses have a broad spectrum of application. An important fermentation product of wood sugar of increasing interest is ethanol.

Ethanol can be used as fuel either blended with traditional hydrocarbon fuel or as pure ethanol. Ethanol is also an important platform chemical for further processing [8].

1.2.2.4 Furfural

Döbereiner was the first to report the formation and separation of furfural by distillation of bran with diluted sulfuric acid in 1831. In 1845 the English Chemist G. Fownes proposed the name "furfurol" (furfur – bran; oleum – oil). Later the suffix "ol" was changed to "al" because of the aldehyde function [9, 10].

Treatment of hemicellulose-rich raw materials with dry steam in the presence of hydrogen chloride gave especially good results [11]. Industrial technology for production of furfural from pentose is based on a development of an Anglo-American company named Quaker Oats. The process was been developed in the nineteen-twenties [E. P. 203691 (1923), F. P. 570531 (1923)]. Since 1922 Quaker Oats Cereal Mill in Cedar Rapids/Iowa, USA, has produced up to 2.5 tons of furfural per day from oat husks. Since 1934 the process had been established as an industrial furfural plant. Furfural was the cheapest aldehyde, at 16–17 cents per lb (lb = pound; 1 metric ton = 1000 kg = 2204.62442 lb; 1 kg = 0.453592 lb) [12]. Until approximately 1960 DuPont used furfural as a precursor of Nylon-6.6. Furfural has since been substituted by fossil based precursors.

1.2.2.5 Cellulose and Pulp

In 1839 the Frenchman A. Payen discovered that after treatment of wood with nitric acid and subsequent treatment with a sodium hydroxide solution a residue remained which he called "les cellules", cellulose [13]. In 1854 caustic soda and steam were used by the Frenchman M. A. C. Mellier to disintegrate cellulose pulp from straw. In 1863 the American B. C. Tilgham registered the first patent for production of cellulose by use of calcium bisulfite. Together with his brother, Tilgham started the first industrial experiments to produce pulp from wood by treatment with hydrogen sulfite. This was 1866 at the paper mill Harding and Sons, Manayunk, close to Philadelphia. In 1872 the Swedish Engineer C. D. Ekman was the first to produce sulfite cellulose by using magnesium sulfite as cooking agent [14]. By 1900 approximately 5200 pulp and paper mills existed worldwide, most in the USA, approximately 1300 in Germany, and 512 in France.

1.2.2.6 Levulinic Acid

In 1840 the Dutch Professor G. J. Mulder (who also introduced the name "protein") synthesized levulinic acid (4-oxopentanoic acid, γ-ketovaleric acid) by heating fructose with hydrochloride for the first time. The former term "levulose" for fructose gave the levulinic acid its name [15]. Although levulinic acid has been well known since the 1870s when many of its reactions (e.g. esters) were established, it has never reached commercial use in any significant volume. In the 1940s commercial levulinic acid production was begun in an autoclave in the United States by A. E. Staley, Dectur, Illinois [16]. At the same time utilization of hexoses from low-cost cellulose products was examined for the production of levulinic acid [17]. As early as 1956 levulinic acid was regarded as a platform chemical with high potential [18].

1.2.2.7 Lipids

From 1850 onward European import of tropical plant fats, for example palm-oil and coconut oil, started. Together with the soda process, invented by the French N. Leblanc in 1791, the industrialization of the soap production began and soap changed from luxury goods into consumer goods. The developing textile industry also demanded fat based products. In 1902 the German chemist W. Normann discovered that liquid plant oils are converting into tempered fat by augmentation of hydrogen. Using nickel as catalyst Norman produced tempered stearic acid by catalytic hydration of liquid fatty acids [19]. The so called "fat hardening" led to the use of European plant oils in the food industry (margarine) and other industries.

1.2.2.8 Vanillin from Lignin

In 1874 the German chemists W. Haarmann and F. Tiemann were the first to synthesize vanillin from the cambial juice of coniferous wood. In 1875 the company Haarmann and Reimer was founded. The first precursor for the production of vanillin was coniferin, the glucoside of coniferyl alcohol. This precursor of lignin made from cambial juice of coniferous trees was isolated, oxidized to glucovanillin, and then cleaved into glucose and vanillin [20]. This patented process [21] opened the way to industrial vanillin production. It was also the first industrial utilization of lignin. Besides the perfume industry, the invention was of great interest to the upcoming chocolate industry. Later, however, eugenol (1-allyl-4-hydroxy-3-methoxybenzene), isolated from clove oil, was used to produce vanillin. Today, vanillin production is based on lignosulfonic acid which is a side product of wood pulping. The lignosulfonic acid is oxidized with air under alkaline conditions [22, 23].

1.2.2.9 Lactic Acid

In 1895 industrial lactic acid fermentation has been developed by the pharmaceutical entrepreneur A. Boehringer. The Swedish pharmacist C. W. Scheele had already discovered lactic acid in 1780 and the conversion of carbohydrates into lactic acid had been known for ages in food preservation (e.g. Sauerkraut) or agriculture (silage fermentation). Because of the activity of Boehringer the German company Boehringer-Ingelheim can be regarded as the pioneer of industrial biotechnology. Both the process and the demand for lactic acid by dyeing factories, and the leather, textile, and food industries made the company the leading supplier. In 1932 W. H. Carothers, who was also the inventor of polyamide-6.6, developed, together with van Natta, a polyester made from lactic acid, poly(lactic acid) [24]. In the late 1990s this poly(lactic acid) was commercialized by the company NatureWorks (Cargill, the former Cargill Dow) [25].

1.2.3
The Origins of Integrated Biobased Production

In the year 1940 the German chemist P. von Walden (noted for his "Inversion of configuration at substitution reactions", the so-called "Walden-Reversion") calculated that in 1940 Germany produced 13 million tons of cellulose leaving 5 to 6 million tons of lignin suitable only as wastage. He then formulated the question: How long can national economy tolerate this [26]? Approaches to integrated production during industrial processing of renewable primary products have a long tradition, starting from the time when industrial cellulose production expanded continuously, as also did the related waste-products. Typical examples of this will be mentioned.

As early as 1878 A. Mitscherlich, a German chemist, started to improve the sulfite pulp process by fermentation of sugar to ethyl alcohol – it should be mentioned that sugar is a substance in the waste liquor during sulfite pulp production. He also put into practice a procedure to obtain paper glue from the waste liquor. Both processes were implemented in his plant located in Hof, Germany, in the year 1898 [27].

In 1927 the American Marathon Corporation assigned a group of chemists and engineers to the task of developing commercial products from the organic solids in the spent sulfite liquor from the Marathon's Rothschild pulp and paper operations close to Wausau, Wisconsin, USA. The first products to show promise were leather tanning agents. Later, the characteristics of lignin as dispersing agents became evident. By the mid 1930s, with a considerable amount of basic research accomplished, Marathon transferred operations from a research pilot plant to full-scale production [28].

One of the most well known examples is the production of furfural by the Quaker Oats Company since 1922, thus coupling food, i.e. oat flakes, production and chemical products obtained from the waste [10] (Section 1.2.2). On the basis of furfural a whole section of chemical production developed – furan chemistry.

Agribusiness, especially, strived to achieve combined production from the very beginning. Modern corn refining started in the middle of the 18th century when T. Kingsford commenced operation of his corn refining plant in Oswego, New York [29]. Corn refining is distinguished from corn milling because the refining process separates corn grain into its components, for example starch, fiber, protein and oil, and starch is further processed into a substantial number of products [30].

The extensive usage of green crops has been aim of industry for decades, because there are several advantages. Particularly worthy of mention is the work of Osborn (1920) and Slade and Birkinshaw (1939) on the extraction of proteins from green crops, for example grass or alfalfa [31].

In 1937 N.W. Pirie developed the technical separation and extraction methods needed for this use of green crops [32, 33]. By means of sophisticated methods all the botanical material should have been used, both for production of animal feed, isolated proteins for human nutrition, and as raw material for further industrial processes, for example glue production. The residual material, juices rich in nutrients, had initially been used as fertilizer; later they were used for generation of fermentation heat based on biogas production [34, 35].

These developments resulted in market-leading technology, for example the Proxan and Alfaprox procedures, used for generation of protein–xanthophyll concentrates, including utilization of the by-products, however, predominantly in agriculture [36].

In the United States commercial production of chlorophyll and carotene by extraction from alfalfa leaf meal had started in 1930 [37, 38]. For example Strong, Cobb and Company produced 0.5 ton chlorophyll per day from alfalfa as early as 1952. The water-soluble chlorophyll, or chlorophyllin, found use as deodorizing agent in toothpastes, soaps, shampoos, candy, deodorants, and pharmaceuticals [39].

A historical important step for today's biorefinery developments was the industry-politics-approach of "Chemurgy", founded in 1925 in the US by the Chemist W.J. Hale, son-in-law of H. Dow, the founder of Dow Chemical, and C.H. Herty, a former President of the American Chemical Society. They soon found prominent support from H. Ford and T.A. Edisons. Chemurgy, an abbreviation of "chemistry" and "ergon", the Greek word for work [40], means by analogy "chemistry from the acre" that is the connection of agriculture with the chemical industry.

Chemurgy was soon shown to have a serious industrial political philosophy – the objective of utilizing agricultural resources, nowadays called renewable resources, in industry. There have been common conferences between agriculture, industry, and science since 1935 with a national council called the "National Farm Chemurgic Council" [41]. The end of Chemurgy started with the flooding of the world market with cheap crude oil after World War II; numerous inventions and production processes remained, however, and are again highly newsworthy. One was a car, introduced by Henry Ford 1941, whose car interior lining and car body consisted 100% of bio-synthetics; to be specific it had been made from a cellulose meal, soy meal, formaldehyde resin composite material in the proportions 70% : 20% : 10%, respectively. The alternative fuel for this car was pyrolysis methanol produced from cannabis. Throughout the thirties more than 30 industrial products based on soy bean were created by researchers from the Ford company; this made it necessary to apply complex conversion methods [42]. Hale was a Pioneer of ethyl alcohol and hydrocarbon fuel mixture (Power Alcohol, Gasohol) [43]. This fuel mixture, nowadays called E10-Fuel, consisting of 10 percent bioethanol and 90 percent hydrocarbon-based fuel, has been the national standard since the beginning of this millennium in the United States.

Associated with the work of Bergius, 1933 [44], and Scholler, 1923 and 1935 [45, 46], wood saccharification was reanimated at the end of WW II. Beside optimization of the process, use of lignocelluloses was of great interest. The continuously growing agribusiness left behind millions of tons of unused straw. Two Americans, Othmer and Katzen, were the main pioneers in the field of wood saccharification [47]. Between the years 1935 and 1960 several hydrolysis plants were built in Germany and the United States; in these deal, wood flour, surplus lumber, and also straw were hydrolyzed [48]. One of the most well known plants are those of Scholler/Tornesch located in Tornesch, Germany, with a production rate of 13,000 tons per year, in Dessau, Germany, production rate 42,000 tons per year, based on wood, in Holzminden, Germany, production rate of 24,000 tons per year, also based on wood, in Ems, Switzerland, with a production rate of 35,000 tons per year, also wood based, and the plants in Madison and Springfield, United States, and the Bergius plants in Rheinau, Germany (Rheinau I, built 1930, with a production rate of 8000 tons per year, based on surplus lumber; Rheinau II, built 1960 with a production rate of 1200 tons per year, based on wood) and the plant in Regensburg, Germany, with a production rate of 36,000 tons per year [49].

During WW II the plant in Springfield, Oregon, US (using the Scholler-Tornesch process as modified by Katzen) produced 15,000 gallons of ethyl alcohol per day from 300 tons wood flour and sawdust, i.e. 50 gallons per ton of wood [50]. The plant in Tornesch, Germany, has been producing approximately 200 liters of ethyl alcohol, purity 100%, per ton wood and approximately 40 kg yeast per ton of wood. In 1965 there were 14 plants in what was then the Soviet Union, with a total capacity of 700,000 tons per year and an overall annual wood consumption of 4 million tons [6].

During the nineteen-sixties wood chemistry had its climax. Projects had been developed, which made it possible to produce nearly all chemical products on the basis of wood. Examples are the complex chemical technological approaches of wood processing from Timell 1961 [51], Stamm 1964 [52], James 1969 [53], Brink and Pohlmann 1972 [54], and the wood-based chemical product trees by Oshima 1965 [55]. Although these developments did not make their way into industrial production, they are an outstanding platform for today's lignocellulose conversions, product family trees, and LCF biorefineries (Section 1.5.2).

Most of the above mentioned technologies and products, some of which were excellent, could not compete with the fossil-based industry and economy; nowadays, however, they are prevailing again. The basis for this revival started in the seventies, when the oil crisis and continuously increasing environmental pollution resulted in a broad awareness that plants could be more than food and animal feed. At the same time the disadvantages of intensive agricultural usage, for example over-fertilization, soil erosion, and the enormous amounts of waste, were revealed. From this situation developed complex concepts, which have been published, in which the aim was, and still is, technological and economical cooperation of agriculture, forestry, the food-production industry, and conventional industry, or at least consideration of integrated utilization of renewable resources.

Typical examples of this thinking were:

- integrated industrial utilization of wood and straw [56];
- industrial utilization of fast growing wood-grass [57, 58];
- complex utilization of green biomass, for example grass and alfalfa, by agriculture and industry [59–61];
- corn wet-grinding procedures with associated biotechnological and chemical product lines [62];
- modern aspects of thermochemical biomass conversion [63];
- discussion of the concept "organic chemicals from biomass" with main focus on biotechnological methods and products (white biotechnology) [64–66] and industrial utilization of biomass [67].

These rich experiences of the industrial utilization of renewable resources, new agricultural technology, biotechnology, and chemistry, and the changes in ecology, economics, and society led inevitably to the topic of complex and integrated substantial and energy utilization of biomass and, finally, to the biorefinery.

1.3
Situation

1.3.1
Some Current Aspects of Biorefinery Research and Development

Since the beginning of the 1990s the utilization of renewable resources for production of non-food products has fostered research and development which has received increasing attention from industry and politicians [68–70]. Integrated processes, biomass refinery technology, and biorefinery technology have become object of research and development. Accordingly, the term "biorefinery" was established in the 1990s [1, 71–80]. The respective biorefinery projects are focused on the fabrication of fuels, solvents, chemicals, plastics, and food for human beings. In some countries these biorefinery products are made from waste biomass. At first the main processes in the biorefinery involved ethanol fermentation for fuels (ethanol-oriented biorefineries) [81–85], lactic acid (LA) fermentation [25, 86], propanediol (PDO) fermentation [87], and the lysine fermentation [88] especially for polymer production. The biobased polymers poly(lactic acid) [25], propandiol-derived polymers [89], and polylysine [88] have been completed by polyhydroxyalkanoates [90] and polymerized oils [91].

Many hybrid technologies were developed from different fields, for example bioengineering, polymer chemistry, food science and agriculture. Biorefinery systems based on cereals [92, 93], lignocelluloses [94, 95], and grass and alfalfa [35, 96], and biorefinery optimization tools are currently being developed [97, 98]. The integration of molecular plant genetics to support the raw material supply is currently being discussed intensely [99, 100].

Broin and Associates has begun the development of a second generation of dry mill refineries and E.I. du Pont de Nemours has developed an integrated corn-based biorefinery. In 2001 NatureWorks LCC (to Cargill, former Cargill Dow LLC) started the industrial production of PLA (PLA-oriented Biorefinery) on the basis of maize.

Biorefineries are of interest ecologically [101], economically, and to business, government, and politicians [102–107]. National programs [108, 109], biobased visions [110], and plans [111] have been developed and the international exchange of information is increasing, for example as a result, among others, of series of international congresses and symposia:

1. BIO World Congress on Industrial Biotechnology and Bioprocessing [112];
2. biomass conferences [113, 114];
3. The Green and Sustainable Chemistry Congress [115]; and
4. the Biorefinica symposia series [116, 117].

Currently, biorefinery systems are in the stage of development world-wide. An overview of the main aspects, activity, and discussions is the content of this book. An attempt to systematize the topic "Biorefinery" will be presented below.

1.3.2
Raw Material Biomass

Nature is a permanently renewing production chain for chemicals, materials, fuels, cosmetics, and pharmaceuticals. Many of the biobased industry products currently used are results of direct physical or chemical treatment and processing of biomass, for example cellulose, starch, oil, protein, lignin, and terpenes. On one hand one must mention that because of the help of biotechnological processes and methods, feedstock chemicals are produced such as ethanol, butanol, acetone, lactic acid, and itaconic acid, as also are amino acids, e.g. glutaminic acid, lysine, tryptophan. On the other hand, only 6 billion tons of the yearly produced biomass, $1.7–2.0\times10^{11}$ tons, are currently used, and only 3 to 3.5% of this amount is used in non-food applications, for example chemistry [118].

The basic reaction of biomass is photosynthesis according to:

$$nCO_2 + nH_2O \quad \rightarrow \quad (CH_2O)_n + nO_2$$

Industrial utilization of raw materials from agriculture, forestry, and agriculture is only just beginning. There are several definitions of the term "biomass" [118]:

- the complete living, organic matter in our ecological system (volume/non-specific)
- the plant material constantly produced by photosynthesis with an annual growth of 170 billion tons (marine plants excluded)
- the cell-mass of plants, animals, and microorganism used as raw materials in microbiological processes

Biomass is defined in a recent US program [108, 109]: "The term "biomass" means any organic matter that is available on a renewable or recurring basis (excluding old-growth timber), including dedicated energy crops and trees, agricultural food and feed crop residues, aquatic plants, wood and wood residues, animal wastes, and other waste materials."

For this reason it is essential to define biomass in the context of the industrial utilization. A suggestion for a definition of "industrial biomass" [108, 109] is: "The term "industrial biomass" means any organic matter that is available on a renewable or recurring basis (excluding old-growth timber), including dedicated energy crops and trees, agricultural food and feed crop residues, aquatic plants, wood and wood residues, animal wastes, and other waste materials usable for industrial purposes (energy, fuels, chemicals, materials) and include wastes and co-wastes of food and feed processing."

Most biological raw material is produced in agriculture and forestry and by microbial systems. Forestry plants are excellent raw materials for the paper and

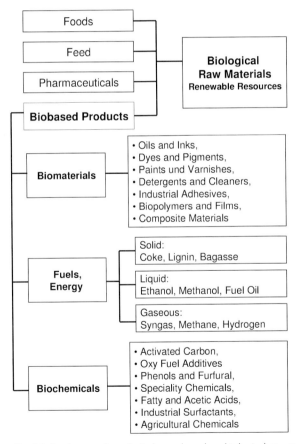

Fig. 1.2 Products and product classes based on biological raw materials [78].

cardboard, construction, and chemical industries. Field fruits are an pool of organic chemicals from which fuels, chemicals, chemical products, and biomaterials are produced (Fig. 1.2), [69]. Waste biomass and biomass of nature and agricultural cultivation are valuable organic reservoirs of raw material and must be used in accordance with their organic composition. During the development of biorefinery systems the term "waste biomass" will become obsolete in the medium-term [119].

1.3.3
National Vision and Goals and Plan for Biomass Technology in the United States

Industrial development was pushed by the US President [108] and by the US congress [109], initially in 2000. In the USA it is intended that by 2020 at least 25% of organic-carbon-based industrial feedstock chemicals and 10% of liquid fuels (compared with levels in 1994) will be produced by biobased industry. This would mean that more than 90% of the consumption of organic chemicals in the US and up to 50% of liquid fuel needs would be biobased products [1].

The Biomass Technical Advisory Committee (BTAC) of the USA in which leading representatives of industrial companies, for example Dow Chemical, E. I. du Pont de Nemours, Cargill Dow LLC, and Genencor International, and Corn growers associations and the Natural Resources Defense Council are involved and which acts as advisor to the US government, has made a detailed plan with steps toward targets of 2030 with regard to bioenergy, biofuels, and bioproducts (Table 1.1) [110].

Simultaneously, the plan *Biomass Technology in the United States* has been published [111] in which research, development, and construction of biorefinery

Table 1.1 The US national vision goals for biomass technologies by the Biomass Technical Advisory Committee [110].

Year	Current	2010	2020	2030
BioPower (BioEnergy) Biomass share of electricity and heat demand in utilities and industry	2.8% (2.7 quad)[a]	4% (3.2 quad)	5% (4.0 quad)	5% (5.0 quad)
BioFuels Biomass share of demand for transportation fuels	0.5% (0.15 quad)	4% (1.3 quad)	10% (4.0 quad)	20% (9.5 quad)
BioProducts Share of target chemicals that are biobased	5%	12%	18%	25%

a) 1 quad = 1 quadrillion BTU = 1 German billiarde BTU;
   BTU = British thermal unit; 1 BTU = 0.252 kcal,
   1 kW = 3413 BTU, 1 kcal = 4.186 kJ

demonstration plants are determined. Research and development are necessary to:

1. increase scientific understanding of biomass resources and improve the tailoring of those resources;
2. improve sustainable systems to develop, harvest, and process biomass resources;
3. improve efficiency and performance in conversion and distribution processes and technologies for development of a host of biobased products and
4. create the regulatory and market environment necessary for increased development and use of biobased products.

The Biomass Advisory Committee has established specific research and development objectives for feedstock production research. Target crops should include oil and cellulose-producing crops that can provide optimum energy content and usable plant components. Currently, however, there is a lack of understanding of plant biochemistry and inadequate genomic and metabolic information about many potential crops. Specific research to produce enhanced enzymes and chemical catalysts could advance biotechnology capabilities.

1.3.4
Vision and Goals and Plan for Biomass Technology in the European Union and Germany

In Europe there are already regulations about substitution of nonrenewable resources by biomass in the field of biofuels for transportation [120] and the "Renewable energy law" of 2000 [121]. According to the EC Directive "On the promotion of the use of biofuels" the following products are regarded as "biofuels":
(a) "bioethanol", (b) "biodiesel", (c) "biogas", (d) "biomethanol", (e) "biodimethyl ether",
(f) "bio-ETBE (ethyl tertiary-butyl ether)" on the basis of bioethanol,
(g) "bio-MTBE (methyl tertiary butyl ether)" on the basis of biomethanol, and
(h) "synthetic biofuels", (i) "biohydrogen", (j) pure vegetable oil

Member States of the EU have been requested to define national guidelines for a minimum amounts of biofuels and other renewable fuels (with a reference value of 2% by 2005 and 5.75% by 2010 calculated on the basis of energy content of all petrol and diesel fuels for transport purposes). Table 1.2 summarizes this goal of the EU and also those of Germany with regard to establishment of renewable energy and biofuel [122, 123].

Today there are no guidelines concerning "biobased products" in the European Union and in Germany. After passing directives relating to bioenergy and biofuels, however, such a decision is on the political agenda. The "biofuels" directive already includes ethanol, methanol, dimethyl ether, hydrogen, and biomass pyrolysis which are fundamental product lines of the future biobased chemical industry.

Table 1.2 Targets of the EU and Germany with regard to the introduction of technologies based on renewable resources.

Year	2001	2005	2010	2020–2050
Bioenergy Share of wind power, photovoltaics, biomass and geothermal electricity and heat demand in utilities and industry	7.5%	–	12.5%	26% (2030) 58% (2050)
Biofuels Biomass share of demand in transportation fuels (petrol and diesel fuels)	1.4%	2.8%	5.75%	20% (2020)
Biobased Products Share of target chemicals that are biobased	8%	–	–	–

In the year 2003, an initiative group called "Biobased Industrial Products" consisting of members from industry, small and middle-class businesses, and research, and development facilities met and formulated a strategy paper, called "BioVision 2030" [124]. This strategy paper has been included in the resolution of the German Government (Deutscher Bundestag) on the topic "Accomplish basic conditions for the industrial utilization of renewable resources in Germany" [125]. An advisory committee consisting of members of the chemical industry, related organizations, research facilities, and universities has been established to generate a plan concerning the formulation of the objectives for the third column, bio-products in Europe (Table 1.2) [126].

1.4
Principles of Biorefineries

1.4.1
Fundamentals

Biomass, similar to petroleum, has a complex composition. Its primary separation into main groups of substances is appropriate. Subsequent treatment and processing of those substances lead to a whole range of products. Petrochemistry is based on the principle of generating simple to handle and well defined chemically pure products from hydrocarbons in refineries. In efficient product lines, a system based on family trees has been built, in which basic chemicals, intermediate products, and sophisticated products are produced. This principle of petroleum refineries must be transferred to biorefineries. Biomass contains the synthesis performance of the nature and has different $C:H:O:N$ ratio from petroleum. Biotechnological conversion will become, with chemical conversion, a big player in the future (Fig. 1.3).

Thus biomass can already be modified within the process of genesis in such a way that it is adapted to the purpose of subsequent processing, and particular target products have already been formed. For those products the term "precursors" is used. Plant biomass always consists of the basic products carbohydrates, lignin, proteins, and fats, and a variety of substances such as vitamins, dyes, flavors, aromatic essences of very different chemical structure. Biorefineries combine the essential technologies which convert biological raw materials into the industrial intermediates and final products (Fig. 1.4).

A technically feasible separation operation, which would enable separate use or subsequent processing of all these basic compounds, is currently in its initial stages only. Assuming that of the estimated annual production of biomass by biosynthesis of 170 billion tons 75% is carbohydrates, mainly in the form of cellulose, starch, and saccharose, 20% lignin, and only 5% other natural compounds such as fats (oils), proteins, and other substances [127], the main attention should first be focused on efficient access to carbohydrates, and their subsequent conversion to chemical bulk products and corresponding final products. Glucose, accessible by microbial or chemical methods from starch, sugar, or cellulose, is, among other things, predestined for a key position as a basic chemical, because a broad range of biotechnological or chemical products is accessible from glucose. For starch the advantage of enzymatic compared with chemical hydrolysis is already known [128].

For cellulose this is not yet realized. Cellulose-hydrolyzing enzymes can only act effectively after pretreatment to break up the very stable lignin/cellulose/

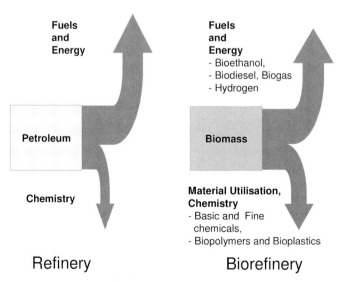

Fig. 1.3 Comparison of the basic-principles of the petroleum refinery and the biorefinery.

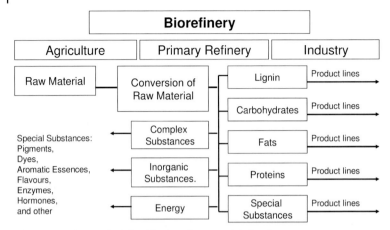

Fig. 1.4 Providing code-defined basic substances (via fractionation) for development of relevant industrial product family trees [78, 79].

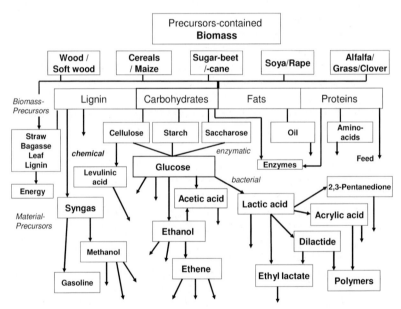

Fig. 1.5 Possible schematic diagram of biorefinery for precursor-containing biomass with preference for carbohydrates [78, 79].

hemicellulose composites [129]. These treatments are still mostly thermal, thermomechanical, or thermochemical, and require considerable input of energy. The arsenal for microbial conversion of substances from glucose is large, and the reactions are energetically profitable. It is necessary to combine degradation processes via glucose to bulk chemicals with the building processes to their subsequent products and materials (Fig. 1.5).

Among the variety of microbial and chemical products possibly accessible from glucose, lactic acid, ethanol, acetic acid, and levulinic acid, in particular, are favorable intermediates for generation of industrially relevant product family trees. Here, two potential strategies are considered: first, development of new, possibly biologically degradable products (follow-up products from lactic and levulinic acids) or, second, entry as intermediates into conventional product lines (acrylic acid, 2,3-pentanedione) of petrochemical refineries [78].

1.4.2
Definition of the Term "Biorefinery"

The young working field "Biorefinery Systems" in combination with "Biobased Industrial Products" is, in various respects, still an open field of knowledge. This is also reflected in the search for an appropriate description. A selection is given below.

The term "Green Biorefinery" was been defined in the year 1997 as: "Green biorefineries represent complex (to fully integrated) systems of sustainable, environmentally and resource-friendly technologies for the comprehensive (holistic) material and energetic utilization as well as exploitation of biological raw materials in form of green and residue biomass from a targeted sustainable regional land utilization" [73]. The original term used in Germany "complex construction and systems" was substituted by "fully integrated systems". The US Department of Energy (DOE) uses the following definition [130]: "A biorefinery is an overall concept of a processing plant where biomass feedstocks are converted and extracted into a spectrum of valuable products. Based on the petrolchemical refinery." The American National Renewable Energy Laboratory (NREL) published the definition [131]: "A biorefinery is a facility that integrates biomass conversion processes and equipment to produce fuels, power, and chemicals from biomass. The biorefinery concept is analogous to today's petroleum refineries, which produce multiple fuels and products from petroleum. Industrial biorefineries have been identified as the most promising route to the creation of a new domestic biobased industry."

There is an agreement about the *objective*, which is briefly defined as: "Developed biorefineries, so called "phase III-biorefineries" or "generation III-biorefineries", start with a biomass–feedstock-mix to produce a multiplicity of most various products by a technologies-mix" [74] (Fig. 1.6).

An example of the type "generation-I biorefinery" is a dry milling ethanol plant. It uses grain as a feedstock, has a fixed processing capability, and produces a fixed amount of ethanol, feed co-products, and carbon dioxide. It has almost no flexibility in processing. Therefore, this type can be used for comparable purposes only.

An example of a type "generation-II biorefinery" is the current wet milling technology. This technology uses grain feedstock, yet has the capability to pro-

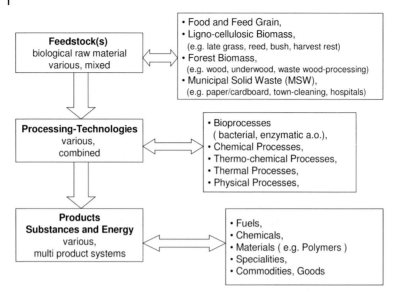

Fig. 1.6 Basic principles of a biorefinery (generation III biorefinery) [78].

duce a variety of end products depending on product demand. Such products include starch, high-fructose corn syrup, ethanol, corn oil, plus corn gluten feed, and meal. This type opens numerous possibilities to connect industrial product lines with existing agricultural production units. "Generation-II biorefineries" are, furthermore, plants like NatureWorks PLA facility [25] (Sections 1.2 and 1.3.1) or ethanol biorefineries, for example Iogen's wheat straw to ethanol plant [132].

Third generation (generation-III) and more advanced biorefineries have not yet been built but will use agricultural or forest biomass to produce multiple products streams, for example ethanol for fuels, chemicals, and plastics.

1.4.3
The Role of Biotechnology

The application of biotechnological methods will be highly important with the development of biorefineries for production of basic chemicals, intermediate chemicals, and polymers [133–135]. The integration of biotechnological methods must be managed intelligently in respect of physical and chemical conversion of the biomass. Therefore the biotechnology cannot remain limited to glucose from sugar plants and starch from starch-producing plants. One main objective is the economic use of biomass containing lignocellulose and provision of glucose in the family tree system. Glucose is a key chemical for microbial processes. The preparation of a large number of family tree-capable basic chemicals is shown in subsequent sections.

1.4.3.1 Guidelines of Fermentation Section within Glucose-product Family Tree

Among the variety of chemical products, and derivatives of these, accessible microbially from glucose a product family tree can be developed, for example (C-1)-chemicals methane, carbon dioxide, methanol; (C-2)-chemicals ethanol, acetic acid, acetaldehyde, ethylene, (C-3)-chemicals lactic acid, propanediol, propylene, propylene oxide, acetone, acrylic acid, (C-4)-chemicals diethyl ether, acetic acid anhydride, malic acid, vinyl acetate, *n*-butanol, crotonaldehyde, butadiene, 2,3-butanediol, (C-5)-chemicals itaconic acid, 2,3-pentane dione, ethyl lactate, (C-6)-chemicals sorbic acid, parasorbic acid, citric acid, aconitic acid, isoascorbic acid, kojic acid, maltol, dilactide, (C-8)-chemicals 2-ethyl hexanol (Fig. 1.7).

Guidelines are currently being developed for the fermentation section of a biorefinery. The question of efficient arrangement of the technological design for production of bulk chemicals needs an answer. Considering the manufacture of lactic acid and ethanol, the basic technological operations are very similar. Selection of biotechnologically based products from biorefineries should be done in a way such that they can be produced from the substrates glucose or pentoses. Furthermore the fermentation products should be extracellular. Fermenters should have batch, feed batch, or CSTR design. Preliminary product recovery should require steps like filtration, distillation, or extraction. Final product recovery and purification steps should possibly be product-unique. In addi-

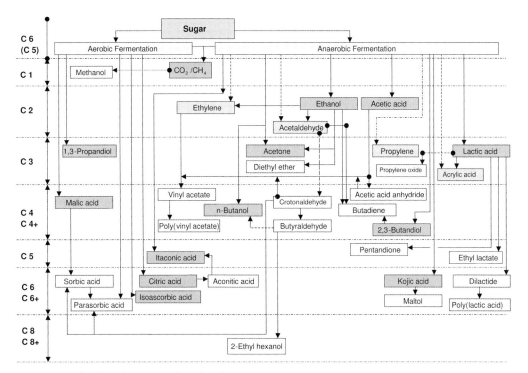

Fig. 1.7 Biotechnological sugar-based product family tree.

tion, biochemical and chemical processing steps should be advantageously connected.

Unresolved questions for the fermentation facility include:

1. whether or not the entire fermentation facility can/should be able to change from one product to another;
2. whether multiple products can be run in parallel, with shared use of common unit operations;
3. how to manage scheduling of unit operations; and
4. how to minimize in-plant inventories, while accommodating necessary change-overs between different products in the same piece of equipment [95].

1.4.4
Building Blocks, Chemicals and Potential Screening

A team from Pacific Northwest National Laboratory (PNNL) and NREL submitted a list of twelve potential biobased chemicals [98]. A key area of the investigation as biomass precursors, platforms, building blocks, secondary chemicals, intermediates, products and uses (Fig. 1.8).

The final selection of 12 building blocks began with a list of more than 300 candidates. A shorter list of 30 potential candidates was selected by using an iterative review process based on the petrochemical model of building blocks, chemical data, known market data, properties, performance of the potential candidates, and previous industry experience of the team at PNNL and NREL. This list of 30 was ultimately reduced to 12 by examining the potential markets for the building blocks and their derivatives and the technical complexity of the synthetic pathways.

The reported block chemicals can be produced from sugar by biological and chemical conversions. The building blocks can be subsequently converted to several high-value biobased chemicals or materials. Building-block chemicals, as considered for this analysis, are molecules with multiple functional groups with the potential to be transformed into new families of useful molecules. The twelve sugar-based building blocks are 1,4-diacids (succinic, fumaric, and malic), 2,5-furandicarboxylic acid, 3-hydroxypropionic acid, aspartic acid, glucaric acid, glutamic acid, itaconic acid, levulinic acid, 3-hydroxybutyrolactone, glycerol, sorbitol, and xylitol/arabinitol [98].

A second-tier group of building blocks was also identified as viable candidates. These include gluconic acid, lactic acid, malonic acid, propionic acid, the triacids citric and aconitic, xylonic acid, acetoin, furfural, levuglucosan, lysine, serine, and threonine. Recommendations for moving forward include:

- examining top value products from biomass components, for example aromatic compounds, polysaccharides, and oils;
- evaluating technical challenges in more detail in relation to chemical and biological conversion; and
- increasing the suites of potential pathways to these candidates.

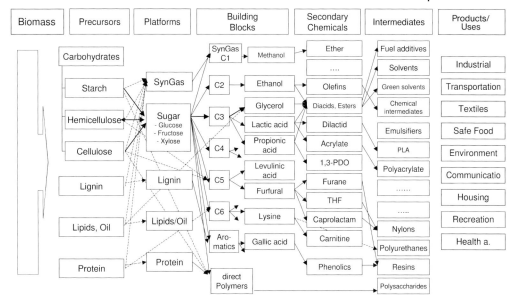

Biomass	Precursors	Platforms	Building Blocks	Secondary Chemicals	Intermediates	Products/ Uses

Fig. 1.8 Model of a biobased product flow-chart for biomass feedstock [98].

No products simpler than syngas were selected. For the purposes of this study hydrogen and methanol comprise the best short-term prospects for biobased commodity chemical production, because obtaining simple alcohols, aldehydes, mixed alcohols, and Fischer-Tropsch liquids from biomass is not economically viable and requires additional development [98].

1.5
Biorefinery Systems and Design

1.5.1
Introduction

Biobased products are prepared for a usable economic use by meaningful combination of different methods and processes (physical, chemical, biological, and thermal). It is therefore necessary that basic biorefinery technologies are developed. For this reason profound interdisciplinary cooperation of various disciplines in research and development is inevitable. It seems reasonable, therefore, to refer to the term "biorefinery design", which means: "bringing together well founded scientific and technological basics, with similar technologies, products, and product lines, inside biorefineries". The basic conversions of each biorefinery can be summarized as follows. In the first step, the precursor-containing biomass is separated by physical methods. The main products (M_1–M_n) and the by-products (B_1–B_n) will subsequently be subjected to microbiological or chemical methods. The follow-up products (F_1–F_n) of the main and by-products can also be converted or enter the conventional refinery (Fig. 1.6).

Currently four complex biorefinery systems are used in research and development:

1. the "lignocellulosic feedstock biorefinery" which use "nature-dry" raw material, for example cellulose-containing biomass and waste;
2. the "whole crop biorefinery" which uses raw material such as cereals or maize;
3. the "green biorefineries" which use "nature-wet" biomasses such as green grass, alfalfa, clover, or immature cereal [78, 79]; and
4. the "biorefinery two platforms concept" includes the sugar platform and the syngas platform [98].

1.5.2
Lignocellulosic Feedstock Biorefinery

Among the potential large-scale industrial biorefineries the lignocellulose feedstock (LCF) biorefinery will most probably be pushed through with the greatest success. On the one side the raw material situation is optimum (straw, reed, grass, wood, paper-waste, etc.), on the other side conversion products have a good position on both the traditional petrochemical and future biobased product market. An important point for utilization of biomass as chemical raw material is the cost of raw material. Currently the cost of corn stover or straw is 30 US$/ ton and that of corn is 110 US$/ton (3 US$/ bushel; US bushel corn =25.4012 kg=56 lb) [136].

Lignocellulose materials consist of three primary chemical fractions or precursors:

- hemicellulose/polyoses, sugar polymers of, predominantly, pentoses;
- cellulose, a glucose polymer; and
- lignin, a polymer of phenols (Fig. 1.9).

The lignocellulosic biorefinery-regime is distinctly suitable for genealogical compound trees. The main advantages of this method is that the natural structures and structural elements are preserved, the raw materials are inexpensive, and large product varieties are possible (Fig. 1.10). Nevertheless there is still a demand for development and optimization of these technologies, e.g. in the field of separation of cellulose, hemicellulose and lignin, and utilization of the lignin in the chemical industry.

$$\text{Lignocellulose} + H_2O \rightarrow \text{Lignin} + \text{Cellulose} + \text{Hemicellulose}$$
$$\text{Hemicellulose} + H_2O \rightarrow \text{Xylose}$$
$$\text{Xylose } (C_5H_{10}O_5) + \text{acid Catalyst} \rightarrow \text{Furfural } (C_5H_4O_2) + 3H_2O$$
$$\text{Cellulose}(C_6H_{10}O_5) + H_2O \rightarrow \text{Glucose } (C_6H_{12}O_6)$$

Fig. 1.9 A possible general equation for conversion at the LCF biorefinery.

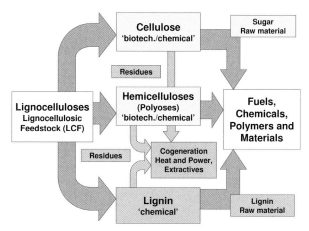

Fig. 1.10 Lignocellulosic feedstock biorefinery.

An overview of potential products of an LCF biorefinery is shown in Fig. 1.11. In particular furfural and hydroxymethylfurfural are interesting products. Furfural is a starting material for production of Nylon 6,6 and Nylon 6. The original process for production of Nylon-6,6 was based on furfural (see also Section 1.2.2). The last of these production plants was closed in 1961 in the USA, for economic reasons (the artificially low price of petroleum). Nevertheless the market for Nylon 6 is huge.

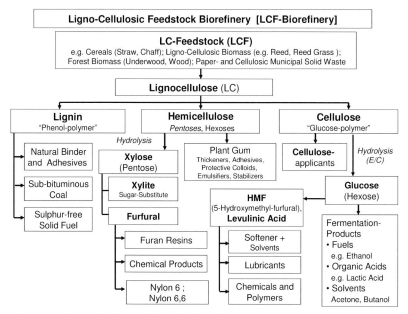

Fig. 1.11 Products of a lignocellulosic feedstock biorefinery (LCF-biorefinery, Phase III) [78, 79, 95].

There are, however, still some unsatisfactory aspects of the LCF, for example the utilization of lignin as fuel, adhesive, or binder. Unsatisfactory because the lignin scaffold contains substantial amounts of mono-aromatic hydrocarbons, which, if isolated in an economically efficient way, could add a significant increase in value to the primary processes. It should be noticed there are no natural enzymes capable of splitting the naturally formed lignin into basic monomers as easily as is possible for natural polymeric carbohydrates or proteins [137].

An attractive process accompanying the biomass-nylon-process is the already mentioned hydrolysis of the cellulose to glucose and the production of ethanol. Some yeasts cause disproportionation of the glucose molecule during their generation of ethanol from glucose, which shifts almost all its metabolism into ethanol production, making the compound obtainable in 90% yield (*w/w*, with regard to the chemical equation for the process).

On the basis of recent technology a plant has been conceived for production of the main products furfural and ethanol from LC feedstock from West Central Missouri (USA). Optimal profitability can be achieved with a daily consumption of approximately 4360 tons of feedstock. The plant produces 47.5 million gallon of ethanol and 323,000 tons of furfural annually [74].

Ethanol can be used as a fuel additive. It is also a connecting product to the petrochemical refinery, because it can be converted into ethene by chemical methods and it is well-known that ethene is at the start of a series of large-scale technical chemical syntheses for production of important commodities such as polyethylene or poly(vinyl acetate). Other petrochemically produced substances, for example hydrogen, methane, propanol, acetone, butanol, butandiol, itaconic acid, and succinic acid, can also be manufactured by microbial conversion of glucose [138, 139].

1.5.3
Whole-crop Biorefinery

Raw materials for the "whole crop biorefinery" are cereals such as rye, wheat, triticale, and maize. The first step is mechanical separation into corn and straw, approximately 10 and 90% (*w/w*), respectively [140]. Straw is a mixture of chaff, nodes, ears, and leaves. The straw is an LC feedstock and may further be processed in a LCF biorefinery.

There is the possibility of separation into cellulose, hemicellulose, and lignin and their further conversion in separate product lines which are shown in the LCF biorefinery. The straw is also a starting material for production of syngas by pyrolysis technology. Syngas is the basic material for synthesis of fuels and methanol (Fig. 1.13).

The corn may either be converted into starch or used directly after grinding to meal. Further processing may be conducted by four processes – breaking up, plasticization, chemical modification, or biotechnological conversion via glucose. The meal can be treated and finished by extrusion into binder, adhesives, and filler.

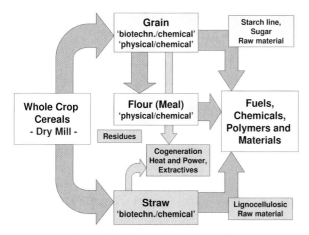

Fig. 1.12 Whole-crop biorefinery based on dry milling.

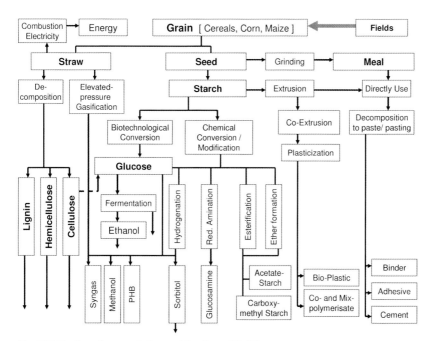

Fig. 1.13 Products from a whole-crop biorefinery [78, 79].

Starch can be finished by plasticization (co- and mix-polymerization, compounding with other polymers), chemical modification (etherification into carboxymethyl starch; esterification and re-esterification into fatty acid esters via acetic starch; splitting reductive amination into ethylenediamine, etc., hydrogenative splitting into sorbitol, ethylene glycol, propylene glycol, and glycerin), and biotechnological conversion into poly-3-hydroxybutyric acid [69, 76, 92, 93, 141].

An alternative to traditional dry fractionation of mature cereals into grains and straw only was been developed by Kockums Construction (Sweden), which later became Scandinavian Farming. In this crop-harvest system whole immature cereal plants are harvested. The whole harvested biomass is conserved or dried for long-term storage. When convenient, it can be processed and fractionated into kernels, straw chips of internodes, and straw meal (leaves, ears, chaff, and nodes) (see also green biorefinery).

Fractions are suitable as raw materials for the starch polymer industry, the feed industry, the cellulose industry, and particle board producers, gluten can be used by the chemical industry and as a solid fuel. Such dry fractionation of the whole crop to optimize the utilization of all botanical components of the biomass has been described [142, 143]. A biorefinery and its profitability has been described elsewhere [144].

One expansion of the product lines in grain processing is the "whole crop wet mill-based biorefinery". The grain is swelled and the grain germ is pressed, releasing high-value oils. The advantages of whole-crop biorefinery based on wet milling are that production of natural structures and structure elements such as starch, cellulose, oil, and amino acids (proteins) are kept high yet well known basic technology and processing lines can still be used. High raw material costs and, for industrial utilization, the necessary costly source technology are the disadvantages. Some of the products formed command high prices in, e.g., the pharmaceutical and cosmetics industries (Figs. 1.14 and 1.15). The basic biorefinery technology of corn wet mills used 11% of the US corn harvest in 1992, made products worth $7.0 billion, and employed almost 10,000 people [1a].

Wet milling of corn yields corn oil, corn fiber, and corn starch. The starch products of the US corn wet milling industry are fuel alcohol (31%), high-fructose corn syrup (36%), starch (16%), and dextrose (17%). Corn wet milling also

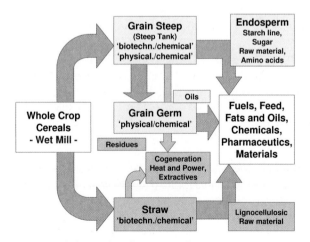

Fig. 1.14 Whole-crop biorefinery, wet-milling.

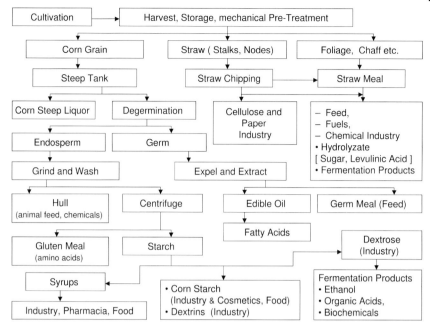

Fig. 1.15 Products from a whole-crop wet mill-based biorefinery.

generates other products (e.g. gluten meal, gluten feed, oil) [62]. An overview about the product range is shown in Fig. 1.15.

1.5.4
Green Biorefinery

Green biorefineries are also multi-product systems and furnish cuts, fractions, and products in accordance with the physiology of the corresponding plant material, which maintains and utilizes the diversity of syntheses achieved by nature. Most green biomass is green crops, for example grass from cultivation of permanent grass land, closure fields, nature reserves, or green crops, such as lucerne, clover, and immature cereals from extensive land cultivation. Green crops are a natural chemical factory and food plant and are primarily used as forage and as a source of leafy vegetables. A process called wet-fractionation of green biomass, green crop fractionation, can be used for simultaneous manufacture of both food and non food items [145].

Scientists in several countries, in Europe and elsewhere, have developed green crop fractionation [146–148]. Green crop fractionation is now studied in approximately 80 countries [149]. Several hundred temperate and tropical plant species have been investigated for green crop fractionation [148, 150, 151] and more than 300,000 higher plants species have still to be investigated. The subject has been covered by several reviews [73, 146–148, 151–155]. Green biorefineries can, by fractionation of green plants, process from a few tonnes of green crops per hour (farm scale process) to more than 100 tonnes per hour (industrial scale commercial process).

Careful wet fractionation technology is used as a first step (primary refinery) to isolate the contents of the green crop (or humid organic waste goods) in their natural form. Thus, they are separated into a fiber-rich press cake (PC) and a nutrient-rich green juice (GJ).

The advantages of the green biorefinery are high biomass profit per hectare, good coupling with agricultural production, and low price of the raw materials. Simple technology can be used and there is good biotechnical and chemical potential for further conversion (Fig. 1.16). Rapid primary processing or use of preservation methods, for example silage production or drying, are necessary, both for the raw materials and the primary products, although each method of preservation changes the content of the materials.

In addition to cellulose and starch, the press cake contains valuable dyes and pigments, crude drugs and other organic compounds. The green juice contains proteins, free amino acids, organic acids, dyes, enzymes, hormones, other organic substances, and minerals. Application of the methods of biotechnology results in conversion, because the plant water can simultaneously be used for further treatment. In addition, the lignin–cellulose composite is not as intractable as lignocellulose-feedstock materials. Starting from green juice the main focus is directed toward products such as lactic acid and its derivatives, amino acids, ethanol, and proteins. The press cake can be used for production of green feed pellets, as raw material for production of chemicals, for example levulinic acid, and for conversion to syngas and hydrocarbons (synthetic biofuels). The residues of substantial conversion are suitable for production of biogas combined with generation of heat and electricity (Fig. 1.17). Reviews have been published on the concepts, contents, and goals of the green biorefinery [73, 75, 119].

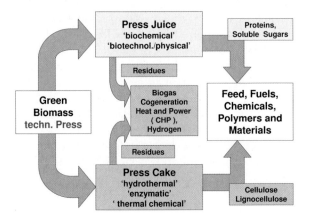

Fig. 1.16 A "green biorefinery" system.

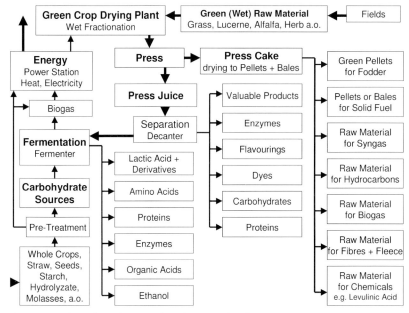

Fig. 1.17 Products from the green biorefinery. In this illustration a green biorefinery has been combined with a green crop-drying plant [78, 79].

1.5.5
Two-platform Concept and Syngas

The "two-platform concept" is one which uses biomass consisting, on average, of 75% carbohydrates which can be standardized as a "intermediate sugar platform", as a basis for further conversion, but which can also be converted thermochemically into synthesis gas and the products made from this. The "sugar platform" is based on biochemical conversion processes and focuses on fermentation of sugars extracted from biomass feedstocks. The "syngas platform" is based on thermochemical conversion processes and focuses on the gasification of biomass feedstocks and by-products from conversion processes [63, 98, 131]. In addition to the gasification other thermal and thermochemical biomass conversion methods have also been described – hydrothermolysis, pyrolysis, thermolysis, and burning. The application chosen depends on the water content of biomass [156].

The gasification and other thermochemical conversions concentrate on utilization of the precursor carbohydrates and their intrinsic carbon and hydrogen content. The proteins, lignin, oils and lipids, amino acids, and other nitrogen and sulfur-containing compounds occurring in all biomass are not taken into account (Fig. 1.18).

The advantage of this concept is that the production of energy, fuels, and bio-based products is possible using only slightly complex and low-tech technology,

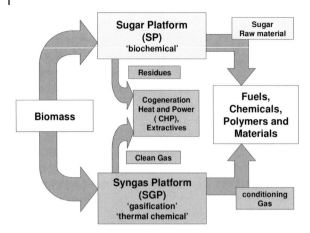

Fig. 1.18 The sugar platform and the syngas platform [131].

for example saccharification and syngas technology. The sugar platform also enables access to a huge range of family tree-capable chemicals (Figs. 1.7 and 1.8).

In-situ conversion of biomass feedstock into liquid or gas could be one way of using existing infrastructure (developed pipe network), but with the disadvantages of the need to remove hetero-atoms (O, N, S) and minerals present in the biomass and the highly endothermic nature of the syngas process [157]. Currently, production of simple alcohols, aldehydes, mixed alcohols, and Fischer-Tropsch liquids from biomass is not economically viable and additional developments are required [98] (Fig. 1.19).

1.6
Outlook and Perspectives

Biorefineries are the production plants in which biomass is economically and ecologically converted to chemicals, materials, fuels, and energy. For successful development of "industrial biorefinery technologies" and "biobased products" several problems must be solved. It will be necessary to increase the production of substances (cellulose, starch, sugar, oil) from basic biogenic raw materials and to promote the introduction and establishment of biorefinery demonstration plants. Ecological transport of biomass must also be developed, for example utilization of already developed pipe networks.

Another important aspect is committing chemists, biotechnologists, and engineers to the concept of biobased products and biorefinery systems and promoting the combined biotechnological and chemical conversion of substances. Last, but not least, the development of systematic approaches to new synthesis and technologies is required to meet the sustainable principles of "ideal synthesis" and "principles of green chemistry and process engineering" [159–161].

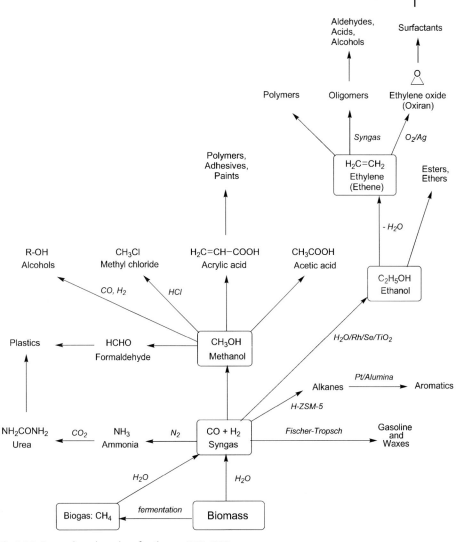

Fig. 1.19 Syngas-based product family tree [157, 158].

References

1 National Research Council; Biobased Industrial Products, Priorities for Research
and Commercialization [National Academic Press, Washington D.C., **2000**,
ISBN 0-309-05392-7] a) 74

2 Marggraf, A. S.; In: Histoire de l'Académie Royale des Sciences et Belles Let-
tres, Anné 1748 [Preußische Akademie,
Berlin, **1749**]

3 Marggraf, A. S.; Chym. Schriften (Chemische Schriften) 2 Bd., Berlin **1761** till
1767

4 Kirchhoff, G. S. C.; *Schweigers Journal für
Chemie und Physik*, **4** (1812) 108

5 Graebe, C.; History of Organic Chemistry. Bd 1 [Verlag Julius Springer, Berlin, **1920**, germ.] a) 28, b) 122 f

6 Kosaric, N.; Vardar-Sukan, F.; Potential Sources of Energy and Chemical Products; In: The Biotechnology of Ethanol [M. Roehr (ed.), Wiley–VCH, Weinheim et al, **2001** ISBN 3-527-30199-2] 132

7 Prescott, S. C.; Dunn, C. G.; Industrial Microbiology. 3rd Ed. [McGraw-Hill, New York, Toronto, London, **1959**]

8 Osteroth, D.; From Coal to Biomass [Springer, New York, **1989**, ISBN 0-387-50712-4, germ.] 192 ff

9 McKillip, W. J.; Furan and Derivatives in Ullmann's Encyclopedia of Industrial Chemistry. 6th Ed., Vol. 15 [Wiley–VCH, Weinheim, **2003**] 187 ff

10 www.furan.com

11 Pringsheim, H.; *Cellulosechemie*, **2** (1921) 123

12 Ullmann, F.; Enzyklopädie der Technischen Chemie. 2. Aufl., 5. Bd. [Urban und Schwarzenberg, Berlin und Wien, **1930**] 442 ff

13 Payen, A.; *Comptes rendus de l'Académie des Sciences* (C. r.), **8** (1839) 51

14 Gruber, E.; Krause Th., Schurz, J.: Cellulose; In: Ullmann, Enzyklopädie der technischen Chemie, 4. Aufl. Bd. 9 [Verlag Chemie, Weinheim, **1975**] 184–191

15 Mulder, G. J.; *J. Prakt. Chem.*, **21** (1840) 219

16 A. E. Staley, Mfg. Co. A. E. (Decatur Ill.); Levulinic Acid **1942** [C.A. 36, 1612]

17 Kitano et al., Levulinic Acid, A New Chemical Raw Material – Its Chemistry and Use. *Chemical Economy and Engineering Review* (**1975**) 25–29

18 Leonard, R. H.; Levulinic acid as a Basic Chemical Raw Material. *Ind. Eng. Chem.*, 1956, 1331–1341

19 Norman, W.; Process for Converting Unsaturated Fatty Acids or their Glycerides into Saturated Compounds. BP 1515 , 1903

20 Sandermann, W.; Grundlagen der Chemie und chemischen Technologie des Holzes [Akademische Verlagsgesellschaft, Leipzig, **1956**] 147

21 Tiemann, F., Haarmann, W., Ueber das Coniferin und seine Umwandlung in das aromatische Princip der Vanille. *Ber. dt. chem. Ges.*, **7** (1874) 608–623

22 Dignum, M. J. W.; Kerler, J., Verpoorte, R.; Vanilla Production: Technological, Chemical and Biosynthetic Aspects. *Food Rev. Intern.*, **17** (2001) 199–219.

23 Vaupel, L., Vanille and Vanillin. *Pharm. Zeit.*, **38** (2002)

24 Carothers, H.; Dorough, G. L.; and Van Natta, F. J.; *J. Am. Chem. Soc.*, **54** (1932) 761

25 Gruber, P. R.; O'Brien, M.; Polylactides "Nature Works" PLA; In: Biopolymers, Polyester III [Y. Doi, A. Steinbüchel (eds.), Wiley-VCH, Weinheim, **2002**]

26 Walden, P., History of Organic Chemistry since 1880. Bd. 2 [Graebe, C. (Ed.), Verlag Julius Springer, Berlin, **1941**, germ.] 686

27 Pötsch, W. R.; Lexicon of famous Chemists. [Bibliographisches Institut, Leipzig, **1988**, ISBN 3-323-00185-0, germ.] a) 305

28 Borregaard LignoTech; marathon co.; http://www.ltus.com.

29 Peckham; B. W.; The First Hundred Years of Corn Refining in the United States. In Corn Annual 2000 [Corn Refiners Association, Washington, DC, **2000**]

30 Johnson, D. L.; The Corn Wet milling and Corn Dry milling industry [in this book, **2005**]

31 Slade, R. E.; Birkinshaw, J. H. (ICI); Improvement in or related to the utilization of grass and other green crops. *Brit. Pat.* **BP 511,525** (1939)

32 Pirie, N. W.; *Chem. Ind.*, **61** (1942) 45

33 Pirie, N. W.; *Nature*, **149** (1942) 251

34 Heier, W.; *Grundlagen der Landtechnik* **33** (1983) 45–55

35 Kamm, B.; Kamm, M.; The Green Biorefinery – Principles, Technologies and Products. In: Proceed. 2nd Intern. Symp. Green Biorefinery, October, 13–14, 1999 [SUSTAIN (eds), Feldbach, Austria, **1999**] S. 46–69

36 Knuckles, B. E.; Bickoff, E. M.; Kohler, G. O.; *J. Agric. Food Chem.*, **20** (1972) 1055

37 Schertz, F. M.; *Ind. Eng. Chem.*, **30** (1938) 1073–1075

38 Shearon, W. H.; Gee, O. F.; *Ind. Eng. Chem.*, **41** (1949) 218–226

39 Judah, M.A.; Burdack, E.M.; Caroll, R.G.; *Ind. Eng. Chem.*, **46** (1954) 2262–2271

40 Hale, W.J.: The Farm Chemurgic [The Stratford Co., Boston, **1934**]

41 Borth, Ch.; Pioneers of Plenthy [Bobbs-Merril Co, Indianapolis, New York, **1939**]

42 Lewis, D.L.; The Public Image of Henry Ford [Wayne State University Press, Detroit, **1976**]

43 Brandt, E.N.; Growth Company – Dow Chemical's First Century [Michigan State University press, East Lansing, **1997**]

44 Bergius, F.; *Trans. Inst. Chem. Eng.* (London), **11** (1933) 162

45 Scholler, H.; Dissertation, Technical University of Munich, Germany **1923**

46 Scholler, H.; French Patent, **F.P. 777,824** (1935)

47 Katzen, R.; Tsao, G.T.; A View of the History of Biochemical Engineering IN. Advances in Biochemical Engineering/ Biotechnology, Vol. 70 [Springer, Berlin, **2000**]

48 Conrad, T.F.; Holzzuckerbrennerei; In: Die Hefen, Vol. II 8 F. Reiff, R. Kautzmann, H. Lüers, M. Lindemann (eds.) [Verlag Hans Carl, Nürnberg, 1962] 437–444

49 Prescott, S.C.; Dunn, C.G.; Industrial Microbiology. 3rd Ed. [McGraw-Hill, New York, Toronto, London, **1959**]

50 Harris, E.E. et al; Madison Wood Sugar Process. *Ind. Eng. Chem.*, **38** (1946) 896–904

51 Timell, T.E.; *Tappi*, **44** (1961) 99

52 Stamm, A.J.; Wood and Cellulose Science [Ronald Press, New York, **1964**]

53 James, R.L.; In: The pulping of wood, 2nd edn., vol. 1 [McGraw-Hill, New York, **1969**] 34

54 Brink, D.L.; Pohlmann, A.A.; *Tappi*, **55** (1972) 381 ff.

55 Oshima, M.; Wood Chemistry – Process Engineering Aspects [Noyes development Corp. New York, **1965**, No. 10965]

56 Puls, J.; Dietrichs, H.H.; In: Energy from Biomass. Proceed. of First European Comm. Inter. Conf. on Biomass, Brighton, UK, November 1980 [W. Palz, P. Chartier, D.O. Hall (eds), Elsevier, **1981**, ISBN: 0-85334-970-3] 348

57 Shen, S.Y.; Wood Grass Production Systems for Biomass. Proceed. Midwest Forest Economist Meeting, Duluth, Minnesota, April **1982**

58 Shen, S.Y.; Biological Engineering for Sustainable Biomass Production; In: Biodiversity [E.O. Wilson, Harvard University (ed.), National Academy of Sciences/ Smithsonian Institution, National Academic Press, Washington DC, **1988**, German Edition: "Ende der biologischen Vielfalt?", 1992, ISBN 3-89330-661-7] 404–416

59 Carlsson, R.; Trends for future applications of green crops. In: Forage Protein Conservation and Utilization. Proceed. of EFC Conf. 1982 [EFC Press, Dublin, Ireland, **1982**] 57–81

60 Carlsson, R.; Green Biomass of Native Plants and new Cultivated Crops for Multiple Use: Food, Fodder, Fuel, Fibre for Industry, Photochemical Products and Medicine. In: New Crops for Food and Industry [G.E. Wickens, N. Haq, and P. Day (eds.), Chapman and Hall, London, **1989**]

61 Dale, B.E.; Biomass refining: protein and ethanol from alfalfa. *Ind. Eng. Product Research and Development*, **22** (1983) 446

62 Hacking, A.J.; The American wet milling industry. In: Economic Aspects of Biotechnology [Cambridge University Press, New York, **1986**] 214–221

63 White, D.H.; Wolf, D.; Research in Thermochemical Biomass Conversion [A.V. Bridgewater, J.L. Kuester (eds.), Elsevier Applied Science, New York, **1988**]

64 Lipinsky, E.S.; Chemicals from Biomass: petrochemical substitution options. *Science*, **212** (1981) 1465–1471

65 Wise, D.L. (ed.); Organic Chemical from Biomass [The Benjamin/Cummings Publishing Co., Inc., Menlo Park, California, **1983**]

66 Bailey, J.E.; Ollis, D.F.; Biochemical Engineering Fundamentals. 2nd edition. [McGraw-Hill, New York, **1986**]

67 Szmant, H.H.; Industrial Utilization of Renewable Resources [Technomic Publishing, Lancaster, Pa., **1987**]

68 Eggersdorfer, M.; Meyer J.; Eckes, P.; Use of renewable resources for non-food materials. *FEMS Microbiolol. Rev.*, **103** (1992) 355–364

69 Morris D. J.; Ahmed I.; The carbohydrate Economy: Making Chemicals and Industrial Materials from Plant Matter [Institute of Local Self Reliance, Washington D.C. **1992**]

70 Bozell, J. J.; Landucci, R.; Alternative feedstock program – technical and economic assessment [US Department of Energy, **1992**]

71 Schilling, L. B.; Chemicals from alternative feedstock in the United States. *FEMS Microbiol. Rev.*, **16** (1995) 1001–1110

72 de la Ross, L. B.; Dale, B. E.; Reshamwala, S. T.; Latimer, V. M.; Stuart, E. D.; Shawky, B. T.; An integrated process for protein and ethanol from coastal Bermuda grass. *Appl. Biochem. Biotechnol.*, **45/46** (1994) 483–497

73 Soyez, K.; Kamm, B.; Kamm, M. (eds.); The Green Biorefinery, Proceedings of. 1st International Green Biorefinery Conference, Neuruppin, Germany, 1997 [Verlag GÖT, Berlin, **1998**, ISBN 3-929672-06-5, German and English]

74 Van Dyne D. L.; Blasé M. G.; Clements L. D.; A strategy for returning agriculture and rural America to long-term full employment using biomass refineries. In: Perspectives on new crops and new uses. [J. Janeck (ed), ASHS Press, Alexandria, Va., **1999**] pp 114–123

75 Narodoslawsky, M.; The Green Biorefinery, Proceedings 2nd Intern. Symp. Green Biorefinery, Feldbach, Austria [SUSTAIN, (ed.), TU Graz, **1999**]

76 Nonato R. V.; Mantellato, P. E.; Rossel C. E. V.; Integrated production of biodegradable plastic, sugar and ethanol. *Appl. Microbiol. Biotechnol.*, **57** (2001) 1–5

77 Ohara, H. Biorefinery. *Appl. Microb. Biotechn.* (AMB), **62** (2003) 474–477

78 Kamm, B.; Kamm, M.; Principles of Biorefineries. *Appl. Microbiol., Biotechnol., (AMB)*, **64** (2004) 137–145

79 Kamm, B.; Kamm, M.; Biorefinery-Systems. *Chem. Biochem. Eng. Q.*, **18** (2004) 1–6

80 U.S. Department of Energy (DEO); National Biomass Initiative and Energy, Environmental and Economics (E3) Handbook [www.bioproducts-bioenergy.gov]

81 Lynd L. R.; Cushman J. H.; Nichols R. J.; Wyman C. E.; Fuel Ethanol from Cellulosic Biomass. *Science*, **251** (1991) 1318.

82 Keller, F. A. Integrated bioprocess development for bioethanol production. In: handbook ob bioethanol: production and utilization. [C. E. Wyman (ed), Taylor and Francis, Bristol, Pa. **1996**] 351–379

83 Wyman C. E.; Handbook on Bioethanol: Production and Utilization. Applied Energy Technology Series [Taylor and Francis, **1996**]

84 Lynd, L.; Overview and evaluation of fuel ethanol from cellulosics biomass: technology, economics, the environment, and policy. *Annual Review of Energy and the Environment*, **21** (1996) 403–465

85 Galbe, M.; Zacci, G.; A review of the production of ethanol from softwood. *Appl. Microbiol. Biotechnol.*, **59** (2002) 618–628

86 Datta, R.; Tasi, S.-P.; Bonsignore, P.; Moon, S. H.; Frank, J. R.; Technological and economics potential of poly (lactic acid) and lactic acid derivatives. *FEMS Microbiol. Rev.*, **16** (1995) 221–231

87 Witt, U.; Müller R. J.; Widdecke, H.; Deckwer, W.-D.; Synthesis, properties and biodegradability of polyesters based on 1,3-propanediol. *Macrom. Chem. Phys.*, **195** (1994) 793–802

88 Yosida, T.; Nagasawa, T.; ε-Poly-L-lysine: microbial production, biodegradation and application potential. *Appl. Microbiol. Biotechnol.*, **62** (2003) 21–26

89 Potera, C.; Genencor and DuPont create "green" polyester. *Genet. Eng. News*, **17** (1997) 17

90 Poirier, Y.; Nawrath, C.; Somerville, C.; Production of polyhydroxyalkanoates, a family of biodegradable plastics. *Bio/technology*, **13** (1995) 142–150

91 Warwel, S.; Brüse, F.; Demes, C.; Kunz, M.; Rüsch gen Klaas, M.; Polymers and Surfactants on the basis of renewable resources. *Chemosphere*, **43** (2001) 39–48

92 Bozell, J. J.; Alternative Feedstocks for Bioprocessing; In: Encyclopedia of Plant and Crop Science [R.M. Goodman (ed.), Dekker, New York, 2004, 0-8247-4268-0]

93 Webb, C.; Koutinas, A.A.; Wang, R.; Developing a Sustainable Bioprocessing Strategy Based on a Generic Feedstock. *Adv. Biochem Eng./Biotechn.*, **87** (2004) 195–268

94 Gravitis, J.; Suzuki, M.; Biomass Refinery – A Way to produce Value Added Products and Base for Agricultural Zero Emissions Systems; In: Proc. 99 Intern. Conference on Agric. Engineering, Beijing, China 1999 [United Nations University Press, Tokyo, **1999**] III-9–III-23

95 Van Dyne, D.L., et al., Estimating the Economic Feasibility of Converting Ligno-Cellulosic Feedstocks to Ethanol and Higher Value Chemicals under the refinery concept: A Phase II Study [University of Missouri, **1999**, OR22072-58]

96 Kurtanjek, Z. (ed.); *Chemical and Biochemical Engineering Quarterly, Special Issue*, **18** (2004) 1–88

97 Marano, J.J.; Jechura, J.L.; Biorefinery Optimization Tools – Development and Validation. In: 25th. Symposium on Biotechnology for Fuels and Chemicals: Program and Abstracts [National Renewable Energy Laboratory, Golden, CO, No. NREL/BK-510-33708, **2003**] 104

98 T. Werpy, G. Petersen (eds.); Top Value Added Chemicals from biomass (ed) [U.S. Department of Energy, Office of scientific and technical information, **2004**, No.: DOE/GO-102004-1992, www.osti.gov/bridge]

99 Goddijn, O.J.M.; Plants as bioreactors. *Trends Biotechnol.*, **13** (1995) 379–387

100 Wilke, D.; Chemicals from biotechnology: molecular plant genetic will challenge the chemical and the fermentation industry. *Appl. Microbiol. Biotechnol.*, (AMB), **52** (1999) 135–145

101 Anex, R. (ed.).; *Journal of Ind. Ecology, Special Issue,* **7** (2003) 1–235

102 Ludgar, R.G.; Woolsey, R.J.; The new petroleum. *Foreign Affairs*, **78** (1999) 88–102

103 Wyman, C.E.; Production of Low Cost Sugars from Biomass: Progress, Opportunities, and Challenges; In: Biomass: A Growth Opportunity in Green Energy and Value-Added Products [R.P. Overend and E. Chornet (eds.), Pergamon Press, Oxford, UK, 1999] 867–872

104 Bachmann, R.; Bastianelli, E.; Riese, J.; Schlenzka, W.; Using plants as plants. Biotechnology will transform the production of chemicals. *The McKinsey Quarterly*, **2** (2000) 92–99

105 Hettenhaus, J.R.; Wooley, B.; Biomass Commercialization: Prospect in the Next 2 to 5 Years [NREL, Golden Colorado, **2000**, No. NREL/ACO-9-29-039-01]

106 Woolsey, J.; Hydrocarbons to Carbohydrates, The strategic Dimension; In: The Biobased Economy of the 21st Century: Agriculture Expanding into Health, Energy, Chemicals, and Materials. NABC Report 12 [National Agricultural Biotechnology Council, Ithaca, New York, **2000**, No. 14853]

107 Eaglesham, A.; Brown, W.F.; Hardy, R.W.F. (eds.); The Biobased Economy of the 21st Century: Agriculture Expanding into Health, Energy, Chemicals, and Materials. NABC Report 12 [National Agricultural Biotechnology Council, Ithaca, New York, **2000**, No. 14853]

108 US President: Developing and Promoting Biobased Products and Bioenergy, Executive Order 13101/13134 [William J. Clinton, The White House, Washington D.C. **1999**]

109 US Congress; Biomass Research and Development, Act of 2000 [Washington D.C., **2000**]

110 Biomass R&D, Technical Advisory Committee; Vision for Bioenergy and Biobased Products in the United States [Washington D.C. Oct. **2002**, www.bioproducts-bioenergy.gov/pdfs/BioVision_03_Web.pd]

111 Biomass R&D, Technical Advisory Committee; Roadmap for Biomass Technologies in the United States [Washington D.C., Dec. **2002**, www.bioproducts-bioenergy.gov/pdfs/FinalBiomassRoadmap.pdf]

112 Biotechnology Industrial Organisation; World Congress on Industrial biotechnology and Bioprocessing, http://www.bio.org/World%20Congress

113 Biomass Conferences of the Americas; http://www.nrel.gov/bioam/

114 Biomass, a growth opportunity in green energy and value-added products, Proceedings of the 4th Biomass Conference of the Americas, Oakland California, USA, August 29–September 2, 1999 [Elsevier Science Ltd, Overend, R.P.; Chornet, E. (ed.)], ISBN: 0080430198, Oxford, UK, 1999]

115 Green and Sustainable Chemistry Congress; http://www.chemistry.org

116 Biorefinica – International Symposia Biobased Products and Biorefineries; www.biorefinica.de

117 Kamm, B.; Hempel, M.; Kamm, M. (eds.); biorefinica 2004, International Symposium Biobased Products and Biorefineries, Proceedings and Papers, October, 27 and 28, 2004, [biopos e.V., Teltow, **2004**, ISBN 3-00-015166-4]

118 Zoebelin, H. (ed.); Dictionary of Renewable Resources [Wiley-VCH, Weinheim, **2001**]

119 Kamm B, et al.; Green Biorefinery Brandenburg, Article to development of products and of technologies and assessment. *Brandenburgische Umweltberichte*, **8** (2000) 260–269

120 European parliament and Council; Directive 2003/30/EC on the promotion of the use of biofuels or other renewable fuels for transport [Official Journal of the European Union L123/42, 17. 05. 2003, Brussels, **2003**]

121 Gesetz für den Vorrang erneuerbarer Energien; Erneuerbare Energiegesetz, EEG/EnWGuaÄndG., 29. 03.2000, BGBI, 305, **(2000)**

122 European parliament and Council; Green Paper "Towards a European strategy for the security of energy supply" KOM2002/321, 26. 06. 2002, **(2002)**

123 Umweltbundesamt; Klimaschutz durch Nutzung erneuerbarer Energien, Report 2 [Erich Schmidt Verlag, Berlin, 2000]

124 BioVision2030-Group: Strategiepapier "Industrielle stoffliche Nutzung von Nachwachsenden Rohstoffen in Deutschland", Nov. **2003**, www.biorefinica.de/bibliothek

125 Deutscher Bundestag; Rahmenbedingungen für die industrielle stoffliche Nutzung von Nachwachsenden Rohstoffen in Deutschland schaffen, Antrag 15/4943, Berlin **(2005)**

126 Busch, R.; Hirth, Th.; Kamm, B.; Kamm, M.; Thoen, J.; Biomasse-Industrie – Wie aus "Bio" Chemie wird. *Nachrichten aus der Chemie*, **53** (2005) 130–134

127 Röper, H.; Perspektiven der industriellen Nutzung nachwachsender Rohstoffe, insbesondere von Stärke und Zucker. *Mitteilung der Fachgruppe Umweltchemie und Ökotoxikologie der Gesellschaft Deutscher Chemiker*, **7(2)** (2001) 6–12

128 Kamm, B.; Kamm, M.; Richter, K.; Entwicklung eines Verfahrens zur Konversion von hexosenhaltigen Rohstoffen zu biogenen Wirk- und Werkstoffen – Polylactid aus fermentiertem Roggenschrot über organische Aluminiumlactate als alternative Kuppler biotechnischer und chemischer Stoffwandlungen. In: Chemie nachwachsender Rohstoffe [P.B. Czedik-Eysenberg (ed.), Österreichisches Bundesministerium für Umwelt (BMUJF) Wien, **1997**] 83–87

129 Kamm, B.; Kamm, M.; Schmidt, M.; Starke, I.; Kleinpeter, E.; Chemical and biochemical generation of carbohydrates from lignocellulose-feedstock (*Lupinus nootkatensis*), Quantification of glucose, *Chemosphere* (in press)

130 US Department of Energy; http://www.oit.doe.gov/e3handbook

131 National Renewable Energy Laboratory (NREL); http://www.nrel.gov/biomass/biorefinery.html

132 Tolan, J.S.; Iogen's Demonstration Process for Producing Ethanol from Cellulosic Biomass. In this book, **2005**

133 EuropaBio; White Biotechnology: Gateway to a more sustainable future [EuropaBio, Lyon, April **2003**]

134 BIO Biotechnology Industry Organisation: New Biotech Tools for a cleaner Environment – Industrial Biotechnology for Pollution Prevention, Resource Conservation and Cost Reduction,

2004; http://www.bio.org/ind/pubs/cleaner2004/cleanerReport.pdf

135 Dti Global Watch Mission Report: Impact of the industrial biotechnology on sustainability of the manufacturing base – the Japanese Perspective, **2004**

136 Dale, B.; Encyclopedia of Physical Science and Technology, Third Edition, Volume 2: (**2002**) 141–157

137 Ringpfeil M.; Biobased Industrial Products and Biorefinery Systems – Industrielle Zukunft des 21. Jahrhunderts? [**2001**, www.biopract.de]

138 Zeikus, J.G.; Jain, M.K.; Elankovan, P.; Biotechnology of succinic acid production and markets for derived industrial products. *Appl. Microbiol. Biotechnol.*, **51** (1999) 545–552

139 Vorlop, K.-D.; Wilke, Th.; Prüße, U.; Biocatalytic and catalytic routes for the production of bulk and fine chemicals from renewable resources: [in this book], **2005**

140 Wurz, O.; Zellstoff- und Papierherstellung aus Einjahrespflanzen [Eduard Roether Verlag, Darmstadt, **1960**]

141 Rossel C.E.V.; Mantellato, P.E.; Agnelli, A.M.; Nascimento, J.; Sugar-based Biorefinery – Technology for an integrated production of Poly(3-hydroxybutyrate), Sugar and Ethanol, in this book, **2005**

142 Rexen, F.; New industrial application possibilities for straw. Documentation of Svebio Phytochemistry Group (Danish) [Fytokemi i Norden, Stockholm, Sweden, 1986-03-06, **1986**] 12

143 Coombs, J.; Hall, K.; The potential of cereals as industrial raw materials: Legal technical, commercial considerations; In: Cereals – Novel Uses And Processes [G.M. Campbell, C. Webb, and S.L. McKee (eds.), Plenum Publ. Corp., New York, USA, **1997**] 1–12.

144 Audsley, E.; Sells, J.E.; Determining the profitability of a whole crop biorefinery; In: Cereals – Novel Uses and Processes [G.M. Campbell, C. Webb, and S.L. McKee (eds.), Plenum Publ. Corp.; New York, USA; **1997**] 191–294

145 Carlsson, R.; Sustainable primary production – Green crop fractionation: Effects of species, growth conditions, and physiological development; In: Handbook of Plant and Crop Physiology [M. Pessarakli (ed.), Marcel Dekker Inc., N.Y., USA, **1994**] 941–963.

146 Pirie, N.W.; Leaf Protein – Its agronomy, preparation, quality, and use [Blackwell Scientific Publications, Oxford/Cambridge, UK, **1971**]

147 Pirie, N.W.; Leaf Protein and Its By-Products in Human and Animal Nutrition [Cambridge Univ. Press, UK, **1987**]

148 Carlsson, R.; Status quo of the utilization of green biomass. In: The Green Biorefinery, Proceedings of 1st International Green Biorefinery Conference, Neuruppin, Germany, 1997 [S. Soyez, B. Kamm, M. Kamm (eds.), Verlag GÖT, Berlin, **1998**, ISBN 3-929672-06-5]

149 Carlsson, R.; Food and non-food uses of immature cereals; In: Cereals – Novel Uses and Processes [G.M. Campbell, C. Webb, S.L. McKee (eds), Plenum Publ. Corp., New York, USA, **1997**], pp. 159–167

150 Carlsson, R.; Leaf protein concentrate from plant sources in temperate climates. In: Leaf Protein Concentrates [L. Telek, H.D. Graham (eds.), AVI Publ. Co., Inc., Westport, Conn., USA, **1983**] 52–80

151 Telek, L.; Graham, H.D. (eds.); Leaf Protein Concentrates [AVI Publ., Co., Inc., Westport, Conn., USA, **1983**]

152 Wilkins, R.J. (ed.); Green Crop Fractionation [The British Grassland Society, c/o Grassland Research Institute, Hurley, Maidenhead, SL6 5LR, UK, **1977**]

153 Tasaki, I. (ed.); Recent Advances in Leaf Protein Research, Proc. 2nd Int. Leaf Protein Res. Conf. [Nagoya, Japan, **1985**]

154 Fantozzi, P. (ed.); Proc. 3rd Int. Leaf Protein Res. Conf., Pisa-Perugia-Viterbo, Italy, **1989**

155 Singh, N. (ed.); Green Vegetation Fractionation Technology [Science Publ. Inc., Lebanon, NH 03767, USA, **1996**]

156 Okkerse, C.; van Bekkum, H.; From fossil to green. *Green Chemistry*, **4** (1999) 107–114

157 Lancaster, M.; The Syngas Economy; In: Green Chemistry [The Royal Society of Chemistry, Cambridge, UK, **2002**, ISBN: 0-85404-620-8] 205

158 Matlack, A. S.; The Use of Synthesis Gas from Biomass; In: Introduction to Green Chemistry [Marcel Dekker, New York, **2001**, ISBN: 0824704118] 369

159 Clark, J. H.; Green Chemistry. Challenges and opportunities. *Green Chemistry*, **1** (1999) 1–8

160 Lancaster, M.; The Biorefinery. In: Green Chemistry [The Royal Society of Chemistry, Cambridge, UK, **2002**, ISBN: 0-85404-620-8] 207

161 Anastas, P. T.; Warner, J. C.; Green Chemistry. Theory and Practice [Oxford University Press, New York, **1998**]

2
Biomass Refining Global Impact –
The Biobased Economy of the 21st Century

Bruce E. Dale and Seungdo Kim

2.1
Introduction

We are in the early phases of a truly historic transition – from an economy based largely on petroleum to a more diversified economy in which renewable plant biomass will become a significant feedstock for both fuel and chemical production. The development of the petroleum refining industry over the past century provides many instructive lessons for the future biobased economy and also many reasons for supposing that the new biobased economy will be different from the hydrocarbon economy in crucial ways. This paper explores the similarities and differences between the petroleum refining and biorefining industries in a historical context and the implications of these similarities and differences for the biobased economy in the long term.

We assume a mature biobased economy – as the petroleum economy is mature today – and from that assumption we extrapolate likely features of the mature biobased economy. Among the technical, social, and economic forces that will drive the mature biobased economy are:

1. yield (using the whole "barrel of biomass");
2. gradual diversification of biobased products, probably starting with higher-value chemical products and trending toward fuels over time;
3. the great diversity of biomass resources combined with their considerable compositional similarity;
4. possible/likely limits on agricultural productivity;
5. integration of biorefining and agricultural ecosystems in a local social and political context (the "all biomass is local" paradigm); and
6. the sustainability of the mature biobased economy and its most important underlying resource – productive soils.

Biorefineries – Industrial Processes and Products. Status Quo and Future Directions. Vol. 1
Edited by Birgit Kamm, Patrick R. Gruber, Michael Kamm
Copyright © 2006 WILEY-VCH Verlag GmbH & Co. KGaA, Weinheim
ISBN: 3-527-31027-4

2.2
Historical Outline

2.2.1
Background and Development of the Fossil Carbon-processing Industries

Materials that contain carbon, including the primary commercial fuels, virtually all food and fiber products, and most commodity chemicals, pharmaceuticals, and nondurable manufactured goods, play an integral role in the world economy [1]. Carbon-rich raw materials originate through the process of photosynthesis in which plants and some bacteria use solar energy to convert atmospheric carbon dioxide into organic substances including simple sugars, polysaccharides, amino acids, proteins, lipids, and aromatic compounds such as lignin. Some carbon-rich raw materials are derived from fossil sources such as petroleum, coal, and natural gas. Fossil sources result from photosynthesis in ancient times and comprise a large, but nonrenewable, reserve. In contrast, present day photosynthesis provides a potentially renewable source of carbon.

Renewable agricultural and forestry resources have been used since ancient times as fuels and raw materials for numerous products. Starting in the late 1700s, at the beginning of the Industrial Revolution, coal began to displace wood as a fuel. In the mid 1800s the large-scale processing of petroleum to fuel and chemical products began, taking away some markets from coal and many more from renewable carbon sources. In the last half of the 20th century, uses of natural gas began to expand greatly, both as a fuel and as a feedstock for chemical production [Ref. 1, Chapter 1]. Currently petroleum provides 40% of the United States' and 35% of the world's direct primary energy supply whereas plant material in all forms provides approximately 10% of the world's energy supply.

Although remaining supplies of petroleum, coal, and natural gas are very large, it is, nonetheless, obvious that the world is using these essentially nonrenewable resources at a huge and growing rate. Natural processes are simply not replacing fossil carbon at even a minute fraction of the rate at which we are using it. For example, some experts believe that the peak rate of production of conventional oil will occur within this decade whereas others predict this will occur before mid-century [2, 3]. After that point, conventional, inexpensive oil production will irreversibly decline. Natural gas production will peak later than conventional oil, but will still begin permanent decline within the next few decades. Although other sources of petroleum exist (e.g., tar sands, deep-water oil), they will be more difficult and much more expensive to produce. Whatever the exact date of peak oil production, we are approaching a major change in the way we must provide energy and other services to the world's population.

This paper addresses two related questions:

1. is it realistic to believe that renewable sources of carbon can provide a large share of the energy and other services currently provided by fossil carbon, particularly petroleum?

2. what might be the salient characteristics of a mature biobased economy producing not only food and fiber but also fuels and chemicals?

We will touch somewhat on question 1 but will treat question 2 more extensively.

An extensive ongoing project called the Role of Biomass in America's Energy Future (RBAEF Project) sponsored by the US Department of Energy and the Energy Foundation is attempting to address the first question with considerable breadth and depth. The RBAEF Project is led by Professor Lee R. Lynd of Dartmouth College (Hanover, New Hampshire, USA), Dr John Sheehan of the National Renewable Energy Laboratory (Golden, Colorado, USA), and Mr Nathanael Greene of the Natural Resources Defense Council (New York, New York, USA). We encourage all readers of this article to make themselves aware of the findings of the RBAEF team as these findings become available. Dr Lynd provides an outline of some of the expected results in another article in this volume.

2.2.2
The Existing Biobased Economy: Renewable Carbon

Renewable carbon-based raw materials are produced in agriculture, silviculture and microbial systems, including managed and unmanaged systems. Although estimates are necessarily imprecise, the total amount of new carbon-based plant material fixed yearly by terrestrial plants is of the order of 100×10^{12} kg (assuming biomass is on average 50% by weight carbon) [4, 5]. This amount of plant material has an energy content (via heat of combustion) roughly five times the energy value of all forms of energy used worldwide and over ten times the energy content of all petroleum used worldwide [6]. Although this plant resource is dispersed, has competing uses, and, as a solid, is not in an ideal form for easy transporting and processing, the size of the renewable carbon resource and its associated energy content clearly suggest significant potential to provide raw material and energy services.

The amount of new plant biomass dwarfs the use of fossil carbon to produce organic chemicals. For example, the United States produces about 100×10^9 kg fine, specialty, intermediate, and commodity organic chemicals each year, or approximately 0.1% of total world biomass production [7]. Less than 10% of this total is produced from renewable carbon [1]. The total mass of these organic chemicals is roughly equal to 40% of US production of corn grain, about twice the grain that the United States exports each year. In fact, there is pressure on the US (and the EU) from developing countries to reduce export and other subsidies of their agricultural products. As this occurs, more US grain may rather quickly find its way into fuel and chemical production. Already approximately 9 billion kg (3 billion gallons) annually of fuel ethanol are produced primarily from corn in the US, consuming approximately 12% of domestic corn production. There is, however, no reasonable expectation that grain will be able to provide the approximately 750 billion kilograms per year of refined petroleum products used in the United States [8]. That quantity of renewable carbon must come from crop and forestry residues and energy crops (crops grown specifically to produce energy products) – not from food/feed grain.

In addition to existing uses of renewable carbon to produce organic chemicals and fuels, renewable carbon sources provide about 90% of organic materials such as lumber and paper, natural fibers, and composites, cellulosics, and some proteins [Ref. 1, Chapter 2]. Finally, renewable carbon provides nearly all of our food and animal feed. There is no reasonable alternative to using renewable carbon to meet food/feed demand, although the efficiency with which this demand is met is certainly subject to change and innovation. We briefly explore some possible innovations for food and feed production in this paper – a much more complete discussion will be available in the RBAEF reports.

In total, the organic chemical, fuels (solid, liquid, and gaseous), carbon-based materials, food, and feed components of the US domestic economy exceed US $ 2 trillion per year. Much of this economic activity is already based on renewable carbon. The question which naturally arises is: could the fraction of fuels and chemicals from renewable carbon be significantly increased without interfering with other essential uses of plant material?

Before addressing this issue, we wish to point out two important facts that we will explore in more detail below. First, there are several largely unexplored alternatives for coproducing animal feed and human food with fuels. Doing so would make the whole enterprise more efficient, and very probably more economically competitive. Second, both US and European agriculture are currently constrained by demand, not by ability to produce. Respective national governments have been paying farmers not to produce to capacity for many years. If large new demands for renewable carbon were to arise, there is every reason to believe that much more plant material could be produced on the same or similar acreages.

2.2.3
Toward a Much Larger Biobased Economy

Given the amount of grain available in the US and the EU and the ability to supply very pure dextrose in large quantities for around US $ 0.20 per kg at corn wet mills, we suggest that material supply, convenience, and purity considerations favor dextrose derived from corn (and perhaps other grain) as a feedstock for organic chemical manufacture. The supply of grain dextrose is more than adequate to produce all organic chemicals that conceivably can be made from dextrose. Furthermore, corn yields are tending to increase with time. Given historical yield increases, each year US agriculture produces an additional 3.5×10^9 kg new dextrose equivalents. The biobased products industry will need to grow very rapidly even to consume the additional dextrose made available from new corn production. A switch from fossil carbon to renewable carbon for organic chemicals will occur as conversion technologies improve, conversion costs decline, and various barriers to entry are overcome.

In most situations it will be difficult for plant biomass to compete economically with coal as a solid fuel for stand alone electricity generation and we do not consider this case. However, electricity generation from biomass processing residues in an integrated processing facility producing liquid fuels and other products is very attractive. Biomass gasification to produce a natural gas substitute is also a much more attractive possibility than direct combustion, but likewise we do not treat it here because of space limitations. Gasification (and even direct combustion) seem most useful when applied to forest products and residues. US forest growth has exceeded harvest since the 1940s. Harvested timber, pulp, and paper have increased from private forestlands at the same time interest in preserving public forests in more or less "unmanaged" conditions has reduced the timber, pulp, and paper available from these public lands.

Thus the land and other agricultural resources of the US seem more than adequate to satisfy current domestic and export demands for food, feed, and fiber and still produce ample raw materials for a much larger biobased economy. Because the US consumes a disproportionate amount of fuel and chemicals compared with the rest of the world, there is reason to hope that other countries can also provide much more of their fuel and chemical needs from renewable carbon sources. We offer further evidence below that this is so. The only situation for which biobased feedstock supply adequacy for materials and chemicals does not seem to be the obvious conclusion is a massive increase of liquid fuel production from renewable carbon. The remainder of this paper deals with the concept of liquid fuel production from renewable carbon (specifically agricultural crops and crop residues) in mature, integrated processing facilities called "biorefineries".

2.3
Supplying the Biorefinery

2.3.1
What Raw Materials do Biorefineries Require and What Products Can They Make?

Although petroleum feedstocks vary somewhat in composition, their compositional variety is much less than for biomass feedstocks. Biomass compositional variety is both an advantage and disadvantage. Biomass feedstocks consist of grain, crop residues, oilseeds, sugar crops, forage crops, and a wide variety of woody crops. Figure 2.1 depicts typical compositions of some of these biomass feedstocks. The major components of biomass include carbohydrates (cellulose and hemicellulose for crop residues, forage crops and woody crops – called lignocellulosic materials, starch for grain, and primarily sucrose for sugar crops), lipids (fats, waxes and oils), proteins of many types, aromatic compounds (primarily lignin), and ash (non carbon minerals such as calcium, phosphorus, potassium, etc.).

An advantage of biomass compositional variety is that biorefineries can make more classes of products than can petroleum refineries, thus providing addi-

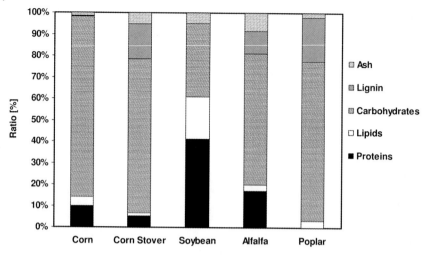

Fig. 2.1 Composition of several biomass species.

tional economic stability and opportunities for new product development. Biorefineries can also use a wider range of raw materials than can petroleum refineries. Among the products that might be produced from biomass are liquid transportation fuels (including both gasoline and diesel substitutes), electricity and steam, a tremendous variety of chemicals containing carbon, oxygen, hydrogen, and nitrogen and combinations of these elements, monomers and polymers, lubricants, adhesives, fertilizers and, significantly, animal feeds and human foods. Some of these products are summarized in Fig. 2.2 in their life cycle context as possible replacements for petroleum-based or petroleum-dependent products [9].

A disadvantage of biorefineries compared with petroleum refineries is that a relatively larger range of processing technologies is needed. This is particularly true for conversion and/or separation of the wider range of components of the renewable feedstock raw materials, as shown in Fig. 2.1. It is important to note in Fig. 2.2 that biorefineries will probably operate by first preprocessing (separating and reacting) the inlet raw materials to a relatively small range of intermediate products including carbohydrates, protein, syngas (mixtures of carbon monoxide, hydrogen and carbon dioxide) and a few other products. These intermediate products will then be upgraded by further reaction and separation steps to a very wide variety of final products. Some of these reaction and separation steps are well developed, others remain to be developed. In particular, the processing technologies to convert lignocellulosic materials economically and in high yield to carbohydrates and other products are not yet fully available. Once these and other processing technologies are developed and deployed, however, they will find use for a much wider variety and much more geographically dispersed set of renewable raw materials than is true for petroleum.

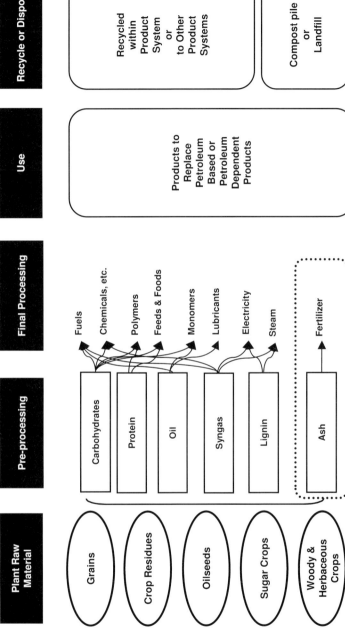

Fig. 2.2 Life cycle overview of biobased products [9].

Prototype biorefineries already exist, including corn wet and dry mills, pulp and paper mills, and other renewable carbon-based processing facilities. Corn wet mills perhaps best exemplify many of the features that are likely to be found in mature biorefineries for large-scale fuel production. Wet mills are large, highly integrated facilities producing a wide range of chemical, biochemical, feed, food, and fuel products, as outlined in Fig. 2.2. Over 90% of the inlet corn leaves as value-added products (selling price per kilogram greater than corn feedstock) [Ref. 1, Chapter 3]. Corn wet mills have continued to add products with time, particularly higher value chemical/biochemical products. Similarly to petroleum refineries, wet mills alter their product mix to meet changing market conditions, including seasonal variations in demand.

2.3.2
Comparing Biomass Feedstock Costs with Petroleum Costs

Of course, the widely dispersed and renewable nature of biomass feedstocks is of little practical importance unless we can reasonably expect to convert these feedstocks to products that will compete economically with petroleum-derived products. Fortunately, this is an entirely reasonable and feasible goal. To support this statement, we note that competitive pressures and continually improving conversion technologies gradually force many high margin new products to eventually become mature, commodity products with narrow margins. This process has occurred with products as diverse as penicillin, Nylon and, of course, gasoline.

Experience shows that approximately 60–70% of the cost of manufacturing commodity products depends on the cost of the raw materials from which these commodities are made [10, 11]. This is true for petroleum-derived commodities in particular, and explains the large swings in gasoline prices as crude oil prices change. We envisage a mature biorefining industry producing liquid biofuels to replace gasoline and diesel fuel. In such a mature biorefining industry the cost of manufacturing biofuels will also depend very highly on raw material cost. The question therefore arises: how does the cost of renewable plant biomass compare with the cost of petroleum? I am indebted to Professors Lee Lynd and Charles Wyman of Dartmouth College (Hanover, New Hampshire, USA) for suggesting the approach outlined in Fig. 2.3 below.

Figure 2.3 shows the cost of plant biomass relative to the cost of petroleum on two different bases – cost per kilogram of material and cost per unit of energy. Three different horizontal lines are drawn representing different classes of plant biomass available at three different prices. Crop residues are valued at $ 20 per ton (US) in Fig. 2.3, hays and forage crops such as low quality alfalfa are valued at $ 50 per ton, and corn grain at $ 120 per 1000 kg is roughly equivalent to current US Corn Belt prices of corn at about $ 2.75 per bushel. Historically, corn grain has been priced at closer to $ 2.00 per bushel in constant dollars, see Fig. 2.4 below.

Figures 2.3 and 2.4 teach several important lessons. First, corn grain at $ 3 per bushel is roughly equivalent to petroleum at $ 35 per barrel on an energy basis

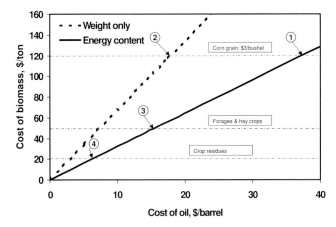

Fig. 2.3 Relative costs of biomass and petroleum by mass and energy content.

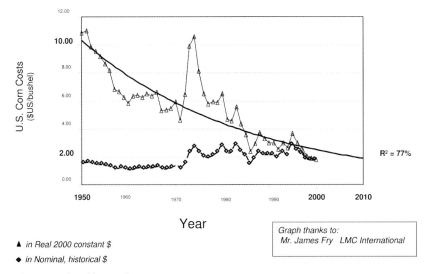

Fig. 2.4 Real and historial corn prices.

(arrow #1 in Fig. 2.3). On a mass basis, however, corn is less than half the cost of petroleum (arrow #2) – giving corn starch and other corn components real potential as a feedstock for chemical production to replace petroleum-derived chemicals. Corn wet millers often use net corn cost to reflect the cost of starch available for chemical and fuel production after coproduct credits (e.g. for protein and oil) are subtracted. Typical net corn costs are roughly 70% of the purchase cost of corn, further reducing the actual cost of corn starch for chemical or fuel production.

Ethanol production from corn grain currently requires various financial incentives to be competitive with gasoline from oil. No such incentives are required for chemicals from corn starch. Very large efforts are currently in progress to

Table 2.1 Ten required biomass feedstock properties.

1. **Economical**
2. Stable price and availability
3. Consistent composition
4. **Low cost**
5. Favorable co-products and by-products
6. Multiple product opportunities
7. **Inexpensive**
8. Environmentally benign or beneficial
9. Storable
10. **Inexpensive**

produce chemicals (e.g. lactic acid, 1,3 propanediol, etc.) from corn starch by either wet milling or dry milling. This is precisely how the petroleum refining industry developed. Additional valuable products such as plastics were added to the refinery over a period of decades as these products and processes were invented or improved and economics became attractive for the new products.

Second, lignocellulosic biomass such as crop residues and herbaceous species (grasses, hays, forage crops) is available at prices that are a fraction (one fifth to one half) of petroleum costs (at $ 35 per barrel) on an energy basis, and even less on a mass basis (arrows #3 and #4 in Fig. 2.3). Therefore, given processing technology that economically and efficiently converts the energy content of lignocellulosic biomass to liquid fuels, we can reasonably expect to derive fuel products that are available at prices similar to current gasoline and diesel prices. Sugar fermentation to ethanol is one such process. Over 90% of the energy content of glucose is captured in the ethanol product from high-yield fermentations.

Feedstock costs are absolutely critical to commodity chemicals and fuels, and biomass feedstocks are already much less expensive than petroleum on both a mass and energy basis. It is impossible to overstate the importance of low cost renewable carbon feedstocks to the eventual commercial success of large-scale, integrated biorefineries. Dr Paul Roessler of Dow Chemical (US) makes this point in a humorous and effective way in his list of ten required biomass feedstock properties, given as Table 2.1. In line with the historical development of other processing industries, as the biomass processing industry develops and the related technology matures, raw material costs will become dominant in the cost of manufacture.

2.3.3
How Much Biomass Feedstock Can be Provided at What Cost?

Renewable carbon feedstock prices are critical to the economic success of biorefineries. Although we believe data on likely biomass prices are encouraging, the ultimate possible scale of the industry, and hence its ability to displace petroleum, will also be determined by the amount of biomass available at these prices. We now briefly examine this subject using Table 2.2 to frame our discussion.

Table 2.2 summarizes world production of crop residues. In all, approximately 1.55×10^{12} kg residue are produced annually, the equivalent of approximately 600 billion liters of bioethanol at expected ethanol yields for mature technology of about 400 liters per 1000 kg residue [12]. The figure of 600 billion liters is close to the volume of gasoline and diesel consumed each year in the US, a very significant figure indeed.

Rice straw must be removed from fields before planting of the next crop and is probably available close to collection costs, given the demand for the straw. Currently most rice straw is field-burned to remove it, a practice becoming less and less tolerated everywhere. Worldwide, over 700×10^9 kg rice straw are produced annually, mostly in Asia. Almost 200×10^9 kg sugar-cane bagasse is collected annually in many locations worldwide. Bagasse is probably available at its fuel cost or below, because it has only limited value to provide energy for the sugar mill. Thus nearly one thousand billion kilograms of rice straw and sugar cane bagasse are probably available at nominal costs.

Considering other residues, approximately 100 billion kg per year corn stover and wheat straw in the Corn Belt and Great Plains regions of the United States are probably available at delivered prices of $ 20 per 1000 kg and less [14]. Similar amounts of residue, mostly wheat straw and barley straw, are available in Europe, probably at costs comparable with those in the United States. At $ 50 per 1000 kg, crop residue availability increases significantly. Approximately 150 billion kg US crop residues are available at this price compared with 100 billion kg at $ 20 per 1000 kg [14]. Other countries should also experience increased incentives to collect and utilize crop residues at higher prices. At about $ 50 per 1000 kg, farmers will also begin to produce hays and grasses specifically for biorefineries [15], and lignocellulosic biomass supplies will expand greatly. The extent to which supplies expand at a price of $ 50 per 1000 kg depends

Table 2.2 Worldwide availability of crop residues [13].

Material (billion kg)	Africa	Asia	Europe	North America	Central America	Oceania	South America	Subtotal
Corn stover	0.0	33.9	28.6	134	0.0	0.2	7.2	204
Barley straw	0.0	2.0	44.2	9.9	0.2	1.9	0.3	58.5
Oat straw	0.0	0.3	6.8	2.8	0.0	0.5	0.2	10.6
Rice straw	20.9	668	3.9	10.9	2.8	1.7	23.5	731
Wheat straw	5.3	145	133	50.1	2.8	8.6	9.8	354
Sorghum straw	0.0	0.0	0.4	6.9	1.2	0.3	1.5	10.3
Bagasse	11.7	74.9	0.0	4.6	19.2	6.5	63.8	181
Subtotal	38.0	924	217	219	26.1	19.7	106	1549

largely on the productivity of crop and pasture lands. The RBAEF Project will treat this subject of productivity in great detail. We simply observe here that the US has nearly 16 million ha in its Conservation Reserve Program (CRP), land which is removed from grain crop production but which would be very suitable for grass and hay production.

In the US, pasture lands (including crop land used as pasture) average about 5600 kg of biomass per ha per year [16]. There is little incentive to increase production on these lands, because there are no markets for increased hay production. Biomass production for energy would provide increased incentive to use these lands efficiently and a severalfold increase in average yield over time seems entirely likely. For example, some lands supporting dairy cattle in Michigan are managed intensively for maximum biomass production, including the use of winter cover crops and corn harvested as silage. Such lands are currently yielding 20000 kg dry biomass per ha per year. Double these yields (40000 kg ha^{-1} per year) of other species such as sugarcane and elephant grass have also been achieved on degraded lands [17]. If all the CRP lands and one half of crop land used as pasture (15 million ha) achieved 20000 kg ha^{-1}, an additional 600×10^9 kg biomass would be produced annually in the US.

We believe the large scale conversion of cellulosic biomass to fuel will be based first on crop residues, given their low cost and availability. There is more than enough low-cost crop residue in the US and elsewhere to begin such an industry. As the industry expands, and processing economics improve with research and experience, the "demand pull" for additional biomass will cause the agricultural research and production sector to learn how to produce much larger amounts of herbaceous biomass profitably at costs approximating $ 50 per 1000 kg on lands that compete only modestly or not at all with food crop production. In addition, biorefineries producing fuels will also produce both protein and energy feeds for animals, just as corn wet and dry mills producing ethanol fuel do today. Coproduction of animal feeds with fuel and chemical products in biorefineries will increase feed supplies and reduce pressure on cropland.

Before concluding this treatment of biomass feedstock costs, we note that the wide geographic availability, abundance and variety of biomass will tend to reduce the risks of raw material supply availability and reduce price swings. Uncertain availability and price volatility are major features of the current petroleum economy. As an essentially fixed world endowment of easily recoverable petroleum is gradually consumed, these risks will only grow and an increasing price paid in terms of national security and stability [2, 18]. Therefore, this economic and energy security issue can only grow in importance. Furthermore, many developed and developing nations which lack petroleum can grow large quantities of plant biomass, and thereby begin to escape the "development trap" that petroleum dependence brings in an era of decreasing petroleum supplies and high and volatile prices [18].

2.4
How Will Biorefineries Develop Technologically?

2.4.1
Product Yield: The Dominant Technoeconomic Factor

Yield (kg salable products per kg purchased raw materials) is usually the dominant factor governing the economics of a given reaction/separation system to produce commercial products. Because, essentially, all chemical and biological reactions produce multiple products, the yield of salable products influences the economics of the system in the following ways.

1. Raw material cost increases per unit of product as yield declines. For example, at $ 0.10 per pound of glucose and 90% yield of lactic acid produced by fermentation of this glucose, the glucose raw material cost is $ 0.11 per pound of lactic acid. At 50% yield, the raw material cost is $ 0.20 per pound of lactic acid. Because the cost of manufacturing commodity fuels and chemicals is very dependent on raw material costs, a lower yield significantly increases the cost of manufacture.
2. The cost of the reaction system increases. If a fixed total annual production rate is required, then at 50% yield almost twice the total reactor volume is needed compared with 90% yield to provide that amount of product.
3. The cost of the separation system increases even more rapidly than the reaction system. The cost of separation is proportional to the volume of fluid handled. Under similar reaction conditions, a lower yield means lower concentration of product and, therefore, a greater volume of reaction fluid must be handled for a given production rate. The cost of separation also increases with the number of components needing separation. Decreasing yield usually means there are more components that must be separated.
4. The cost of waste treatment increases. Either markets for byproducts must be found, which is not always possible, or the resulting waste streams must be treated before disposal, adding to both the capital and operating expense of the overall system.

Given the dominance of yield in process economics for commodities, several conclusions regarding biorefinery development for fuels and commodity chemicals arise.

First, fuel production in biorefineries will tend to be performed first in existing facilities where the yield of products can be improved by adding fuel production and where substantial capital investment has already been made, reducing the risk to innovators. Second, given the mild conditions (moderate pH and temperature) of biological catalysts, bioprocessing and biotechnology will tend to be used in biorefineries instead of harsh chemical or thermal processing to avoid degradation (and thereby the loss of value) of sugars, proteins and other labile biomolecules. Third, there will be continuing pressure to use all of the components of the biomass feedstock at their highest possible value. Thus the number of products will increase over time as will the yield of salable products per unit of raw material(s) consumed. This is precisely the trend that has occurred historically in the petroleum refining industry.

Because we have pointed out several probable similarities between petroleum refineries and biorefineries, it is worth pointing out here a very significant difference between them. Both genetic tools and conventional plant breeding can be used to develop biomass feedstocks that are particularly designed for processing in the biorefinery. For example, lignin content can be altered to make lignocellulosic biomass easier to process. Also, valuable products such as enzymes can be produced in plants and recovered in the biorefinery [Ref. 1, Chapter 1]. This capability has no parallel in petroleum refining and is a major advantage for biorefineries. Continuing advances in the life sciences virtually guarantee that this advantage will grow with time.

2.4.2
Product Diversification: Using the Whole Barrel of Biomass

The importance of finding valuable uses for all biomass components is illustrated by the following example based on the composition outlined in Fig. 2.1. Assume a corn stover-based biorefinery producing 378 million liters per year of fuel ethanol at a yield of 420 liters of ethanol per 1000 kg stover. At a 50% removal rate for stover, approximately 200000 ha corn will be required to provide the stover. Such a biorefinery will also produce nearly 21×10^6 kg minerals (Ca, K, Mg and P), 20×10^6 kg lipids, fats, and waxes, 52×10^6 kg protein (equivalent to the protein produced from nearly 70000 ha soybeans), electricity from burning the lignin residue and probably residual sugars for animal feeding. These conclusions arise directly from the chemical nature of the components of biomass and the realities of chemical and biological processing outlined in Section 2.4.1, above. A biorefinery will be in many businesses (fuels, chemicals, power, feed, etc.) simultaneously. This fact cannot be evaded, but must be faced and dealt with, hopefully to the benefit of the overall biorefining system.

One significant potential benefit that arises from this analysis is that the net requirement for agricultural land to provide feed protein decreases by 70000 ha, or about 1/3 of the land from which stover is harvested. Put another way, 3 ha of corn production are now able to replace 1 ha of soybean production, while still providing all the grain these corn acres produced before and 900×10^6 kg stover for liquid fuel production. If herbaceous biomass species, for example switchgrass, are grown for energy production, they will probably be higher yielding and will also contain significantly more protein than corn stover. Thus such crops should provide even greater net savings of crop land required to meet protein needs. For example, if switchgrass or another herbaceous species such as coastal Bermuda grass is produced at dry matter yields of 20000 kg ha^{-1} per year (about 9 tons acre^{-1} year^{-1}) and contains 10% protein of which 80% is recovered [19, 20], the system will produce 1,600 kg ha^{-1} protein, over twice the amount of protein produced per ha of soybeans. Because the United States currently devotes approximately 30 million ha to soybean production, this emphasis on using the whole barrel of biomass could lead to substantial coproduction of energy and protein, but without devoting any new acreage to energy crop production.

As described in Section 2.4.1 above, if the various components of biomass are not used in salable products, they must be disposed of at a cost. If they are not used in products, they must also be carried along with all the other streams in the process, adding to the capital and operating costs of all the related processing equipment. Likewise, if these components are not used in products, the remaining products must bear a larger portion of the overall costs, particularly the crucial feedstock costs. Thus many forces converge on a single objective: utilizing the entire "barrel of biomass". The overall result of this convergence is quite simple: there is strong and unrelenting pressure to increase the yield and value of the multiple products of biomass and not to waste even a fraction of the raw materials.

Because of this driving force, continuous, incremental process improvement is a key feature of both oil refineries and existing biorefineries. There are, however, many improvements and innovations that cannot occur until a refinery is actually operating and producing products and will not result from laboratory discoveries. We expect this pattern of continuous, incremental improvement in existing facilities will continue both with existing, starch-based biorefineries. It will also occur with the next generation of cellulose biorefineries that will come when key breakthroughs occur. We now briefly discuss breakthroughs required for cellulose biorefineries.

2.4.3
Process Development and a Technical Prerequisite for Cellulosic Biorefineries

If plant raw material is already inexpensive compared with petroleum and sufficiently abundant to support a large scale biorefining industry, one may legitimately ask: "Why has such an industry not already emerged?" We note that such industries have arisen: corn wet and dry mills and pulp and paper mills are examples. For these industries, inexpensive raw materials are coupled with well developed and efficient processing technology to convert the plant raw materials to products. For large scale liquid fuel production from cellulosic materials, however, the missing part of the equation is *demonstrated, inexpensive processing technology* to convert inexpensive and abundant cellulosic raw materials to fuels.

While we believe that the entire barrel of biomass must be used effectively, use of the carbohydrate component (cellulose and hemicellulose represent approximately 70% of cellulosic biomass) is the sine qua non for cellulosic biorefineries [Ref. 1, Chapters 4 and 21]. The accessibility (reactivity) of cellulose and hemicellulose must be increased without significantly degrading these components. These carbohydrate polymers must somehow be converted into chemically reactive intermediate species, as shown in Fig. 2.2. Achieving this objective requires some sort of pretreatment before enzymatic, biological, or chemical upgrading of these sugar polymers to more valuable products such as ethanol fuel. Overcoming the recalcitrance of cellulosic biomass is therefore arguably the single most important research/process development obstacle confronting biorefineries processing cellulosic biomass to fuels.

A closely related research objective for cellulose biorefineries is significantly reducing the cost of enzymes (called "cellulases") required to convert pretreated biomass into fermentable sugars. An even more powerful impact on the economics of cellulose biorefineries than inexpensive enzymes would occur given the high yield, one step biological conversion of pretreated biomass to useful products. This process by which cellulase production, cellulose hydrolysis, and fermentation of soluble sugars to desired products occur in a single process step is called "consolidated bioprocessing" [21].

If viable, inexpensive pretreatments to overcome the recalcitrance of cellulosic biomass are developed, it seems likely they will first be demonstrated in existing facilities where a cellulose/hemicellulose-containing stream is available for upgrading to fuels and chemicals. Such existing facilities include pulp and paper mills, corn wet and dry mills, and perhaps flour mills. When this key piece of technology is available, the first generation of cellulose biorefineries will be launched. These pioneer plants will become the loci for further improvements, both incremental and transformational, in converting cellulosic biomass to a wide variety of fuels, chemicals, animal feeds, and other products.

2.5
Sustainability of Integrated Biorefining Systems

2.5.1
Integrated Biorefining Systems: "All Biomass is Local"

Because biomass feedstocks are solids and tend to be bulky, there is considerable incentive to refine them close to where they are grown. Likewise the waste streams from biorefineries will tend to be high in organic material and therefore biological oxygen demand. But these biorefinery wastes will not be particularly toxic. Many of these waste streams are therefore suitable candidates for returning to agricultural land. Given the capital and operating costs associated with waste handling in the biorefinery, there is a strong economic incentive to apply these wastes to land.

Furthermore, agriculture is, by nature, a regional or local activity because of differences in soil and climate. Therefore crops grown for biorefineries can be or will be adapted to local conditions. The relatively smaller scale of biorefineries (compared with petroleum refineries) also enhances the likelihood that the farmers who produce the crops will have some sort of formal or informal "ownership" of the biorefinery. This pattern of local ownership of the biorefinery, or at least participation in ownership, is observed in many corn dry mills in the US. Corn wet mills are, however, much larger than dry mills (the largest wet mills approach the mass throughput rate of petroleum refineries) and are not farmer-owned. Local ownership of the biorefinery will give farmers an additional incentive to utilize animal feeds, mineral fertilizers, and organic waste streams from the biorefinery. We call this framework the "All Biomass is Local" concept; it is illustrated in Fig. 2.5.

We envisage farmers using locally appropriate agricultural systems growing biomass specifically for the biorefinery. In the biorefinery, biomass is separated into its major components. Some of these components (e.g., protein and minerals or "ash") may be salable or usable without further upgrading. The ash is returned as fertilizer to the land. Protein is fed to animals, preferably in a nearby location to avoid costs of drying and transportation. Animal wastes and organic waste streams from the biorefinery are used in the agricultural system. The nature of these waste streams makes them particularly appropriate for land application to perennial grass systems, where the potential for runoff and leaching to groundwater is minimized.

Therefore, the convergence of these factors:
- local ownership/participation in biorefineries,
- the widespread geographical distribution of these refineries,
- the fact that biorefineries will be intimately involved with land use practices, and
- society's continuing concern with the environment

virtually guarantee that biorefineries will be conceived, designed, built, and operated with an unprecedented emphasis on their local and global environmental impact. Petroleum refineries largely avoided environmental/social issues when that industry was in its infancy, but now are being forced to do so at great cost. Biorefineries that do not adequately address appropriate environmental and social issues will be at substantial risk of failure.

We believe these environmental and social issues surrounding biorefineries are best addressed using the concept of sustainability as an organizing framework and life cycle analysis as a powerful analytical methodology [22]. As we illustrate below, we believe that thoughtful, intelligent design and implementation of integrated agricultural production and biorefining systems can do much more than simply maintain the environmental status quo. Rather, we believe it is possible to effect significant improvements in the local, regional, and global environment by using life cycle analysis of integrated crop production and refining systems.

2.5.2
Agricultural/Forestry Ecosystem Modeling: New Tools for an Age of Sustainability

Sustainability is a very broad subject. In this paper we do not have the scope to treat all aspects of sustainability in relation to crop production and biorefining systems such as those represented in Fig. 2.6. To illustrate an approach that

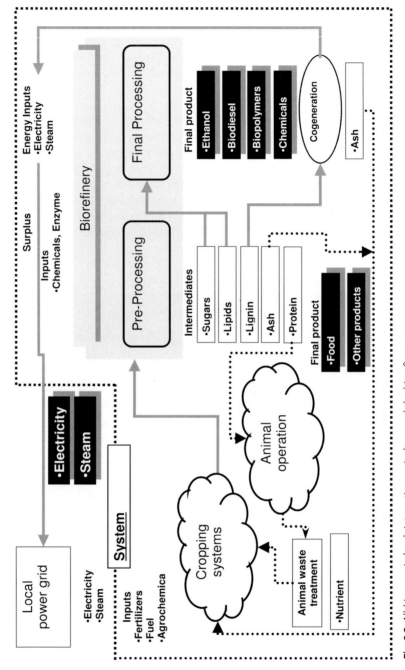

Fig. 2.5 All biomass is local: integrating agriculture and the biorefinery.

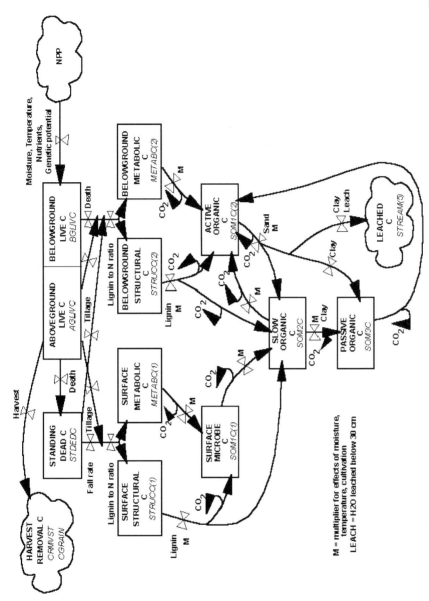

Fig. 2.6 Carbon flows in the CENTURY model [25].

might be taken, however, we consider the dynamics of carbon and nitrogen flow in agricultural ecosystems. We then analyze how those flows might be manipulated to enhance the sustainability of the agricultural production and biorefining system when taken as an integrated whole. We also point out what seem to be some emerging principles for understanding the sustainability of these systems.

Analyzing and modeling carbon and nitrogen flows in agricultural ecosystems has been an active area of research for over thirty years [23, 24]. Researchers have studied a variety of biological and nonbiological processes connected with plant growth. These processes occur in the soil, on the surface and above the surface of the ground. Researchers have estimated the rates of these processes based on local factors such as temperature, soil type, rainfall, plant genetic potential and existing pools of carbon such as microbial carbon, standing dead plant, carbon, etc. Tillage and harvesting practices have also been taken into account, as have other human inputs such as fertilizers and irrigation. As a result of such work, flexible, powerful agricultural ecosystem models such as the CENTURY model have been developed [25, 26]. To illustrate the breadth of processes considered in such ecosystem level studies, a diagram for carbon flow in the CENTURY model is given below.

Similar agricultural ecosystem models have been developed for nitrogen-containing species and are being developed for phosphorus-containing compounds. When these ecosystem models are combined with models of the biorefinery processes, we can use them to evaluate and then improve the sustainability of integrated biorefining systems. We illustrate this approach below.

2.5.3
Analyzing the Sustainability of Integrated Biorefining Systems: Some Results

We envisaged an integrated biorefining system based on corn grain, soybeans, and corn stover, i.e. the cellulosic residue remaining after grain is harvested. We assume that a second harvesting trip through the field is required to cut, bale, and remove the corn stover. Fuel ethanol is assumed to be produced from the corn grain by wet milling and additional ethanol from corn stover by acid hydrolysis and fermentation [27]. Residual fermentation solids are burned to produce electricity and steam. Steam is used in the plant and excess electricity is exported to the grid. Soybean oil is converted to biodiesel. To satisfy soil erosion prevention guidelines, a minimum of 1070 kg ha^{-1} corn stover are left behind. None of the soybean stover is removed. Several different agricultural scenarios are investigated to determine the effect of cropping system management on environmental performance. The cropping system assumptions for sustainability analysis are summarized below in Table 2.3. The acronyms given to each scenario in Table 2.3 are used in subsequent figures to identify simulation results.

In all, six different scenarios are modeled and analyzed. Because "all biomass is local" we choose a particular location, Washington County, Illinois, USA, for our analysis. Climate and soil data and cropping practices are available for this

Table 2.3 Assumptions for cropping system sustainability analysis.

Basic cropping system
– Corn (plow till) – soybean (no-till): CPSN (grain)

Effect of winter cover crop under no-till corn continuous cultivation
– 0% of corn stover removed: CC (grain) (No winter cover crop)
– Average 56% of corn stover removed: CC (56%) (No winter cover crop)
– Wheat and oat as winter cover crops with 70% corn stover removal: CwCo (70%)

Effect of winter cover crop under no-till corn–soybean rotation
– Wheat and oat as winter cover crops after corn cultivation with 70% corn stover removal:
  CwCo (70%)
– Average 54% of corn stover removed: CS (54%) (No winter cover crop)
Cover crop not harvested

location. The agricultural base is conventional midwestern US corn–soybean rotation with only corn grain and soybean harvested, using plow till for corn and no till cultivation for soybeans (CPSN in Table 2.3). For all other scenarios both corn and soybeans are grown under no-till cultivation practices, in which soil is left undisturbed from harvest to planting. A second scenario is the continuous cultivation of corn (CC), again with only corn grain harvested. A third scenario includes the harvest and removal of 56% of the corn stover and all the grain under continuous corn cultivation (CC 56%). A fourth scenario is rotation of corn with soybeans and removal of 54% of the corn stover and all the corn grain and soybeans (CS 54%).

We explore the use of cover crops in the two final scenarios. In some areas it is common to plant another crop such as wheat or oats in the late fall after the corn is harvested. These young plants grow a few centimeters, survive over the winter and then resume growth in the spring once conditions permit. Cover crops can be harvested, killed with herbicide or plowed under to increase soil organic matter. In this analysis we assume that the cover crop is not harvested by rather is killed with herbicide and the corn or soybean is planted in the dead cover crop.

Cover crops help eliminate wind and water erosion and are also effective in removing excess nitrogen fertilizer left behind in the previous cropping cycle. This excess nitrogen is vulnerable to conversion by various processes to soluble nitrogen species that leach through soil and are transported to streams, lakes, rivers and the ocean. This excess nitrogen can also be converted by anaerobic soil bacteria to nitrous oxide, a potent greenhouse gas. The fifth scenario therefore considers continuous corn with 70% removal of stover plus winter wheat or oats as a cover crop (CwCo 70%). The sixth and last scenario assumes a corn–soybean rotation from which 70% of the corn stover is harvested and winter cover crops are grown (CwSo 70%).

Soil organic carbon levels were predicted over time using the six scenarios modeled. Depending on conditions chosen, either static or increasing soil organic carbon levels are possible as shown in Fig. 2.7, below, as long as cultivation is no till. The use of winter cover crops enables very substantial removal of corn stover for industrial uses while still enhancing soil quality over time.

The total amount of protein, lipids, lignin and carbohydrate (including starch, cellulose and hemicellulose) produced by each of the cropping systems above was estimated over a 40 year period. Based on data from biorefinery operations and crop production databases, greenhouse gases were also calculated in kilogram carbon dioxide equivalents per kilogram of each of these species produced. Figure 2.8 shows greenhouse gas production per kilogram of carbohydrate for each of the six scenarios.

Once again, the cropping system chosen has a significant effect on the results. The results range from a net production of 560 g of CO_2 kg^{-1} carbohydrate for conventional corn–soybean rotation to 9 g (net carbon sequestration) kg^{-1} carbohydrate for continuous corn cultivation under no-till conditions with winter wheat and 70% stover removal.

A similar life-cycle approach is taken to estimate the greenhouse gas reduction when ethanol produced using the biorefinery systems outlined above is consumed in a mid-sized passenger vehicle. Figure 2.9 summarizes these results. All of the cropping systems result in net greenhouse gas reduction, but there are substantial differences between cropping systems. Aggressive corn stover removal when coupled with winter cover crops can result in over 70% reduction in greenhouse gas formation compared with a gasoline fueled vehicle. But as Fig. 2.7 shows, soil health can continue to improve even when large amounts of stover are removed.

Finally, even more dramatic reductions in leached nitrogen (inorganic nitrogen species escaping the root zone of plants) are possible by judicious choice of cropping systems and agricultural system management. Using the nitrogen flow submodel of the CENTURY model to predict the effects of different agricultural practices, it seems possible to reduce inorganic nitrogen losses more

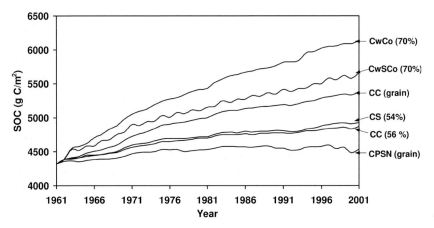

Fig. 2.7 Soil organic carbon trends under different agricultural practices.

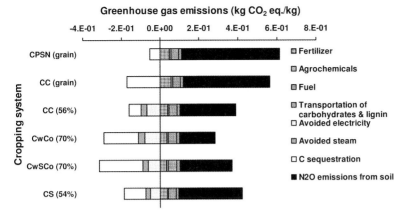

Fig. 2.8 Greenhouse gas emissions per kg carbohydrate.

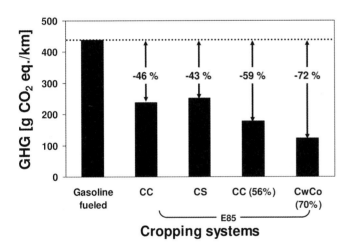

Fig. 2.9 Greenhouse gas reductions under different cropping systems.

than a factor of ten by use of conventional corn production as the base case. These results are summarized in Fig. 2.10. The results are for a 40 year period in which these practices are used in a specific geographic location – Washington County, Illinois, USA.

As expected, the use of winter cover crops greatly reduces nitrogen leaching. It is also interesting to note that stover removal seems to reduce nitrogen leaching – compare CC with CC (56%). One mechanistic explanation of these results is that the nitrogen content of the corn stover (approx. 1% by weight) is not available for conversion to soluble inorganic nitrogen species when the stover is removed, thereby reducing leaching. Also, the carbohydrates in harvested stover are not then available to provide metabolic energy for microbial processes that

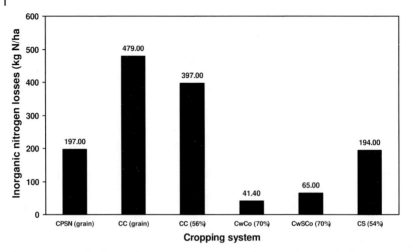

Fig. 2.10 Inorganic nitrogen losses over 40 years – Washington Country, Illinois.

convert organic nitrogen into inorganic nitrogen. Although stover removal must be carefully managed to maintain soil fertility, stover removal has powerful environmental benefits. These benefits include providing renewable carbon for biorefining to fuels and chemicals and reduced inorganic nitrogen leaching.

On the basis of these and other results, we believe that a combination of creative system design, careful planning and use of powerful ecosystem and biorefinery modeling tools can help us achieve very significant environmental improvements as we develop the biobased economy of the 21st century. We need not be content with maintaining the environmental status quo or even with modest improvements. Instead, very significant improvements are possible if we are both wise and informed.

2.6
Conclusions

The biobased economy will grow rapidly during the 21st century. A combination of low-cost plant raw materials and gradually improving biorefinery process technology for converting these raw materials into a variety of fuels, chemicals, materials, food, and feed will drive the adoption of the biobased economy. The biological sciences will have a particularly powerful impact on both the raw materials and the processing technologies underlying the biobased economy. The biobased economy, and its associated biorefineries, will be shaped by many of the same forces that shaped the development of the hydrocarbon economy and its refineries over the past century. These similarities include the importance of yield (using the whole "barrel of biomass"), continuing diversification of products, and gradual process improvement in functioning biorefineries.

However, significant differences between the biobased economy and the hydrocarbon economy are also apparent. Among these are the great compositional variety of plant raw material, requiring a greater range of processing technologies to add value to the basic components, and the much wider geographic distribution of both raw materials and the associated refineries. This wide geographic distribution of both raw materials and biorefineries will promote greater economic/national security and more equitable distribution of wealth. We believe that supposed limits on agricultural productivity to support the biobased economy are mostly illusory. There is no "food vs. fuel" conflict. Economic profitability and process efficiency will force the adoption of "food and fuel" scenarios. Biorefineries and their associated crop production systems will be highly integrated. Furthermore, integrated biorefining systems will be designed to achieve not only economic profitability but also environmental benefits. Truly transformational environmental benefits can be achieved by creative design of these integrated biorefining systems.

Acknowledgements

The authors gratefully acknowledge support from Cargill Dow, LLP, from DuPont Biobased Materials, Inc., and from the Center for Plant Products and Technology at Michigan State University.

References

1 C. J. Arntzen, B. E. Dale (Eds.), *Biobased Industrial Products: Research and Commercialization Priorities*, National Academy Press, USA, **2000**, 26–54.
2 C. J. Campbell, J. H. Laherrere, *Scientific American*. **1998**, 278 (3), 78–83.
3 L. F. Ivanhoe, *World Oil* **1996**, 217(11), 91–94.
4 J. T. Houghton, *Ency. Energy Tech. Environ.* **1995**, 1, 491–504.
5 M. Graboski, R. Bain, *Biomass Gasification: Principles and Technology*, T. B. Reed (Ed.), Noyes Data Corporation, USA, **1981**, 41–71.
6 Energy Information Agency, http://www.eia.doe.gov/pub/international/iealf/table18.xls, United States Dept. of Energy, **2002**.
7 Anon., Chem. Eng. News **2002**, 22, 55–63.
8 Statistical Abstract of the United States, Table #958 (http://www.census.gov/prod/2001pubs/statab/sec19.pdf), **2000**.
9 S. Kim, B. E. Dale, *J. Ind. Ecol.* **2004**, 7(3/4), 147–162.
10 B. E. Dale, *TIBTECH*. **1987**, October 287–291.
11 G. E. Tong, *Chem. Eng. Prog.* **1978**, April 70–83.
12 C. E. Wyman, *Ann. Rev. Energy Environ.* **1999**, 24, 189–226.
13 S. Kim, B. E. Dale, *Biomass & Bioenergy* **2004**, 26, 361–375.
14 P. Gallagher, et al., *Biomass from Crop Residues: Cost and Supply Estimates*, US Dept of Agriculture Economic Report 819, USA, **2003**.
15 United States Dept. of Agriculture Hay Reporter http://www.ams.usda.gov/mnreports/DC_GR310.txt. **2004**.
16 United States Dept. of Agriculture Agricultural Statistics Table 6.1 http://www.usda.gov/nass/pubs/agr04/04_ch6.pdf. **2003**.

17 J. A. Stricker, et al., *Production and Management of Biomass/Energy Crops on Phosphatic Clay in Central Florida*, Univ. of Florida Cooperative Extension Service Circular 1084, USA, **1993**.

18 R. G. Lugar, R. J. Woolsey, *Foreign Affairs*. **1999**, 78(1), 88–102.

19 M. E. Ensminger, C. G. Olentine, Jr., *Feeds and Nutrition – Complete*, The Ensminger Publishing Company, USA, **1978**.

20 L. B. de la Rosa, et al., *Appl. Biochem. & Biotech*. **1994**, 45/46, 483–497.

21 L. R. Lynd, C. E. Wyman, T. U. Gerngross, *Biotech. Prog.* **1999**, 15, 777–793.

22 R. Anex (Ed.), *J. Ind. Ecol.* **2004**, 7(3/4). See articles on pages 75–92, 93–116, 117–146 and 147–162.

23 L. Kristen, et al., *Parameterizing Century to model cultivated and noncultivated sites in the loess region of western Iowa*, US Geological Survey Report 00-508, US Department of the Interior, USA, **2000**.

24 P. Smith, et al., *Quantifying the change in greenhouse gas emissions due to natural resource conservation practice application in Indiana*, Final report to the Indiana Conservation Partnership, Colorado State University Natural Resource Ecology Laboratory and USDA Natural Resources Conservation Service, USA, **2002**.

25 A. K. Metherall, L. A. Harding, C. V. Cole, W. J. Parton, CENTURY Soil organic matter model environment. Technical documentation. Agroecosystem version 4.0. Great Plains System Research Unit Technical Report No. 4. UDSA-ARS, USA, **1993**.

26 R. H. Kelly, et al., *Geoderma* **1999**, 81, 75–90.

27 J. Sheehan, et al., *Is ethanol from corn stover sustainable?*, National Renewable Energy Laboratory Draft Report, USA, December 2002.

3
Development of Biorefineries –
Technical and Economic Considerations

Bill Dean, Tim Dodge, Fernando Valle, and Gopal Chotani

3.1
Introduction

As the world's population and economy continue to grow, so does the demand for goods to sustain that growth. Growth has come at the expense of our non-renewable resources. It is only a matter of time before the price of petroleum, upon which the world economy is heavily dependent, will rise to a point where we will be forced by economic factors to find alternatives. We suspect this time is not far off in the future and the time is now to explore viable alternatives.

Our nation is fortunate to have abundant agricultural and forest renewable resources and a climate that is amenable to their productive use. If we put our mind to it, these renewable assets can go a long way to replace our heavy dependence on petroleum and other non-renewables. That process has, in a way, already begun, as we have been in the business of "bio-refining" in the broader sense for quite some time. Our forests are harvested to produce a host of products including paper, solvents, building materials, and many more. Our agriculture industry can produce large quantities of grain and other crops, which can and are being used to produce a host of materials. Starch from grain crops and sucrose from beet, sugar cane, and other materials are being converted to an increasing number of products and chemicals. Some of the chemicals now being produced include ethanol, 1,3-propanediol, lactic acid, and ascorbic acid. As the technology of pathway engineering advances, one can expect many more chemicals (and polymers) to be produced from sugar as a carbon source [1, 2].

Increasing demand for sugars will eventually result in increasing sugar prices and, ultimately, supply problems. It is logical to assume that as more chemicals and materials are produced from fermentable sugars as the carbon source, market forces will inevitably drive fundamental changes in the agriculture and chemical sectors.

Genencor International has been active in developing technologies that have affected the evolution of biorefineries. As part of our efforts in this area, we have actively explored the concept of using cellulosic biomass to provide the car-

Biorefineries – Industrial Processes and Products. Status Quo and Future Directions. Vol. 1
Edited by Birgit Kamm, Patrick R. Gruber, Michael Kamm
Copyright © 2006 WILEY-VCH Verlag GmbH & Co. KGaA, Weinheim
ISBN: 3-527-31027-4

bon source for such future refineries. In this pursuit, we have focused on the conversion of cellulosic biomass into fermentable sugars and on the challenges of biocatalysis in utilizing those sugar streams [3, 4].

Advances in pathway engineering will result in commercially viable and competitive processes based on renewable feedstocks which in many cases will provide the low-cost route to production. The cost of carbon to feed biocatalysis is often more than 50% of the total direct cost of production, and therefore efforts to reduce this cost play an important role in the overall development of the biorefinery concept. It is not surprising that many have focused on cellulosic biomass (e.g., agricultural waste) as the ultimate low cost source of the fermentable sugar in the biorefinery. Much knowledge has been gained and progress made on the understanding of cellulosic biomass saccharification to fermentable sugars to be used for bioconversion to chemicals.

The challenge before us is to develop the technologies that will be required to enable this upcoming industry. We will focus here two of these technologies:
1. enzymes required for conversion of cellulosic biomass to fermentable sugars within an enabling cost structure; and
2. engineered organisms to produce chemicals competitively.

3.2
Overview: The Biorefinery Model

Biorefineries, often referred to as integrated biorefineries, are processing facilities that use renewable plant materials as feedstocks. Plant materials, comprising carbohydrates and associated oil, protein, lignin, and other components, are converted in the biorefinery into higher-value chemicals and materials. Our broad definition of biorefineries includes a initial process that utilizes renewable carbon feedstocks containing sucrose, starch, and cellulose as shown in Fig. 3.1.

Essential elements of a biorefinery are:
1. multiple feedstock capability and a tolerance of wide variation in those feedstocks;
2. feedstock-processing by enzymes to fermentable sugars (and by-product streams);
3. biocatalyst, which converts sugars to desired product(s), and
4. co-products which are used in the process, recycled through the process, or sold.

3.3
Feedstock and Conversion to Fermentable Sugar

Three basic biorefinery approaches, as portrayed in Fig. 3.2, are evolving on the basis of the nature of the feedstock, i.e. sucrose, starch, or cellulose.

On a fermentable-carbon-cost basis, the sucrose-based Biorefinery I is currently the most cost-competitive. In recent years, however, the starch-based Bio-

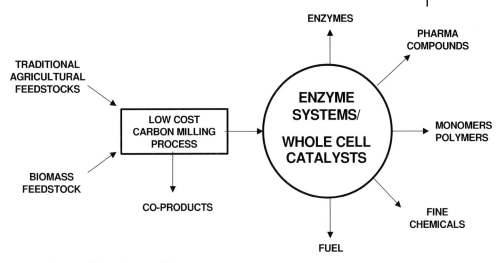

Fig. 3.1 The overall biorefinery model.

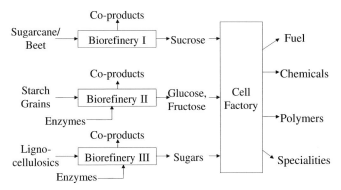

Fig. 3.2 Biorefinery evolution.

refinery II has become more cost competitive as a result of innovations in farming and milling grain like corn. In principle, the cellulose-based Biorefinery III will become more competitive as technical and economic challenges are addressed. As illustrated in Fig. 3.3, fermentable sugars, whether derived from sucrose, starch, or cellulose, will become cost competitive with petroleum-derived carbon for production of fuel, chemicals, polymeric materials, and specialty intermediates.

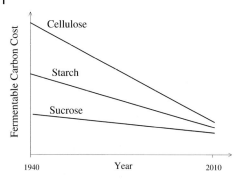

Fig. 3.3 Change of cost of fermentable carbon with time for different carbohydrate sources.

3.3.1
Sucrose

The simplest biorefinery system uses sucrose as feedstock (sugar beet, cane, etc.). Sugar is first extracted from the feedstock. Lignin and cellulosic residuals, if sugar cane is used, are utilized separately or burned for energy to run the operation. The sucrose-based industry is a significant biorefinery opportunity today and into the future. Sucrose is second only to cellulose in availability and current output far exceeds all other commercial carbohydrates combined. It is estimated that only 1.7% of annual sucrose production goes to non-food uses. It is possible to imagine a sugar biorefinery as an integrated producer, not only of sucrose and ethanol, but of important high-value products whose manufacture could be scaled up or down depending on circumstances, economics, and demand [5]. Not surprisingly, more than 50% of ethanol volume produced in the world today has sucrose as feedstock.

3.3.2
Starch

The grain wet-milling industry as it exists today is an excellent example of the biorefinery concept. The grain kernel, e.g. corn, is processed through a series of steps resulting in a glucose (or multimers of glucose) stream and co-products such as oil, protein, fiber, and nutrients (e.g. carotenoids and corn steep liquor). The glucose can be further converted to ethanol, 1,3-propanediol, lactic acid, etc., by fermentation, and to sweeteners, for example high-fructose syrup, by enzymatic conversion. The starch-based biorefinery has been enabled by the development of highly efficient and thermostable amylases and the development of isomerization processes to convert glucose to fructose by immobilized glucose isomerase enzyme systems.

The corn (and other grain) dry mill is a highly specialized abbreviated version of the wet mill whereby many of the initial steeping and extraction steps have been removed and starch is enzymatically converted to glucose and fermented to ethanol in a process called simultaneous saccharification and fermentation (SSF). The capital cost of building these less complex bio-refineries is significantly lower than for wet mills, but the trade-off is that dry mill co-product streams (distillers dried grains and solubles, or DDGS, sold into select animal feed markets) have relatively lower value.

Thermal energy consumption is significant in the milling process. A wet corn mill is very effective in extracting maximum value, because of the multiplicity of products and co-products mentioned above. In general, however, a wet grain mill is capital-intensive, and therefore new ethanol production plants coming on-line in recent years are mainly of the dry grain mill type. New enzyme technology developments hold considerable promise for impact here and these refineries will continue to evolve.

3.3.3
Cellulose

Considering the amount of cellulosic biomass available for saccharification to fermentable sugar, there is a clear opportunity to develop commercial processes that could generate products that are needed at very high volumes and low selling price. Most of such products are now being made from non-renewable resources, mainly through oil refineries. These refineries, starting from a complex mixture (petroleum), use a wide range of unit operations to generate an impressive variety of products that are sold directly or transformed into value-added products like plastics, fibers, etc. Approximately 17% of the volumes of products derived from petroleum in the US are classified as chemicals. If these chemicals could be obtained from renewable resources like biomass in a biorefinery, it would reduce our petroleum dependence and also have a positive environmental impact.

Supplies of starch and sucrose feedstock will probably not be sufficient to meet the feedstock needs of future biorefineries. As an example, the gasoline market in the US alone is 150 billion gallons per year. MTBE (methyl tertiary-butyl ether) replacement at 6% would result in approximately 10 billion gallons per year of ethanol, which would require about 30% of the US farmland currently growing corn. Given that ethanol is only one of many compounds that can flow out of a corn biorefinery, it is likely that other sources of carbon feedstock will also be required. Brazil and a few other tropical and sub-tropical countries use sucrose in biorefineries that produce ethanol. Because it is widely believed that it is not feasible to produce enough sugarcane (and other sugar crops) to meet potential fuel ethanol volume requirements, there has been a 50-plus year effort to develop technologies to convert cellulose from biomass into a carbon feedstock for the biorefinery of the future.

Cellulosic biomass conversion to fermentable sugars has been explored as the potentially lowest cost feedstock for the biorefinery of the future. Unlike sugar energy storage compounds like starch, which can be converted to fermentable sugar with relative ease, cellulosic biomass is a complicated structure of cellulose (β1–4 glucose linkage), hemicellulose (linked C5 sugars including mannose, galactose, xylose, and arabinose), lignin, and numerous minor components. This structure has evolved as a support element of plants, and therefore is not meant to be readily accessible as a carbon source.

Currently, the most promising approach for using this feedstock is enzymatic hydrolysis of the cellulose content after pretreatment of the fiber to make the cellulose more accessible to enzymatic attack. The process for conversion of cellulosic biomass to fermentable sugars faces major technical and engineering challenges that have so far prevented large-scale commercial use of cellulose as a source of fermentable sugar.

A significant cost component in the overall process to break down cellulosic biomass has been the cost of cellulase enzymes required to carry out the process. As much as 100-fold more native cellulase protein (compared with amylase protein for breakdown of starch) is required for conversion of pretreated substrate, e.g. corn stover, into fermentable sugars. Given the relatively high cost of the enzymes and the amount required to produce fermentable sugars, the process has not been viable. In addition, the pretreatment of cellulosic biomass, making cellulose available for the enzymatic hydrolysis, has been a significant challenge. Many approaches have been explored; however, all suffer from their capital intensity because of the extreme conditions of the process. The cost impact of processing differences between corn and stover is reflected in Fig. 3.4.

The cost of cellulose-hydrolyzing enzymes, or cellulases, is not included in this analysis. Through a three-year DOE funded program administered by the National Renewable Energy Laboratory (NREL), and a one year extension of that program, major advances have been made toward reducing the cost of enzymes in ethanol production from pretreated corn stover. The impact of these improvements on cellulase cost, estimated as $ per gallon of ethanol (EtOH) produced in a bench-scale NREL assay, can be seen in Fig. 3.5.

This improvement has come from reducing the cost of producing the enzymes, enhancing the mix of enzymes, and altering, or recruiting, key enzymes to enable operation at elevated temperatures. However, enzyme requirement remains high, even under the higher-temperature operating conditions engineered into the multi-enzyme system. It is anticipated that enzymatic hydrolysis cost will be further reduced by continued improvement in the enzymes and new processes that use elevated temperatures and more effective pre-treatment processes.

One strategy to minimize ethanol production cost is to run simultaneous saccharification and fermentation, or SSF, which would use ethanologens engineered to operate in high temperature environments. Also, the fermentation organism's ability to utilize C5 sugars derived from the hemicellulose component, and have acceptable productivity in the presence of numerous byproducts of the biomass pretreatment process, would lead to lower overall production cost.

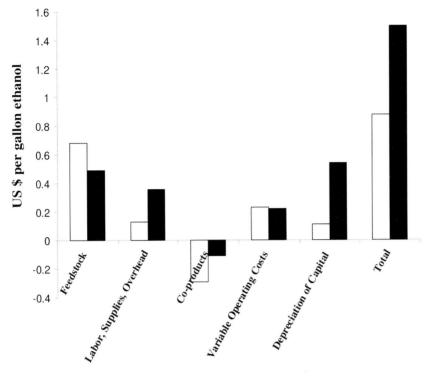

Fig. 3.4 Cost components production of fuel ethanol from corn and corn stover [6].

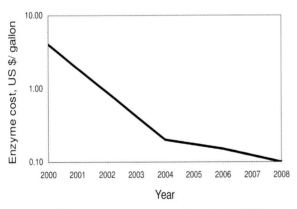

Fig. 3.5 Cellulase enzyme cost estimate based on the NREL assay [6].

3.4
Technical Challenges

3.4.1
Cellulase Enzymes

The challenge of improving cellulase enzymes is significant. Lignocellulose is not a pure compound on which cellulase activity can be optimized. The composition and structure of the biomass substrate can vary dramatically depending on the source of the lignocellulose. Corn stover structure is different from sugarcane bagasse, which in turn is different from municipal solid waste. In addition, corn stover from one part of the country can differ significantly from that from another, because of soil, weather, and other conditions. Finally, different pretreatment processes affect biomass in unique ways, resulting in even further differences between structure and composition. Thus the enzyme system required may need to be optimized for each specific combination of substrate and pretreatment that would be employed.

In 2000, Genencor International was awarded a three-year US Department of Energy (DOE) subcontract through the National Renewable Energy Laboratory (NREL) to reduce the cost of cellulase, on a "per gallon of ethanol produced by NREL process and assay basis", by a factor of ten. That goal was achieved within the three-year timeframe, and the program was extended to further reduce costs to a factor of twenty. These aggressive goals were approached from two directions by making significant improvements in cellulase production economics (reduced cost/gram enzyme) and in cellulase enzyme performance (reduced grams of enzyme needed).

$$\text{Enzyme cost in assay}\left(\frac{\$}{\text{gallons EtOH}}\right) = \text{enzyme cost}\left(\frac{\$}{\text{g enyzme}}\right)$$
$$\times \text{enyzme loading}\left(\frac{\text{g enzyme}}{\text{gallons EtOH}}\right) \tag{1}$$

3.4.1.1 **Improved Cellulase Production Economics**
An understanding of the components of production cost is a necessary prerequisite for effectively reducing the cost. A simplistic, but highly useful, model would identify fixed and direct costs for each of the three major production processes fermentation, enzyme recovery, and formulation:

$$\text{Total cost} = \text{Fermentation cost (fixed + direct)} + \text{Recovery cost (fixed + direct)}$$
$$+ \text{Formulation cost (fixed + direct)} \tag{2}$$

Most current commercial cellulase products are sold as cell-free, stabilized concentrates. Although these formulations meet market needs with regard to application and cost, for many enzyme products it is not uncommon for the recovery and formulation costs to be a major portion of the overall cost. It then follows that reduced post-fermentation processing would possibly lead to reduced cost, with no post-fermentation processing being the lowest cost. This is, however, only practical if the resulting product still meets the needs of the application.

Fermentation broth with no processing was tested in saccharification of pre-treated corn stover. Performance in the saccharification was indistinguishable among fresh whole fermentation broth, fresh fully-recovered and formulated product, and 28-day old fermentation broth. These results suggest that typical recovery and formulation costs can be eliminated for use in biorefinery operations, especially in an integrated plant that both makes and uses the cellulase enzymes.

This leaves the fermentation costs that can be broken down into fixed costs, for example depreciation and labor, and direct costs, for example utilities and raw materials.

$$\begin{aligned} \text{Fermentation cost} = &\text{Fixed cost (labor} + \text{depreciation)} \\ &+ \text{Direct cost (utilities} + \text{other raw materials} \\ &+ \text{carbon/energy source)} \end{aligned} \qquad (3)$$

The single largest cost component for the fermentation process was estimated to be the carbon/energy source for the culture. For *Trichoderma* cellulase, the carbon source has historically been lactose. The cost per unit enzyme produced is a function of the yield of enzyme on the carbon source and the cost of the carbon source itself. When performed in a similar manner, the other costs are proportional to the rate of enzyme production, as measured by volumetric productivity. An integrated plan of action was taken to affect both enzyme expression and the fermentation process. Improvements were made on the production organism, the production process, and in their interactions.

A conventional mutagenesis and screening approach was applied to the existing production strain. The work had several objectives. One was to find strains capable of fast and efficient growth on cellulose. A useful screening method was adapted from the method of Toyama [7]. In this method, mutated spores are poured in large numbers with agar in the bottom of a Petri dish. A second layer is added on top containing cellulose as the sole carbon source. The spores germinate and grow through the agar eventually emerging on top of the cellulose-agar layer. Those that erupt first are more likely to grow quickly and efficiently on cellulose. Another goal was to disrupt existing regulatory mechanisms that result in catabolite repression and the need for induction of cellulase expression. Several plate screening methods were developed that used a high glucose concentration to overcome catabolite repression or glycerol as the carbon source to find expression without induction. A third goal was to improve the secretion of cellulases. Resistance to different chemical agents and selection for hyper-branched morphological mutants were both employed.

Through successive rounds of mutagenesis and selection with different screening methods, an improved host strain was developed. Several new traits were recruited that positively affected fermentation cost. First, the specific growth rate of the strain was increased by 50%. This reduced the growth time needed for the fermentation, positively affecting enzyme productivity. The specific productivity of the strain, enzyme per unit cell mass per unit time, was also improved. This impacted both key metrics, i.e. yield of enzyme from the carbon source and volumetric productivity.

The improvement in yield helped reduce cost of the sugar lactose per unit enzyme produced. Lactose, a by-product of the dairy industry, typically costs significantly more than glucose, a product from sucrose, starch, or cellulose processing. Lactose is a mild inducer of cellulase expression with little to no catabolite repression. Glucose, on the other hand, does not induce cellulase expression and exhibits high catabolite repression. It would thus seem improbable to replace relatively expensive lactose with relatively inexpensive glucose. The disaccharide sophorose (β-1,2 linkage of two glucose units) is one of the most potent inducers of cellulase expression known [8]. It was found that treating a concentrated glucose solution with whole cellulase at elevated temperatures leads to the formation of numerous higher sugars, among them sophorose. This treated solution can then be fed to a cellulase-producing fermentation with performance equal to or better than that obtained using lactose. The small amount of enzyme product that must be recycled to produce sophorose is more than offset by the reduced cost of glucose relative to lactose and by the improved fermentation performance. Traditional fermentation optimization was performed on the improved strain by adjusting the level of salts and other nutrients, temperature, pH, and glucose/sophorose mixture.

The cumulative effect of all these improvements was very significant, and the production cost, per unit of enzyme, was reduced by approximately a factor of seven. These improvements went far beyond what had been deemed probable for an established and mature product such as whole cellulase. Investigations were also made to evaluate pretreated corn stover as a carbon feed for cellulose production; this will be discussed below.

3.4.1.2 Improved Cellulase Enzyme Performance

Reducing enzyme production cost was only part of the solution. As shown in Eq. (1), improving the performance of the cellulase enzymes, resulting in reduced enzyme loading per gallon of ethanol can be equally effective. Several of different approaches have been used to improve enzyme performance, including increasing thermal stability, recruitment of novel cellulolytic activity, and increasing specific activity [9–12].

A major focus was on increasing the thermal stability of the cellulase enzymes. Cellobiohydrolase I (CBH I) is the major component of whole cellulase. It also happens to be the component with the lowest thermal stability, as indicated by T_m, the characteristic "melting" temperature. Successful engineering of

CBH I to improve thermal stability also required several strategies. CBH I structure analysis suggested sites that could affect thermal stability, as did comparing the structures of CBH I homologues. Random mutagenesis and screening were also used. An important part of this effort was the development of a small-scale screening method to quickly and accurately measure the effect of the changes made. By the incorporation of a large number of specific site changes, T_m of CBH I was improved significantly. Placing the engineered CBH I into a production strain in which the native CBH I gene was deleted did not have a negative effect on enzyme production levels.

Along with the ability to engineer proteins for increased thermal stability, it is imperative that the engineered proteins can be expressed at high levels in production strains without negatively affecting the other cellulase components. This has proven to be the case for both *T. reesei*-engineered CBH I and for homologues from other fungi. The homologue from *Humicola grisea var thermoidea* was expressed at levels similar to the wild-type CBH I without negatively affecting the production of the other cellulase components.

By analysis of the CBH I structure, several sites were selected that were hypothesized to affect binding of substrate and products in the active site cleft. Several mutants were made, with significant effects on both K_m, the Michaelis-Menten constant and k_{cat}, the catalytic rate constant.

Many of these improved enzymes have been produced effectively in whole cellulase production strains. As discussed above, improved cellulase production has been maintained with the improved enzymes incorporated. The resulting products have been tested in the NREL process scheme and have resulted in an approximately threefold reduction in enzyme loading.

The work discussed above was performed by Genencor International and collaborators as part of a subcontract funded by the DOE administered by NREL. A similar subcontract was also awarded to Novozymes. The improvements reported to date by both the groups have been quantitatively very similar. The approaches taken have also been similar. Together, it is clear that the cost of enzymes for biomass saccharification has been dramatically reduced from the baseline in 2000. Enzyme cost can no longer be regarded as the largest barrier to commercialization of biorefineries.

3.4.2
Fermentation Organisms

A biorefinery would be a processing factory that would separate biomass into component streams, and transform them into a wide range of products, using enzymatic and/or fermentation processes. This concept has been around for some time, but has not been implemented to its full potential. The utilization of biomass and the development of biorefineries are enormous technological challenges that no doubt require the solution of multiple problems.

3.4.2.1 **Biomass Hydrolyzate as Fermentable Carbon Source**

The use of live cell fermentation to convert sugars into commercial products or intermediates has been exploited successfully for many years. These fermentation processes are based on the use of relatively clean sugar streams that contain few impurities. However, the full use of all the carbon components in biomass is more complicated. After biomass pretreatment, and enzymatic hydrolysis of cellulose (and hemicellulose), a mixture of hexose and pentose sugars and several degradation by-products, for example furfural, hydroxymethylfurfural, phenols, and formic, acetic and other acids is obtained. Several of these pretreatment and hydrolysis by-products are well known inhibitors of fermentation processes. The extent of inhibition depends on the fermentation process. Occasionally it is severe and inhibits cell growth completely. To avoid this, the hydrolyzates must be diluted or fed during fermentation, complicating the fermentation processes and reducing the total amount of hydrolyzed biomass that can be used per unit of time or volume. In other circumstances the impact of the by-products is less severe, because they do not inhibit growth but instead have a negative impact on performance of the cells. For example, at certain concentrations, some organic acids, for example formic or acetic, have a negative effect on cell physiology and increase the amount of energy that cells use to perform their normal functions (cell maintenance). This increase in energy consumption is, in turn, reflected in higher consumption of carbon from sugars, with a consequent decrease in the overall yield of product per unit of biomass [13].

Besides the effects of by-products present in hydrolyzed biomass, the highly concentrated stream of carbohydrates obtained can also be a problem. When exposed to high concentrations of sugars and salts, cells tend to undergo osmotic stress that, depending on its magnitude, can inhibit cell growth or cause an increase in cell maintenance, leading to problems described above.

Another well-known response of cells to the presence of high concentrations of carbon sources is that they tend to use the sugars in a particular order and in an inefficient manner. Cells tend to utilize first the carbon source that is easiest to metabolize and that provides more energy. When this carbon source is completely consumed or reaches a particular concentration, cellular metabolism is re-adjusted to utilize another carbon source present in the mixture. This sequential use of the carbon sources and the associated metabolic adjustments complicates fermentation process design because optimum cell-performance is obtained when some of the growth media components, mainly carbon and nitrogen, are present in certain ratios. From the engineering design perspective of the fermentation process, these ratios are calculated on the basis of total carbon present in the mixtures. From the cells' perspective, however, only one or a few carbon sources at a time are "sensed", and a carbon-to-nitrogen ratio calculated on the basis of total carbon content is detected as an unbalanced mixture by the cells. Very often this leads to poor cell and fermentation process performance.

3.4.2.2 Production Process as a Whole

In addition to addressing problems related to the use of mixtures of complex sugars and inhibitors, development of commercially viable fermentation processes requires proper process integration of the different unit operations to reduce costs and disposal of fermentation by-products. Enzymatic hydrolysis of biomass is currently performed with a mixture of enzymes that work in the 50–60 °C temperature range and 3–5 pH range. However, most of the production strains developed so far to utilize biomass hydrolyzates perform better in the 30–40 °C temperature range and the 6–8 pH range. This means temperature and pH must be adjusted before starting fermentation. pH adjustment is not only expensive but also produces salts that will have an osmotic effect during fermentation and must be disposed of properly at the end of the process. Temperature adjustments also increase fermentation costs.

For these reasons it is highly desirable to develop production strains that can utilize biomass hydrolyzates satisfactorily at 50–60 °C and pH 3–5 [14]. This would enable relatively inexpensive SSF processes. Furthermore, low pH and high-temperature fermentation conditions would retard contamination. On the other hand, it is important to note that at high temperatures the inhibition effects of toxic compounds in biomass hydrolyzates are also magnified.

An SSF process may not always be the best means of obtaining specific products from biomass hydrolyzates, however. Occasionally the physiochemical properties of the product(s) must be considered when designing a process. For example, a study on production of twelve top value-added chemicals from biomass identified eight as acids, three of which must be produced in the free-acid form directly during fermentation. If these are produced in the salt forms first, the cost impact on product purification and disposal of by-product salts is high [15]. As shown in Table 3.1, pK values of several commercially relevant acids are in the 3–5 range. For production of these, therefore, the fermentation pH necessary for a product in the free-acid form must be in the 2–4 range, making SSF an unlikely process choice.

Table 3.1 pK values of some commercially important organic acids that are or potentially can be produced by fermentation.

Acid	pK Value
Pyruvic	2.50
Fumaric	3.03
Malic	3.40
Itaconic	3.84
Lactic	3.86
Aspartic	3.90
Succinic	4.19
Glutamic	4.20
Oxalic	4.21

3.4.2.3 **Emerging Solutions**

On the basis of the challenges discussed above it is evident that future efforts to develop commercial processes utilizing biomass hydrolyzates for fermentation will require production strains different from traditional organisms like yeast, *Bacillus, E. coli, Pseudomonas, Corynebacterium,* etc. [14]. Instead, we will need to find or develop microorganisms capable of performing better at low pH and/or higher temperatures, and under high concentration of carbohydrates. Furthermore, these new microorganisms would also need to be able to resist the by-products generated during biomass pretreatment and hydrolysis.

In the last few years there has been an explosion in our knowledge of nontraditional microorganisms. Today, the genomes of hundreds of bacteria and Archaea are available [16]. In this collection of newly characterized microorganisms we can find almost any physiological trait that we want. These strains can, furthermore, often be manipulated genetically. Some examples of these are shown in Table 3.2. From these microorganisms and many others we can learn the strategies that Nature has selected to deal with high temperatures, high concentrations of toxic compounds, sugars, salts, pH, etc., and in some of the genomes we can also find new enzymes that would enable the use of lignocellulosic materials for fermentation.

On one side, genomics is providing an immense number of physiological solutions. Likewise, advances in other research areas are providing possible solutions to some of the problems mentioned. For example, some mutations have been designed to eliminate the sequential utilization of carbohydrates present in complex mixtures [17–19]. Some of these mutations reduce the ability of the production strains to induce hundreds of genes that could produce undesired phenotypes during fermentation. Also, use of genomic arrays is helping us un-

Table 3.2 Some examples of the sequenced genomes from microorganisms with properties relevant for the development of biorefineries.

Organism name	Relevant properties
Thermoplasma acidophilum	Optimum growth: 59 °C, pH 2.0
Thermatoga maritima	Optimum growth temp. 80 °C. Capable of using starch, cellulose, xylan as carbon sources
Halobacterium sp. NRC-1	Requires 4 M NaCl to grow
Corynebacterium efficiens	Grows and produces glutamic acid above 40 °C
Gluconobacter oxydans	Extracellular oxidation of a wide range of carbohydrates and alcohols. The corresponding products (aldehydes, ketones and organic acids) are secreted almost completely into the medium
Picrophilus torridus	Optimum growth at 60 °C and pH 0.7. Its membrane has very low proton permeability
Sulfolobus sulfataricus P2 and *Sulfolobus tokodaii* strain 7	Grow optimally at 80 °C and pH 2–4

derstand the types of physiological response that occur when cells are exposed to stressful conditions. For example, comparison of *E. coli* strains capable of producing ethanol at different levels has shown that increased ethanol tolerance results from a combination of multiple changes affecting different aspects of cell physiology [20].

3.5
Conclusions

The importance of the biorefinery concept is growing and the recent increased demand for fuel ethanol has in large part driven that growth, as shown in Fig. 3.6.

New products such as the lactic acid and 1,3-propanediol produced from su-gar in engineered organisms are recent examples of the biorefinery concept pro-gressing toward reality. Apart from co-product streams resulting from the pro-cessing of grain or biomass, the resulting sugars are being used as carbon feed to furnish an ever-growing list of products including fuel and the building blocks for the synthesis of chemicals and polymers. Commercial production of 1,3-propanediol for Sorona, based on technology developed in a close collabora-tion between DuPont and Genencor, will mark the emergence of commercial vi-able application of the biorefinery concept for production of basic chemical building blocks in competition with petrochemical-derived materials [21].

Many of the biorefinery elements required for financial success seem to be currently present, for example:
- high-volume, low-cost application (fuel ethanol);
- multiple alternate product streams;
- ability to shift to different products quickly when required; and
- acceptable cost structure (at least for sucrose, starch).

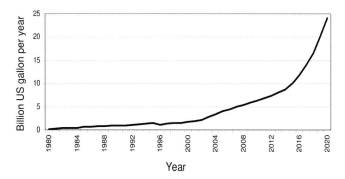

Fig. 3.6 World demand for fuel ethanol over the years.

Several financial requirements will enable the biorefinery concept to become a reality in the near future:

- parts of the overall biorefinery scheme that can operate in a stand-alone manner from a financial perspective, and the ability to evolve from there;
- the potential for multiple product or co-product streams – note that this may ultimately drive efforts to engineer crops to maximize their potential;
- the ability to make use of a variety of feedstocks as a hedging strategy and to take advantage of pricing opportunities;
- manageable capital requirements and favorable investment environment; and
- government enablement (funded demonstration/development pilot plants; reasonable regulation of biorefinery operations; favorable tax treatment; strategic market support to give new biorefinery products a head start).

In summary, the concept of the biorefinery is not new. In its simplistic form, several pieces have been in operation for thousands of years. Biorefineries continue to evolve depending on market needs, and growth now is being driven by the rising demand for fuel ethanol. It will continue to evolve in a manner similar to the petroleum refineries in the 1900s. Ultimately, as technological developments expand and the range of products grows, biorefineries will utilize a wide variety of feedstocks, including cellulosic biomass.

Acknowledgments

This work was supported in part by a subcontract from The Office of Biomass Program, within the DOE Office of Energy Efficiency and Renewable Energy. The authors thank Colin Mitchinson and Mike Knauf of Genencor International for their guidance of the work presented.

References

1 G Chotani, T Dodge, A Hsu, M Kumar, R LaDuca, D Trimbur, W Weyler, and K Sanford. Commercial Production of Chemicals using Pathway Engineering. Biochemica Biophysica Acta, 1543 (2), 434–455, 2000.

2 Manoj Kumar, Jeff Pucci, Gopal Chotani, and Karl Sanford. Biocatalytic Conversion of Renewable Feedstock to Industrial Chemicals. In Lignocellulose Biodegradation (ACS Symposium Series 889) Badal C. Saha and Kiyoshi Hayashi, editors, Oxford Univ. Press, pp 363–376, 2004.

3 Mitchinson, Colin. Improved Cellulases for the BioRefinery: A review of Genencor's progress in the DOE subcontract for cellulase cost reduction for bioethanol. Stanford GCEP Biomass Energy Workshop, April 2004.

4 Michael Knauf and Mohammed Moniruzzaman. Lignocellulosic Biomass Processing: A Perspective. International Sugar Journal, 106#1263, 147–150, April 2004.

5 Mary Ann Godshall, Future Directions For The Sugar Industry, 2003. http://www.spriinc.org/buton10a.html

6 Determining the cost of producing ethanol from corn starch and lignocellulosic feedstocks. NREL/TP-580-28893. Oct 2000.

7 Toyama et al. 2002. Applied Biochemistry and Biotechnology, 98–100:257–263.

8 Mary Mandels, Frederick W. Parrish, and Elwyn T. Reese, J. Bacteriol. 1962 February; 83(2): 400–408.

9 Foreman PK, Brown D, Dankmeyer L, Dean R, Diener S, Dunn-Coleman NS, Goedegebuur F, Houfek TD, England GJ, Kelley AS, Meerman HJ, Mitchell T, Mitchinson C, Olivares HA, Teunissen PJ, Yao J, Ward M. Transcriptional regulation of biomass degrading enzymes in the filamentous fungus *Trichoderma reesei*. J. Biological Chemistry, 278(34): 31988–31997, 2003.

10 M. Sandgren, P. Gualfetti, A. Shaw, A. G. Day, L. Gross, T. Alwyn Jones and C. Mitchinson. Comparison of Homologous Family 12 Glucosyl hydrolases and Recruited Variants Important for Stability. Protein Science, 12(4): 848–860, 2003.

11 F. Goedegebuur, J. Phillips, WAH van der Kley, P. van Solingen, L. Dankmeyer, S.D. Power, T. Fowler. Cloning and Relational Analysis of 15 Novel Fungal Endoglucanases from Family 12 Glycosyl Hydrolase. Current Genetics, 41:2, 89–98, 2002.

12 Sandgren M, Shaw A, Ropp T, Wu S, Bott R, Cameron A, Stahlberg J, Mitchinson C, Jones A. The X-ray crystal structure of the Trichoderma reesei family 12 endoglucanase 3 (Cel12A) at 1.9 Å J. Molecular Biology, 308(2):295–310, 2001.

13 Zaldivar, J., Nielsen J. and Olsson L. Fuel ethanol production from lignocellulose: a challenge for metabolic engineering and process integration. Appl. Microbiol. Biotechnol. (2001) 56: 17–34.

14 Hettenhauss, J. Ethanol fermentation strains: Present and future requirements for biomass to ethanol commercialization. http://www.afdc.nrel.gov/pdfs/4957.pdf.

15 Werpy, T. and Petersen G. Eds. Top value added chemicals from biomass. Volume I. Results of screening for potential candidates from sugars and synthesis gas, NREL, August 2004. http://www.osti.gov/bridge

16 TIGR Microbial Database: a listing of microbial genomes and chromosomes in progress. http://www.tigr.org/tigr-scripts/CMR2/CMRGenomes.spl.

17 Hernandez-Montalvo, V., Valle, F., Bolivar F. and Gosset G. Characterization of sugar mixtures utilization by an *Escherichia coli* mutant devoid of the phosphotransferase system. Appl. Microbiol. Biotechnol. (2001) 57: 186–191.

18 Chatterjee, R., Sanville-Millard, C., Champion, K., Clark D. and Donnelly M. Mutation of the *ptsG* gene results in increased production of succinate in fermentation of glucose by *Escherichia coli*. Appl. Environ. Microbiol. (2001) 67: 148–154.

19 Nichols, N., Dien, B. and Bothast R. Use of catabolite repression mutants for fermentation of sugar mixtures to ethanol. Appl. Microbiol. Biotechnol. (2001) 56: 120–125.

20 Gonzalez, R., Tao, H., Purvis J., York, S., Shanmugam K. and Ingram L. Gene array-based identification of changes that contribute to ethanol tolerance in ethanologenic *Escherichia coli*: comparison of KO11 (parent) to LY01 (resistant mutant). Biotechnol. Prog. (2003) 19: 612–623.

21 C. Nakamura and G. Whited. Metabolic engineering for the microbial production of 1,3 propanediol. Curr. Opin. Biotechnol. 2003 Oct; 14(5): 454–459.

4
Biorefineries for the Chemical Industry –
A Dutch Point of View

Ed de Jong, René van Ree, Robert van Tuil, and Wolter Elbersen

4.1
Introduction

As a major policy goal for 2020, the Dutch government has stipulated that 10% of its energy use should be provided by renewable sources to meet its Kyoto objectives. Biomass is expected to be a major contributor with an expected share of more than 50% of the policy goal mentioned. Further, the Ministry of Economic Affairs has defined some very ambitious policy targets for biomass in the longer term (2040), namely 30% fossil fuel substitution in the power and transport sector and 20–45% fossil-based raw material substitution in the industrial sector. It has been calculated that the energy-substitution policy goal corresponds to a long-term required biomass substitution volume of about 600–1000 PJ_{th} $annum^{-1}$, in a scenario in which severe energy savings have also been taken into account (Ministry of Economic Affairs 2003). Adding the very ambitious raw material policy goal an additional biomass substitution volume of several hundreds of PJ_{th} $annum^{-1}$ will be required.

Biomass in the Netherlands that is not currently used for food applications is mainly used as animal feed or as fuel for power (and heat) production. Biomass is converted mainly by means of direct/indirect cofiring in conventional coal-fired power plants and also by stand-alone combustion plants (Cuijk, Lelystad). To meet the longer-term policy ambitions biomass must be applied in additional market sectors of the Dutch economy, using new thermochemical and (bio)chemical conversion/production processes, for example advanced gasification and fermentation technology. A current disadvantage of these processes is that final products will be produced that are more expensive than their fossil-based alternatives. Prolonged financial governmental support (e.g. investment subsidies, fiscal measures) necessary to support successful market implementation is currently lacking in the Netherlands. Further, to meet the longer-term policy ambitions, the use of potentially available relatively cheap organic side- and waste streams will not be sufficient. The use of dedicated, relatively expensive "energy" crops grown both in and outside the Netherlands (imports) is therefore inescapable.

Biorefineries – Industrial Processes and Products. Status Quo and Future Directions. Vol. 1
Edited by Birgit Kamm, Patrick R. Gruber, Michael Kamm
Copyright © 2006 WILEY-VCH Verlag GmbH & Co. KGaA, Weinheim
ISBN: 3-527-31027-4

Within this framework it is believed biorefineries will play a major role in the transition to a more sustainable Dutch economy. Realization of high-efficiency biorefining processes at places where biomass can be gathered, grown, and/or imported and where the "green" products can be sold to a cluster of chemical and material industries are believed to be key technologies to meet the longer-term policy goals.

The chemical and material industries are founded on innovation. Because of the emerging interaction between chemistry, biology, and process engineering the industries of 2020 will be significantly different from those of today. Not only does technological development encourage changes in the design of processes and products, however, pressure from consumers and the general public also fuels a transition to a more sustainable industry. This stimulates discussion on if and how the use of renewable resources can add to a future scenario of a continuing innovative chemical industry taking into account the wishes and constraints of all current and future stakeholders.

This paper first provides the societal and institutional context for the transition to sustainability in the evolution of the chemical industry. Second, it reviews different perspectives on the future of a modified chemical industry, partly resulting from emerging technological opportunities. Third, taking into account these emerging technological opportunities, this paper discusses the potential of the use of biomass in the chemical industry of today and tomorrow. Special emphasis will be given to the potential that "biorefineries" offer the chemical industry.

4.2
Historical Outline – The Chemical Industry: Current Situation and Perspectives

The objective of this section is to present an overview of the chemical products that the current industry produces. It also gives an overview of the technological pathways involved in the production of these chemical products. This overview covers the scope of chemical products and chemical intermediates that need to be produced from biomass and also provides an overview of currently produced biomass-based chemical products.

4.2.1
Overview of Products and Markets

The oil industry may be divided into several important refinery sectors and products including: gas for commercial energy supply, heavy gasoline for car fuels, naphtha for the petrochemical industry, kerosene for aviation fuel, and oil residues used in bitumen and lubricating oils. This review focuses on the naphtha fraction in the petrochemical industry and the gamut of chemicals, products, applications, and markets that can be derived from it.

The current chemical industry's most important feedstock is naphtha which can be cracked to obtain a range of olefins, for example ethylene and butanes, and other small (un)saturated hydrocarbons and aromatic compounds, for example benzene and alkyl benzenes. These simple hydrocarbons form the back-bone of the possible products that are generated in the chemical industry today. The scope of different chemicals (and transformations) that can be achieved from naphtha for the chemical industry is illustrated schematically in Fig. 4.1. In principal these materials can be transformed to the bulk of chemicals produced by two initial key pathways:

- they may be directly isolated, used, and transformed by a variety of chemical techniques to a range of compounds; or
- they may undergo a gasification process to form synthesis gas (CO and H_2) which on recombination enables access to another branch of alternative chemicals and technologies.

The chemicals described in Fig. 4.1, derived from the small (un)saturated hydro-carbons and synthesis gas, enables an array of chemicals of technological and economically important products, applications, and markets to be obtained. For example:

- vinyl monomers for plastics used in pipe, packaging, and rubber applications;
- monomers for polyester and amide synthesis used in fibers (for textiles), engineering materials, and some container materials;
- solvents for, among others, the paint industry;
- chemicals for the pharmaceutical industry; and
- chemicals for the insecticide and herbicide industry.

4.2.2
Technological Pathways

Closer examination of the chemical transformation steps involved in converting one substance into another (Fig. 4.1), reveals some generic approaches to the types of chemistry and technology used in the chemical industry:

- oxidative and reductive techniques are most prolific;
- introduction of nitrogen into chemical structures is most frequently achieved by initial amination or amidation with ammonia;
- carbonylation reactions are frequently used to make small incremental changes in chain length and for introduction of new functionality;
- extensive use of gaseous reagents;
- high selectivity of chemical steps by utilization of catalytic materials, therefore reducing the need for chemical derivatization for transformation; and
- high conversion in chemical steps by use of catalytic materials

4.2.3
Biomass-based Industrial Products

Although most chemicals are of petrochemical origin an important example of a chemical produced in bulk from a non-petrochemical source is ethanol. Ethanol, produced by fermentation of molasses, etc., has been most extensively used

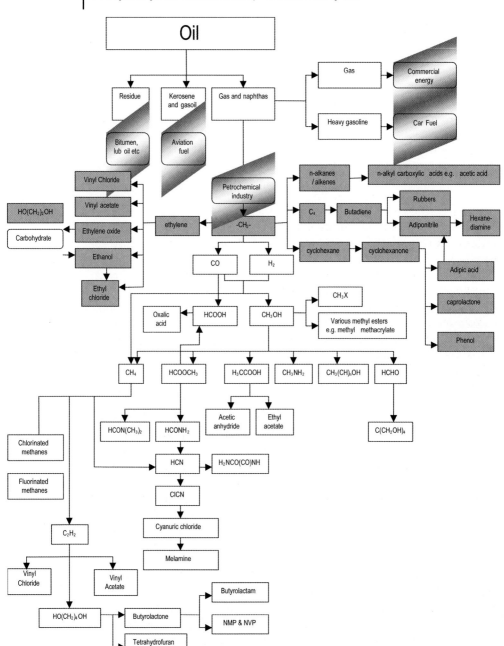

Fig. 4.1 Schematic representation of chemical transformation steps in the (petro)chemical industry.

Table 4.1 Estimated EU potential of major biomass-based products (Ehrenberg 2002).

Market sector	Total consumption market (1998) (kton)	Renewable consumption market (1998) (kton)	Potential of renewables in 2010 (kton)	Potential share in 2010 (%)
Polymers	33 000	25	500	1.5
Lubricants	4240	100	200	5
Solvents	4000	60	235	12.5
Surfactants	2260	1180	1450	52

in the food and beverage industry, although increasing amounts are also used in bio-based transportation fuels and to prepare non-food industrial chemical products. Although ethanol is perhaps the most widely known example of a bio-based chemical product both in the Netherlands and worldwide, a range of other bio-based chemical products is produced and used in a variety of industrial applications. These fall into several generic categories:

- naturally occurring carbohydrate polymers;
- fats and oils of plant origin (and, to a lesser extent, of animal origin);
- terpene-based materials;
- chemical products of carbohydrate-containing materials; and
- fermentation products of carbohydrate-containing sources.

A recent study coordinated by the European Renewable Resources and Materials Association (ERRMA) has evaluated the current situation of biomass use as an industrial feedstock for chemicals and materials (Ehrenberg 2002). Table 4.1 shows the potential of biomass to replace petrochemical-based products in the areas of polymers, lubricants, solvents, and surfactants. Many of those applications, especially lubricants, solvents, and surfactants, can be achieved by direct extraction of the components from the biomass without additional (bio)conversion steps.

4.2.3.1 Carbohydrates

Today's bio-based products include commodity and specialty chemicals, fuels, and materials. Some of these products result from the direct physical or chemical processing of biomass cellulose, starch, oils, protein, lignin, and terpenes. Most biomass consists of natural polymers and most biomass is carbohydrate in nature. This means that most biomass is in the form of carbohydrate polymers (polysaccharides). These natural polymers can be used both as nature provides them and as the skeletal framework of other derived polymers.

By far the most abundant of these carbohydrate polymers is cellulose, the principal component of the cell walls of all higher plants. It is estimated that 75 billion tons of cellulose are biosynthesized and disappear each year, most of the disappearance being through natural decay. Cellulosic plant materials are used as fuel, lumber, mechanical pulp, and textiles. Purified cellulose is currently used to make wood-free paper, cellophane, photographic film, membranes, explosives, textile fibers, water-soluble gums, and organic-solvent-soluble polymers used in lacquers and varnishes.

The principal cellulose derivative is cellulose acetate, which is used to make photographic film, acetate rayon, a variety of thermoplastic products, and lacquers. The world's annual consumption of cellulose acetate is about 750,000 tons. Cellulose acetate products are biodegradable. Commercial production of lyocell, a cellulosic fiber made from a solvent spinning process, has also started recently. Lyocell, which, unlike rayon, does not require dry cleaning but is washable and very strong, is the first new textile fiber to be introduced in 30 years.

Cotton is currently the most important non-wood fiber crop. It is mainly used for weaving and spinning into cloth. Advances in biotechnology and genetic engineering are now enabling development of cotton cultivars with improved pest resistance, yield, and quality, thereby potentially reducing production costs and better matching cotton characteristics to specific applications. Natural fibers other than cotton occupy a variety of niche markets, for example specialty fabrics, fiber-reinforced composites, papers, cordage, and horticultural mulches and mixes.

Heightened environmental concerns are also helping jute, hemp, flax, sisal, abaca, coir fibers, and products derived from these fibers to find their way into new markets. The use of natural fibers in fiber-reinforced composites, especially, has seen tremendous growth in Europe in recent years (van Dam et al. 2004).

4.2.3.2 Fatty Acids

Fatty acids, readily available from plant oils, are used to make soaps, lubricants, chemical intermediates such as esters, ethoxylates, and amides. These three important classes of intermediate are used in the manufacture of surfactants, cosmetics, alkyd resins, polyamides, plasticizers, lubricants and greases, paper, and pharmaceuticals (Ahmed and Morris 1994). Of the approximately 2.5 million tons of fatty acids produced in 1991, about 1.0 million tons (40%) were derived from vegetable and natural oils; the remaining 1.5 million tons were produced from petrochemical sources. Twenty-five percent of all plant-derived fatty acids used in the coatings industry comes from tall oil (a byproduct of kraft paper manufacture). Surfactants are, currently, by far the most important outlet for fatty acids (Table 4.1). In Europe most raw materials used for surfactant production are derived from tropical oils, because of their more suitable chemical structure. Besides oil-based surfactants there is also a relatively small market (< 5%) for starch-derived surfactants.

4.2.3.3 **Other**

Terpenes, derived from woody materials, also give rise to a variety of chemicals and products. Crude turpentine, isolated from the pulping industry, may be used to isolate "pine oil" commonly used in cleaning products, alternatively its components may be isolated and chemically transformed to materials such as dipentene, which can be polymerized to prepare tacky polymers and used in chewing gum and food packaging coatings.

Although not widespread in Western Europe and North America, several Eastern European, Asian, and South American countries use carbohydrate-containing agricultural residues as a raw material in the chemical industry. For example, hydrolysis of starchy materials to glucose with concomitant severe acid-catalyzed degradation can result in oxalic acid, which is used in the leather industry. Alternatively, pentoses, found in bagasse and corncobs, for example, readily undergo acid-catalyzed dehydration to furfural. Furfural is a flexible chemical raw material which can be used as a solvent itself in several applications or can be used to prepare furfuryl alcohol used in resin materials, and tetrahydrofuran, a common organic solvent. Although many other chemical transformations are possible, their current commercial status is unclear.

Carbohydrates remain a flexible raw material, and beside "classical" chemical transformations, biotechnological transformations have also been explored. For example lactic acid can be used to prepare a biodegradable polymer with interesting properties and has a wide range of potential applications including fibers and packaging materials (Sreenath et al. 2001). Other biotech products include citrates to prepare additive chemicals (dyeing, cleaning, and polymer) and fumaric acid in preserving agents and as a component of unsaturated polyesters.

Specialty chemicals can be made using fermentation and enzymatic processes or directly extracted from plants (or aquatic biomass). It has been shown that plants can be altered to produce molecules with functionality and properties not present in existing compounds (e.g. chiral chemicals). Examples of bio-based specialty chemicals include bioherbicides and biopesticides, bulking and thickening agents for food and pharmaceutical products, flavors and fragrances, nutraceuticals (e.g. antioxidants, noncalorific fat replacements, cholesterol-reducing agents, and salt replacements), chiral chemicals, pharmaceuticals (e.g. Taxol), plant-growth promoters, essential amino acids, vitamins, industrial biopolymers such as xanthan gum, and enzymes. Specialty chemical markets currently represent a wide range of high-value products. These chemicals usually sell for more than $4 \in kg^{-1}$. Although the worldwide market for these chemicals is smaller than for bulk and intermediate chemicals, the specialty chemicals market now exceeds \$ 3 billion.

It is expected that advances in biotechnologies will have significant impacts on the growth of the specialty chemicals market.

4.2.4
International Perspectives

In several industrialized countries (i.e. USA, UK, and the Netherlands) government, business, society, and science have been engaged in outlining future developments in the material and chemical industry (American Chemical Society 1996; Molendijk et al. 2004; National Research Council 2000; Okkerse and van Bekkum 1997; Parris 2004; Sims 2004; UK Foresight program Chemicals Panel 2000; US Department of Energy 1998, 1999; Weaver 2000). Most of these foresight exercises are led by the view that an increased demand for chemicals and materials will place additional pressure on the use of resources and on the environment. Accordingly, the thrust is in finding new technologies and creating novel materials, processes, and capabilities to bring this growth in line with society's demand for sustainability.

The perspectives indicate a shared interest in shifting from sole dependence on fossil resources to a chemical and material industry founded on the application of plant-based resources, derived either from secondary streams (i.e. waste and recycling) or from primary streams (i.e. dedicated production). The discussion suggests that changing the resource base of the chemical and material industries will induce cleaner processes, safer products and a more effective use of scarce resources. The shift to a bio-based chemical and material industry will alter the technological basis of the industry quite radically. To substantiate the sustainable credentials of new products and processes, further research and actual implementation will indicate what specific technological routes in fact contribute to sustainability. This will be necessary for communication with NGO, the general public, regulators, and policy makers about, for example, CO_2 emissions.

From the perspective of the chemical industry striving for sustainability with sound economic foundations draws the attention to three key areas.

4.2.4.1 Production
The actual production process has a major environmental impact both on efficient use of energy and resources and on emission and waste production; this is especially so in bulk industries. This links the provision of multi-quality biomass and the industrial production process. Because of the large volumes used, it may have a far-reaching impact on the environment. Cost reduction, because of cheaper raw materials or processes with less extreme conditions, will be an important consideration.

4.2.4.2 Integration
Implementing a strategy for sustainability requires coordination between different levels of a supply chain, product portfolio, and fine-tuning between distributed technological capabilities. Key technologies in conversion, extraction, and separation will lay the foundation for further improvement in bulk production and the development of products with well defined functionality.

This requires an integrated view on resource use and a strategic view on technology development. Linking of life sciences, chemistry, energy technology, and process engineering is required for taking up such a challenge.

4.2.4.3 Use and Re-use

In terms of specific functionality, life cycle and recycling or safety, the actual performance of end-products importantly defines the shape of a market-oriented strategy for sustainable resource use. Increasing revenues by generating high-value products will also be an important consideration. This links production process with product design and defines new terrain for innovative business enterprises. Communicating the sustainability benefits to consumers or users in the (new) end-use market will enable them to make more informed choices.

To develop a sustainable perspective for the chemical industry a combinatorial approach integrating functionality provided by new molecules or materials, improved efficiency and safety of production processes, and use and re-use of materials must be applied. Integrating criteria such as design for functionality or recycling properties of new materials will encourage the search for new sustainable solutions in the chemical industry.

4.3
Biomass: Technology and Sustainability

The chemical industry undergoes rapid and important changes inherent to the turmoil resulting from transitions at the end of an industry's current lifecycle. These changes require new technological, organizational, and commercial answers from the industry. Moreover, the business strategy of the chemical industry will become increasingly dependent on the acceptance or rejection by society and consumers of its activities and its conduct. This section introduces a perspective on a chemical industry that combines technological innovation with a socially acceptable business strategy.

4.3.1
Transition to a Bio-based Industry: Sectoral Integration in the Netherlands

Products from the chemical, material, and power industries have become an integral part of our daily lives and demand for these products is projected to increase. A general concern is the intensive use of finite resources, in particular fossil resources, and, consequently, the industry is in the midst of reconsidering its current resource use. Two major Dutch companies communicated its transition to the general public – the chemical company DSM advertised its transition process to a specialty company while building an image of sustainability and, in 2002, Shell, the energy company, launched a nation-wide advertisement campaign highlighting the future of natural and renewable resources. In this process, industrial research and development seems to (re)discover the variation of quality and specific functionality in renewable resources; this offers the opportunity to meet the demand for healthy and environmentally friendly end-products. The industry must, however, contend with both established paths of research and development and its extensive infrastructure in terms of production facilities and equipment. As a result, transition to a bio-based industry requires the development of new chains and persistent crossing of boundaries between disciplines, departments, and sectors.

Innovation in the energy sector is an important driver of technology development in the chemical and material industries. Hence, petrochemistry is a constant factor in industrial development, although the use of biomass or renewable resources comes to the fore anticipating rises in oil prices or directive measures related to international agreements, for example EU directive 2003/30/EC on promotion of the use of biofuels or other renewable fuels for transport. There are several political drivers for enforcement of such directives. The most important include:

- the widely accepted threat of global warming as a result of the emission of greenhouse gases;
- the unwanted dependency on oil-producing countries;
- the recent enlargement of the EU with associated political issues especially related to agriculture; and
- sustainable development of rural areas and creation of employment.

The question is whether an integrated energy sector and petrochemical industry is the right or only venue for a transition to a bio-based industry.

Two non-exclusive scenarios can be distinguished:

1. The energy sector and the petrochemical industry integrate further and the oil price remains the major driving force in business and in innovation.
2. The chemical and materials industry dissociate themselves from the petrochemical sector and seeks new potentials of bio-based industrial processes using renewable resources supplied by the agro-sector, leading to environmentally friendly modes of production and to healthy and sustainable end-products with specific qualities (Coombs 1995).

Most likely vertically integrated companies, including Sabic and Shell, will tend to stick to the first strategy, whereas companies not involved in exploration, e.g. Dow, DSM, might tend to follow the second strategy. The selling of the polyolefins division of DSM to Sabic and the acquisition of part of Roche can be seen as an example of this strategy. These scenarios (represented in Fig. 4.2), discussed on a number of occasions in the Netherlands, draw the attention to the linking of the agro-sector and the food and feed-processing industry with the chemicals and materials industry (de Klerk et al. 2002).

Although the Dutch economy still has a strong base in manufacturing, both of food and non-food products, the agro-sector and the chemicals sector operate remotely and lack of synergy between these two sectors may hinder progress in

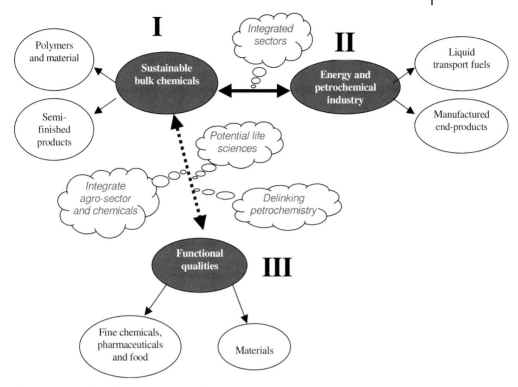

Fig. 4.2 New synthesis between economic clusters.

developing biorefineries with new manufacturing processes and new products. In the 1980s and 1990s the agro-sector was involved in so-called "agrification", i.e. producing industrial crops in rotation with food crops or potatoes, but failed to create ventures with end-users for its resources in the chemical and manufacturing industries (van Roekel and Koster 2000). Pushing the use of renewable resources without identifying a clear demand, either by industry-based end-users or consumers, thus seemed to be unproductive and even counterproductive.

Fine-tuning across sectoral boundaries seems to be an important condition for changing current resource use. In the following discussion we will identify the consequences of this condition for the position of the Dutch agrosector and food industry.

The Dutch agro sector and the food and feed industry are founded not only in primary production of agricultural crops but equally in processing, distributing, and transporting primary and secondary flows of agricultural resources. The combination of intensive agricultural production, the transit of commodities in Rotterdam harbor and an extensive food processing industry is a specific quality of the Dutch economy. Import of resources for the food-processing industry, including starch, sugar, and vegetable oils, results in a high "biomass intensity". A related factor is the opportunity to direct secondary flows, side, and waste streams, to other industries; without the absorption of these secondary flows, mainly by the feed and alcohol producers, the continuity of the processing industry would be in danger (Rabobank International 2001). This sketches a landscape wherein a new synthesis between sectors is possible. This contrasts, however, with the current low-value use of renewable resources, mainly in the feed and power industry. A driver for change in the feed industry might originate in recent scares about the use of slaughter residues and of potentially hazardous fats and oils in feed, bringing these undesired components in the cycle for human consumption. The European debate on genetically modified crops might also result in stricter regulation of the use of these crops in feed and food. Consequently, the composition of feed is affected by public pressures and stricter regulation which, in combination with the tendency to reduce the intensive livestock industry in the Netherlands, might lead to the disappearance of existing markets for secondary flows. This will place high pressure on the food processing industry, because secondary or waste streams will become a cost rather than an income generator (Rabobank International 2001).

The short-term question is where the food processing industry and the agrosector can market their secondary resource flows and/or plant-based resources; this is an environmental and economic problem. Therefore, companies, research institutes, and government try to address the issue of creating new chances for biomass, which includes finding alternative markets for residues and waste streams. A related question is how to find high-value utilization and application of these renewable resources, in addition to low-value energy and bulk products. This will require fine-tuning of the quality, price, and quantity of renewable resources with demand in the end-user market and functionality requirements of new products. We must, therefore, turn round and move from demand and functionality to processing and, eventually, to the production or supply of the raw material.

The next section briefly identifies how different social actors perceive healthy and sustainable products and processes, to provide a guide for formulating technology agendas for the chemicals and materials industry.

4.3.2
Can Sustainability Drive Technology?

One of the more important societal driving forces is the drive for sustainability. Directing innovation and technology development from the perspective of a sustainable, bio-based society is one of the major challenges for the chemicals and materials industries. In response to this widely conceived public concern, companies try to focus their business strategies both on sustainability, including environmental concerns, and on consumer demands for safe products. Most companies trying to address the three Ps (planet, people, profit) are, however, well aware that profit is always the ultimate driving force.

To develop the technology supporting such an ambition still requires a substantive effort, both in terms of innovative research and in terms of bringing together different disciplines, such as chemistry, biology, energy technology, and engineering, and different professional fields, such as design, bulk production of chemicals, and the supply and storage of renewable or plant-based resources. Hence, both from a sustainability and business viewpoint an integral approach to chemical, material, product, and energy outlets must be addressed in biorefineries creating maximum added value from the selected biomass resources.

A sustainable chemical industry must strive for a business strategy that integrates social, safety, health, and environmental objectives with the technological and economic objectives of its activities. Assembling industry, science, and government is one aspect of developing foresight; consulting a wider range of stakeholders, i.e. consumers and citizens, about technology strategies is another. In doing so, interdisciplinary research may be able to contribute to fine-tuning business strategies and technology strategies. Before formulating the shape of such a new perspective, a selected number of international perspectives on technological change in the materials and chemicals industry will be discussed.

4.4
The Chemical Industry: Biomass Opportunities – Biorefineries

The preceding paragraphs have shown the scope of chemical products that are currently produced and therefore the targeted product portfolio of biomass-based chemical products. It was also shown that drivers for a transition to a bio-based economy lie not in technological opportunities alone but are a complex combination of societal, economic, and technological opportunities, challenges, and constraints. This section will focus in more detail on the main technological opportunities to transfer biomass, either directly or via chemical intermediates, into chemical products.

4.4.1
Biomass Opportunities

In the realization of a bio-based chemical industry two distinct approaches can be identified. In the first approach, *the value chain approach*, value-added compounds in biomass are identified and isolated in different processing and (bio)-conversion steps. The remaining biomass is then transformed into a universal substrate from which chemical products can be synthesized. In this approach it is thought that it is technologically and economically beneficial to extract valuable chemicals and polymers from biomass rather than building these compounds from universal building blocks. It can be concluded that the main technological challenges to aid the economic feasibility of this approach lie in the area of biomass refining, separation technology, and bioconversion technology. Far-reaching integration of the food, feed, and chemical industries is, moreover, required, as is a major investment in infrastructure.

The second approach, *the integrated process chain approach*, follows the analog of the petrochemical industry. In this scheme a "universal" substrate is first transformed into universal building blocks, based on which chemical products are produced. In this approach it is thought that it is economically and technologically beneficial to build chemicals in highly integrated production facilities. The main technological challenges for this approach lie in the high-efficiency transformation of biomass into commonly known building blocks for the petrochemical industry (van Tuil 2002).

The main technologies producing chemicals from biomass are:
- biomass refining or pretreatment;
- thermochemical conversion (gasification, pyrolysis, hydrothermal upgrading (HTU));
- fermentation and bioconversion; and
- product separation and upgrading.

Five main categories of building block can be identified as intermediates in the production of chemical products from biomass.
- Refined biomass, i.e. biomass in which the valuable components have been made accessible by physical and/or mild thermochemical treatment. These components are extracted from the refined biomass. The remaining biomass then undergoes further transformation.
- BioSyngas. This gas (mainly CO and H_2) is a multifunctional intermediate in the production of materials, chemicals, transportation fuels, power, and/or heat from biomass; it can easily be used in existing industrial infrastructures to substitute the conventional fossil-based fuels and raw materials.
- Mixed sugars. These C_5 and C_6 sugars are further refined substrates for chemical and bioconversion. These substrates mainly originate from side streams in the food industry and potentially from ligno-cellulosic biomass streams.
- Pyrolysis oil. This oil is produced in fast and flash pyrolysis processes and can be used for indirect cofiring for power production in conventional power plants, for direct decentral heating purposes, and potentially as high energy density intermediate (important for long-distance transportation) bio-based intermediate for the final production of chemicals and/or transportation fuels.
- Biocrude. This material is a fossil oil-like mixture of hydrocarbons with low oxygen content. Biocrude results from severe hydrothermal upgrading (HTU) of (relatively wet) biomass and can, potentially, like its petroleum analog, be used to produce materials, chemicals, transportation fuels, and power and/or heat.

4.4.2
Biorefinery Concept

A biorefinery is a facility that integrates biomass conversion processes and equipment to co-produce fuels, power, and chemicals from diverse biomass sources (Fig. 4.3). The biorefinery concept is analogous to today's petroleum refineries, which produce multiple fuels and products from petroleum (Fig. 4.4).

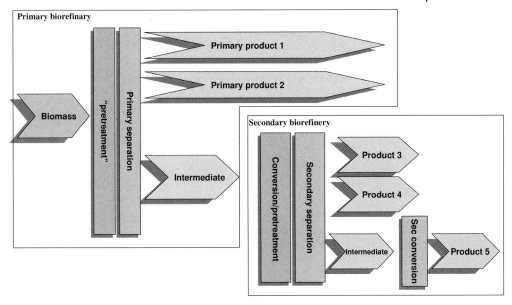

Fig. 4.3 Schematic overview general integrated biorefinery process.

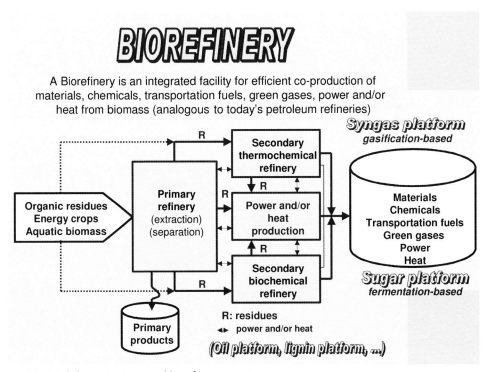

Fig. 4.4 Detailed overview integrated biorefinery process.

Industrial biorefineries have been identified as the most promising routes to the creation of a bio-based economy (Realff and Abbas 2004). Partial biorefineries already exist in some agricultural and forest products facilities (e.g. pulp mills, corn wet milling, starch and sugar beet refining).

These systems can be improved by better utilization of residues and optimization of total added-value creation; new biorefineries can be enhanced by applying the lessons learned from existing facilities to comparable situations.

By producing multiple products, a biorefinery can take advantage of the natural complexity and differences between biomass components and intermediates and therefore maximize the value derived from the biomass feedstock. A biorefinery might, for example, produce one or several low-volume, but high-value, chemical products and a low-value, but high-volume, platform chemical and/or liquid transportation fuel, while generating power and heat for its own use, and probably enough for sale of electricity. The high-value products enhance profitability, the high-volume chemicals and/or transportation fuels help meet European energy needs and CO_2 emission-reduction goals; whereas the power and/or heat both reduce overall production costs and greenhouse gas emissions.

4.4.3
Biomass Availability

The Netherlands is a small country where land is scarce. Although the options for primary crop production are limited, the biomass flux of utilized biomass (organic material) is very high (partially imported). An estimated 42 million dry tons of biomass (13 ton ha^{-1}) (van Dam et al., in preparation) are used and produced in different sectors of the economy (compare with a biomass flux some 5 tonnes for Germany). As markets change this high turnover of biomass does generate many opportunities for reallocating streams toward biorefinery feedstocks.

One of the largest biomass streams is produced in the agri-industrial complex. Many of these streams can be regarded as byproducts. Approximately 10 million tonnes (as received) of byproducts are currently mostly (90%) used for animal feed (Vis 2002; Elbersen et al. 2002). These byproducts vary from slaughterhouse wastes to discarded frying oil, potato peel, etc. As traditional markets change (diminish) and markets for biobased energy and products increase, a large part of these streams can become partially available for biorefinery. This change in market demand for feed is already apparent from the decline in livestock (from 4.6 in 1995 to 3.6 million in 2003), and pigs (14.5 million in 1995 to 10.7 million in 2003), which leads to a smaller demand for feed.

Another estimate has been made of the potentially available (ligno)cellulose biomass feedstocks in The Netherlands that could be used for ethanol production (de Jong et al. 2003). The total amount of these technically suitable feedstocks is approximately 12 million tons (dry weight) per year (about 220 PJ$_{th}$ annum^{-1}), excluding import and biomass energy crops. The potential feedstocks are highly variable, however, and include a range of agro-industrial residues, agricultural wastes, forestry residues, and household organic waste, etc.

As already mentioned, the domestic (primary) biomass energy crop potential is limited with some 2 million ha of agricultural land of which less than 1 million ha is arable land. It is hard to estimate the potential for biomass energy crops as competing demands for land are uncertain. Estimates range from 0 to a maximum of 3 million tonnes (300.000 ha at 10 ton dry weight ha^{-1} $annum^{-1}$, 18 GJ ton^{-1} dry weight) equivalent to 50 PJ_{th} $annum^{-1}$ (Minnesma 2003). In the short term, arable agriculture could be an important source of biorefinery feedstocks with more than 1 million tonnes of crop field residues available.

The maximum total Dutch biomass availability (organic residues and crops) will therefore amount to 300 PJ_{th} $annum^{-1}$ (approx. 15 million tonnes dry weight). Taking the longer-term (2040) policy ambitions into account, requiring a biomass substitution volume of about 600–1000 PJ_{th} $annum^{-1}$, it can be concluded that The Netherlands will have to import at least half, if not more, of its long-term biomass requirements.

The potentially available feedstocks for biorefinery in The Netherlands are highly variable and most streams are dispersed over the country. Though many streams currently have other applications the potential is more than 15 million dry tonnes of biomass. Large-scale biorefinery systems will have to use a variety of feedstocks to secure feedstock availability ("multi-feedstock plant"). The option to import biomass over longer distances should also be available.

For medium-term development (< 10 years) a focus on feedstocks which have the desirable characteristics (for example homogeneous streams low in lignin and/or low in ash) are desirable. For the longer term (> 10 years), as the scale of production increases, the feedstock range should be broadened with additional residues and (woody) energy crops (e.g. willow).

The worldwide average net available biomass potential for non-feed and non-material purposes is expected to amount 200–700 EJ_{th} $annum^{-1}$ (maximum 1100 EJ_{th} $annum^{-1}$) in 2050 (Lysen 2000). Worldwide, enough biomass will be available to fulfill the needs. Because other countries will claim the same biomass, the market price will be internationally settled. Timely participation in the developing international market is a requirement to become an important global player.

4.4.4
Primary Refinery

Deriving a raw material stream with desired specifications (i.e. amount of ash, fermentable sugars, lignin) while simultaneously extracting valuable components from the heterogeneous biomass streams is one of the major biorefinery research and development issues. The main research and development areas which must be addressed before an efficient biomass pretreatment chain can be established are:
- characterization and standardization of raw materials and products;
- development of a cost-effective infrastructure for production, collection, characterization, storage, identity preservation, pre-processing activities, import

and transportation of feedstocks for bio-based products and bioenergy applications; and

- development of economically viable pretreatment processes for commercial use of a range of current and new bio-based feedstocks.

Biorefineries could potentially use complex processing strategies to efficiently produce a diverse and flexible mixture of conventional products, fuels, electricity, heat, chemicals, and material products from all available, environmentally appropriate biomass feedstocks. To achieve economically viable biorefineries it is important that:

- separation and fractionation technologies for high-throughput systems are developed that produce value-added products and no waste streams; and
- generic solutions are identified that will apply across multiple feedstocks while simultaneously achieving a zero-waste production system with either direct use or recycling of all components.

4.4.5
Secondary Thermochemical Refinery

Thermochemical-based refinery processes usually consist of the following interconnected unit operations: pretreatment (i.e. drying, size reduction), feeding, conversion (gasification, pyrolysis, HTU), product clean-up and conditioning, and product end-use. In this subsection only gasification-related aspects are discussed, because it is expected that gasification will be the key technology in (secondary) thermochemical refinery processes.

Atmospheric air-blown gasification processes, based on fixed bed, (circulating) fluidized bed, or indirect dual reactor technology, are commercially available for product gas (mainly CO, H_2, N_2, impurities) production. After gas clean-up this – so called – fuel gas can potentially be used for heat, power, or CHP production in a variety of prime movers. At the moment only direct heat production by coupling of these technologies to conventional (natural gas or diesel fired) furnaces, and power production by indirect cofiring in coal-fired power plants is technically and economically feasible.

The market implementation of fully integrated gasification-based systems for stand-alone power or CHP production is delayed by the high power/CHP production costs, mainly caused by the relatively high investment costs of these new and emerging technologies, and insufficient financial support from the government.

Oxygen-blown gasification processes, especially applicable for the production of BioSyngas (mainly CO and H_2), based on both bubbling fluidized bed and entrained-flow technology, are technically not yet available for biomass applications. Within the framework of the EU Chrisgas-project, TPS et al. are now trying to modify the air-blown pressurized Varnamo gasification plant (Sweden) for oxygen-blown operation.

Within the sixth Framework Program of the EU, ECN et al. are currently (October 2004) preparing a large STREP proposal concerning the modification of existing coal-based slagging oxygen-blown entrained-flow-based gasification technology for 100% biomass use. Main research areas are biomass feeding, gasification/slag behavior, product gas cooling, and the commercial applicability of produced solid waste streams. The final goal is to design, build, and operate several MW_{th} pilot plants within 4 years, so that large commercial implementation can become feasible around 2010. The gasification processes mentioned all require size-reduced and relatively dry (about 15–20% moisture maximum) biomass fuels. "Wet" biomass fuels require rigorous drying before they can be used.

Alternatively these fuels can potentially be converted by means of sub/supercritical gasification processes (or fermentation processes, see Section 4.4.6). Supercritical biomass gasification is performed at conditions above the critical point of water (374 °C, 221 bar), mostly in the temperature range 500–700 °C. Under these conditions an H_2-rich product gas is produced. Under subcritical conditions (temperature range approx. 350–400 °C) a methane-rich gas will be produced. Under these conditions for full carbon conversion very low dry matter concentrations and a catalyst are required. Although bench/pilot facilities are available – FZK (D) 100 $L\,h^{-1}$ (since 2003), University of Twente (NL) 5–30 $L\,h^{-1}$ (since 1998) – the ECN opinion is that some years of laboratory-scale PhD work will be required before the potential commercial implementation of this technology. The technology is expected to be developed for "green natural gas" (SNG) production; for the production of hydrogen, ECN has the opinion that this technology will not become financially competitive in the longer term. Some main research items are: feeding, heat exchange and catalyst behavior.

Within the framework of the biorefinery concept, two gasification-based pathways can be distinguished.

- Application of the biorefinery concept to increase the financial yield of "conventional" gasification processes. By separating highly added-value components from raw biomass fuels before conversion, or afterwards from the raw "products" in product gas clean-up/conditioning, the overall plant economics could be improved, simplifying market implementation (Fig. 4.5).
- Development of highly efficient advanced gasification-based thermochemical secondary biorefining processes. By developing advanced catalyst-supported staged or subcritical gasification processes it is expected that a variety of "products" could be separated from biomass in such a way that the overall process will be market competitive, without the need for substantial governmental support.

4.4.6
Secondary Biochemical Refinery – Fermentative Processes

This section focuses on fermentation as the main form of bioconversion. A large number of chemicals are currently produced by fermentation. These range from bulk chemicals, for example ethanol (for food and fuel purposes) (Reith et al. 2002) and lactic acid (as food ingredient or as monomer of polylactic acid) (Datta et al. 1995), via compounds as amino acids, gluconic acid, and citric acid, to high-value products such as antibiotics.

The efficient conversion of sugars into ethanol and lactate by fermentation increases interest in fermentation technology as a means of production of bulk chemicals. Fermentation has several advantages over conventional chemical reactions.
- Fermentation processes are usually one-step syntheses which could reduce investment costs.
- Microbial biosynthesis offers control over chemical reactions that is unchallenged by state-of-the-art chemical synthesis resulting in highly functional compounds.

Currently, however, fermentation has several disadvantages which have to be solved before it will be able to compete with conventional chemical reactions.

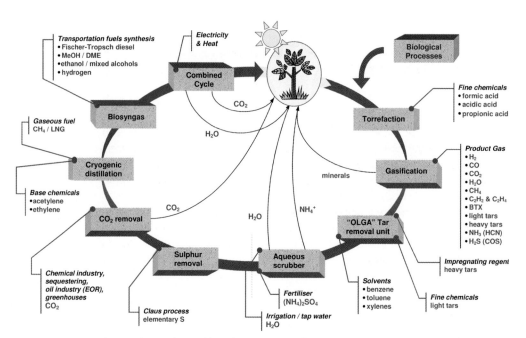

Fig. 4.5 Thermochemical biorefinery concept of ECN to increase the financial yield of "conventional" gasification processes (Boerrigter et al. 2004).

- The costs of fermentation processes for bulk processes are higher than those for the corresponding chemical process.
- The natural product spectrum of microorganisms is limited.
- In fermentation processes several side streams are formed which can be coped with on the small scale but will cause a severe burden on the bulk scale.

4.4.6.1 **Feedstocks**

Most feedstocks currently used for fermentation processes are based on sugar beet, sugar cane, and corn. To reduce feedstock costs other substrates must be used. Several alternative feedstocks are being considered, for example fruit waste, wood, straw, agricultural waste streams, dung, oils, and fatty acids, etc.

Among these the lignocellulosic materials are the most abundant polysaccharide-containing biomass available in the world and are therefore an extensively studied feedstock for fermentation processes. For almost all microorganisms this lignocellulosic material must be hydrolyzed into its component saccharides by mechanical pretreatment, followed by acid, base, or heat treatment, use of organic solvents or wet-oxidation to open the matrix, and, usually, enzymatic hydrolysis of the cellulose. The costs of the hydrolytic enzymes are the main expense in feedstock pretreatment and hydrolysis.

Hydrolysates from lignocellulosic materials contain, beside C_6 sugars such as glucose, also C_5 sugars, for example xylose, and inhibitors. The relative amount depends on the type of feedstock and the process used. Bakers' yeast, used in the production of ethanol, cannot use these C_5 sugars. It has been calculated that for a competitive process these C_5 sugars also must be converted into ethanol. This is probably also true for other, future, processes.

4.4.6.2 **Product Spectrum**

Microorganisms can produce an extremely wide variety of chemical compounds. Most of these compounds are, however, only intermediates in the overall metabolism and will not be produced in significant amounts. Many of the platform chemicals used in the chemical industry are, furthermore, not produced by natural microorganisms. The new fermentation technology must interface directly with existing processes and installations in classical chemistry to reduce investment costs, indicating that the biochemical pathways of the microorganisms must be modified to be able to produce current platform chemicals. Several physiological aspects (yield, productivity, toxicity of product, use of GMO, by-product formation, etc.) must be taken into account if this is to be achieved successfully. This shows that the production of non-natural compounds by microorganisms can be a complex task. Some successful examples of the modification of metabolic pathways, however, are the production of 1,3-propanediol for the production of Sorona by DuPont, the synthesis of muconic acid as a precursor for adipic acid, and the optimization of succinic acid production (Biebl et al. 1999; Chotani et al. 2000; Zeikus et al. 1999).

4.4.6.3 **Side Streams and Recycling**

Fermentation processes are usually regarded as "clean" processes. During fermentation, however, some side-streams are created which could be a severe environmental burden on the bulk scale, for example:

- During ethanol production by bakers' yeast glycerol and fusel oils are produced.
- Lactic acid is removed from the fermentation broth by complexing with calcium ions resulting in the formation of insoluble calcium lactate. This eventually results in the formation of equimolar amounts of gypsum.
- In all fermentations microbial biomass is formed. This can be a considerable fraction. For example in the experimental production of polyhydroxyalkanoates (biopolymers) 20–50% of the product is biomass.

Because gypsum production could also be a problem in the synthesis of other organic acids, much research has been devoted to in the development of other down-stream-processing processes, for example membrane electrodialysis. For the problem of microbial biomass formation another solution must be sought in which the high-added-value components of the microbial biomass, for example pigments, vitamins, and antioxidants are extracted and the remaining material could then be recycled as feedstock in the fermentation process.

4.5
Conclusions, Outlook, and Perspectives

The objective of this section is to draw conclusions from previous sections by presenting an agenda for further activity to facilitate the transition toward the production of chemicals and chemical products from biomass. We believe that if these agendas are addressed the sustainable production of chemicals from biomass will become a realistic option in the future.

4.5.1
Biomass – Sustainability

A transition towards increased use of biomass originates from its possible contribution to sustainable production of energy, fuels, chemicals, and materials. Several chemicals can, moreover, be more easily or energy-efficiently produced from biomass than from other feedstock. Many of these products can be extracted directly from the biomass.

The importance of biomass use towards the sustainability of the production of chemicals is directly linked to the scale of production. It is, moreover, often questioned whether the use of biomass for energy, fuels, and chemicals can form a symbiosis with the use of the same biomass for the production of food, feed, and materials, for example paper and wood. Also mentioned is the uncertainty of the implication of a change in the main feedstock for energy and fuels industry on the chemical industry.

What will be the main feedstock for energy and fuels in 50 years time – water, sunlight, natural gas, or biomass? Are the conversion technologies mentioned in this study elegant ways of waste disposal in the food, feed, and cellulose/paper industry? Is biomass mainly of interest for extraction of valuable chemicals? What will be the impact of a biotechnological revolution on the opportunities and pitfalls of biomass?

Some of these questions have been introduced in this paper. It is, however, suggested that further insight into the role of biomass in chemicals production in the Netherlands will be obtained by scenario evaluation. The result of this evaluation will make it possible to choose feedstock/conversion technology combinations that maximize the potential of biomass use for chemicals and chemical products.

4.5.2
Biomass Refining and Pretreatment

A range of standards is needed to verify performance in the industry and to help improve marketability. These include standards for environmental quality of feedstocks and conversion technologies, and accreditation and standards for energy content and the quality of feedstocks and products. Much of the technology and many of the products developed have not been proven under "real world" conditions and/or face significant certification challenges. These certification challenges are often the result of systems that set standards based on the physical characteristics of petroleum products, rather than on the performance of the end product.

Improved practices in agriculture, silviculture, and aquaculture can play a significant role in increasing yields while reducing required inputs. To achieve great increases in biomass feedstock availability many issues must be resolved in harvesting, collection, storage, import, and transport.

Current methods result in low densities of desired components, high transportation costs, and potential storage stability issues. Pre-processing might be done "on the farm" or even during harvesting or transportation "en route" to densify, dry, and perhaps initially separate biomass components.

New transportation schemes might include pumping a fluid slurry, torrefication, pyrolysis, or "pelletizing" biomass locally. All of these advances must be made while maintaining biodiversity and ensuring the safety and sustainability of the technologies utilized.

Most biomass is solid, requiring improved material handling systems at the front end of conversion operations. Breakthroughs in fractionation and separation technology will be required to produce higher value-added products, to reduce processing costs, waste, and environmental impact.

4.5.3
Conversion Technology

Next to already known conventional thermal, chemical, and bioconversion technologies this report has shown that the potential in conversion technology is enormous, partly as a result of ever-increasing knowledge about thermochemical and biotechnological pathways for the conversion of biomass into chemical products. It is suggested that research efforts be focused on the following areas:

- Optimization of thermochemical conversion technologies. This paper has shown that different technologies have been proposed for thermochemical conversion of biomass. Further improvements lie in: (1) optimization of efficiency and cost reduction of currently employed conventional technologies, and (2) development of new advanced technologies, for example catalytic supported staged or subcritical gasification processes.

- (Bio)catalyst development and bioreactor engineering. Metabolic pathway engineering enables synthesis of very specific catalysts (both whole-cell and enzymes) for transformation of refined biomass (mainly mixed sugars, fatty acids, and syngas) into a variety of chemical intermediates and chemical products. This will lead to the controlled, safe and efficient production of new and existing chemicals and polymers. Important issues for the efficient use of biocatalysts include immobilization, reactor kinetics and design, and separation of the chemical product from the reaction mixture. As in the pretreatment of biomass, separation technology also plays an important role in efficient and cost-effective biocatalytic production processes.

4.5.4
Chemicals and Materials Design

The approaches to the production of chemicals from biomass presented in this section are resource-based forward-integrated approaches. A design approach can also be suggested in which a backward-integrated chemical industry designs chemicals and production methods that fit the application of the chemical product. It is thought that whereas the resource-based approach fits current (petro)-chemical business and production models, the design approach will lead to a real transition in the production and design of chemicals and materials. This backward-integrated approach will initially be applicable in specialty chemical markets but there are also long-term opportunities in bulk chemical markets.

It is thought that with the envisaged development in advanced thermochemical and bioconversion technologies the role of biomass and a biomimetic approach to the design of chemicals and materials may add to sustainable production, use, and reuse or disposal of chemicals and materials. Further examination of the role that chemicals and materials design can have on the sustainable use of biomass and biomass-based resources is therefore suggested.

4.5.5
Dutch Energy Research Strategy ("EOS")

In The Netherlands the Ministry of Economic Affairs has defined a national subsidy program "Energie OnderzoeksStrategie (EOS)" for co-financing long-term (> 10 years) technology developments that support the transition process to a more sustainable society. In this program (2004–2008) an annual subsidy budget of 35 Mio € is available for technology development in pre-defined areas. Biomass-based technology development in direct/indirect cofiring in conventional power plants, gasification, and biorefineries have been selected for co-financing. It is expected that for biorefinery technology development about 10 M € subsidy will be available for project co-funding for the next four years.

The Energy Research Center of the Netherlands (ECN) – Biomass Department, with Agrotechnology and Food Innovations B.V. (A&F), Wageningen University and Research center (WUR), University of Twente (UT), Utrecht University (UU), and Groningen University (RUG), have defined an integral biorefinery-based research and development program for the coming four years. Within this program joint projects will be defined on the basis of a common vision and submitted for co-funding. Research items that will be addressed are: integral chain analysis and scenario studies to identify platform chemicals and provide the framework for technological developments; primary refining processes, including pretreatment; secondary thermochemical and biological refining processes, including product separation and upgrading; and some site-specific case studies to encourage real market implementation.

References

Ahmed, I. and Morris, D. J. (1994) Replacing Petrochemicals with Biochemicals: A Pollution Prevention Strategy for the Great Lakes. Minneapolis: Institute for Local Self-Reliance.

American Chemical Society, American Institute of Chemical Engineers, Chemical Manufacturers Association, Council for Chemical Research, Synthetic Organic Chemical Manufacturers Association (1996) *Technology vision 2020; the U.S. chemical industry* (downloaded at http://www.acs.org)

Biebl, H., Menzel, K., Zeng, A. P., and Deckwer, W. D. (1999) Microbial production of 1,3-propanediol, *Appl. Microbiol. Biotechnol.*, 52, 289–297.

Boerrigter H. et al. (2004). Thermal Biorefinery; high-efficient integrated production of renewable chemicals, (transportation)

fuels, and products from biomass, 2nd World Conference and Technology Exhibition on Biomass for Energy, Industry and Climate Protection, Rome, Italy, 10–14 May 2004.

Chotani, G., Dodge, T., Hsu, A., Kumar, M., LaDuca, R., Trimbur, D., Weyler, W. and Sanford, K. (2000) The commercial production of chemicals using pathway engineering. *Biochim Biophys Acta*, 1543 (2): 434–455.

Coombs, R. (1995) Firm strategies and technological choices. In: Rip et al. (eds) *Managing technology in society: the approach of constructive technology assessment.* Pinter Publishers: London, New York, 331–345.

Dam, J. E. G. van, de Klerk-Engels, B., Struik, P. C. and Rabbinge, R. (2004) Securing renewable resources supplies for changing market demands in a biobased economy. Industrial Crops and Products, in press.

Dam, van J.E.G., C. Boeriu, and J.P.M. Sanders – Sustainable plant production chains for "green chemicals". ACS Symposium: Feedstocks for the Future: Renewables for the Production of Chemicals and Materials, Anaheim, CA, March 28–April 1, 2004 (in preparation).

Datta, R., Stai, S.-P., Bonsignore, P., Moon, S.-H., and Frank, J.R. (1995) Technological and economic potential of poly(lactic acid) and lactic acid derivatives. *FEMS Microbiol. Rev.*, 16, 221–231.

Diamantidis, N.D., and Koukios E.G. (2000) Agricultural crops and residues as feedstock for non-food products in Western Europe. *Ind. Crops Products*, 11, 97–106.

de Jong, E., R.R. Bakker, H.W. Elbersen, R.A. Weusthuis, R.H.W. Maas, J.H. Reith, H. den Uil, and R. van Ree (2003) Perspectives for Bioethanol Production in the Netherlands: feedstock selection and pretreatment options, Poster presentation at the 25th Symposium on Biotechnology for Fuels and chemicals, Breckenridge, Colorado.

de Klerk, B., Vellema, S. and van Tuil, R. (2002) Chemie: de weg naar duurzaamheid? *Chemisch2Weekblad*, 16 Feb. 2002, 14–15.

Ehrenberg, J. (2002) Current situation and future prospects of EU industry using renewable raw materials, (coordinated by the European Renewable Resources & Materials Association (ERRMA), Brussels, February 2002.

Elbersen, H.W., F. Kappen and J. Hiddink (2002) Quickscan value-added applications for byproducts and wastes generated in the Food Processing Industry (Hoogwaardige Toepassingen voor Rest- en Nevenstromen uit de Voedings- en Genotmiddelenindustrie). ATO, Arcadis IMD. For the Ministry of Agriculture.

Lysen, E.H. (2000) GRAIN: Global Restrictions on Biomass Availability for Import to the Netherlands, E2EWAB00.27, Utrecht, The Netherlands, August 2000 (partly in Dutch).

Ministry of Economic Affairs (2003) The Netherlands: Biomass in 2040, The Green Driving Force Behind a Knowledge Economy and Sustainability ... A Vision

Ministry of Economic Affairs (2001) *Catalysis: key to sustainability* (Technology Roadmap Catalysis initiated by Ministry of Economic Affairs and facilitated by PricewaterhouseCoopers Management Consultants) (available at http://www.technologyroadmapping.com).

Minnisma, M. and Hissemoller, M., Biomassa – Een Wenkend Perspectief, IVM, Februari 2003 (in Dutch).

Molendijk, K.G.P., Venselaar, J., Weterings, R.A.P.M. and de Klerk-Engels, B. (2004) Transitie naar een duurzame chemie. TNO-rapport R2004/179.

National Research Council (2000), *Biobased industrial products: priorities for research and commercialization*, Washington D.C.: National Academic Press.

Okkerse C. and van Bekkum, H. (1997) Towards a plant-based economy? In: Van Doren H.A. and van Swaaij A.C. (eds), *Starch 96 – the book*.

Parris, K. (2004) Agriculture, Biomass, Sustainability and Policy: an Overview OECD Workshop on Biomass and Agriculture: Sustainability, Markets and Policies, 10–13 June 2003, Vienna, Austria. OECD Code 512004011P1, pp 27–36.

Rabobank International (2001) *De Nederlandse akkerbouwkolom: het geheel is meer dan de som der delen*. Rabobank Food and Agribusiness Research: Utrecht.

Realff, M.J. and Abbas, C. (2004) Industrial Symbiosis, refining the biorefinery. Journal of Industrial Ecology 7:5–9.

Reit, J.H., den Uil, H., van Veen, H., de Laat, W.T.A.M., Niessen, J.J., de Jong, E., Elbersen, H.W., Weusthuis, R., van Dijken, J.P. and Raamsdonk, L. (2002) Co-production of bio-ethanol, electricity and heat from biomass residues. Proc. of the 12th European Conference and Technology Exhibition on Biomass for Energy, Industry and Climate Protection, June 17–21 2002, Amsterdam, The Netherlands.

Roekel, G.J. van and Koster R. (2000) *Succes – en faalfactoren van de agrificatie in Nederland*. ATO: Wageningen (report for the Dutch Ministry of Agriculture).

Sims, R.E.H. (2004) Biomass, Bioenergy and Biomaterials: Future Prospects. OECD

Workshop on Biomass and Agriculture: 10–13 June 2003, Vienna, Austria. OECD Code 512004011P1, pp 37–62.

Sreenath, H.K., Moldes, A.B., Koegel, R.G. and Straub, R.J. (2001) Lactic acid production from agriculture residues. *Biotechnol. Lett.* 23:179–184.

UK Foresight Programme Chemicals Panel (2000) *A chemicals renaissance* (available at (http://www.foresight.gov.uk)

US Department of Energy (1998) *Plant/Crop-based Renewable Resources 2020: A vision to enhance U.S. economic security through renewable plant/crop-based resource use* (available at http://www.oit.doe.gov/agriculture/).

US Department of Energy (1999) *The Technology Roadmap for Plant/Crop-based Renewable Resources 2020: research priorities*

for fulfilling a vision to enhance U.S. economic security through renewable plant/crop-based resource use (available at http://www.oit.doe.gov/agriculture/).

Vis, M. (2002) Beschikbaarheid van reststromen uit de voedings – en enotmiddelenindustrie voor energieproductie. A report for Novem, Utrecht. DEN nr 2020-01-23-03-0003/4700001071 (in Dutch).

Weaver, P., Jansen, L., van Grootveld, G., van Spiegel, E. and Vergragt, Ph. (2000) *Sustainable technology development.* Greenleaf Publishing: Sheffield.

Zeikus, J.G., Jain, M.K. and Elankovan, P. (1999) Biotechnology of succinic acid production and markets for derived industrial products. *Appl. Microbiol. Biotechnol.* 51, 545–552.

Part II
Biorefinery Systems

Biorefineries – Industrial Processes and Products. Status Quo and Future Directions. Vol. 1
Edited by Birgit Kamm, Patrick R. Gruber, Michael Kamm
Copyright © 2006 WILEY-VCH Verlag GmbH & Co. KGaA, Weinheim
ISBN: 3-527-31027-4

Lignocellulose Feedstock Biorefinery

5
The Lignocellulosic Biorefinery –
A Strategy for Returning to a Sustainable Source of Fuels and Industrial Organic Chemicals

L. Davis Clements and Donald L. Van Dyne

5.1
The Situation

The current, historically high, prices of crude oil are causing economic hardship for families and businesses worldwide, because of the resulting high energy prices. The estimated impacts of increasing energy costs for farmers, truckers, and airlines exceed US $ 13 billion per year for the United States alone. At the same time, it is clear that increasing demand and a finite supply of petroleum will sustain the rising prices and increase competition for secure petroleum supplies.

The strategy outlined here not only addresses these issues, but also provides major benefits to the environment and to farm incomes. This is all accomplished by using known, proven chemical processes (no new research needed) and at very attractive rates of return on investment (ROI) that will *not* require long-term government subsidies when this new industry is established.

5.2
The Strategy

At the most basic level, the strategy is to reduce then, essentially, eliminate dependence on petroleum as the primary source of liquid fuels and industrial organic chemicals (where "industrial organic chemicals" includes those made from both petroleum and biological resources). This is accomplished by replac-

Biorefineries – Industrial Processes and Products. Status Quo and Future Directions. Vol. 1
Edited by Birgit Kamm, Patrick R. Gruber, Michael Kamm
Copyright © 2006 WILEY-VCH Verlag GmbH & Co. KGaA, Weinheim
ISBN: 3-527-31027-4

ing petroleum, the current dominant hydrocarbon source, with hydroxycarbons derived from plant and animal biomass sources. The biomass carbon resources are processed in biorefinery complexes that are analogs of present day petrochemical complexes. These biorefineries will produce the same, or functionally equivalent, fuels and industrial chemicals that are currently obtained from petroleum. The difference is that the biomass resources are renewable and, as will be shown in examples based upon the United States, the biomass resources are largely derived from materials currently regarded as waste.

The United States annually discards *more* tonnes of biomass carbon as "trash" than we consume from petroleum carbon resources. Technologies are, however, available for converting agricultural and forestry residues and municipal solid wastes (MSW), which we now discard, into the fuels and chemicals that we consume. Each year the United States consumes approximately 10 million tonnes of industrial organic chemicals and 325 million tonnes of liquid transportation fuels.

Currently, the United States converts approximately 15 million tonnes of agricultural products into liquid fuels (ethanol and biodiesel) and discards approximately 270 million tonnes of agriculturally derived residues in the form of harvestable crop residues, animal manure, forest residues, and the organic fraction of municipal solid wastes.

Since 1933, an average of 15 million hectares of crop land have laid idle annually in the US, representing an additional 75 million tonnes of potential agriculturally produced biomass. There is no technical or economic reason why the US demand for carbon resources could not be met by biomass replacing petroleum as the primary carbon source.

The functional equivalent of the petrochemical complex for processing agriculturally derived raw and residue materials and MSW processing is a biorefinery. Here the term "biorefinery" is defined as "a production facility that uses multiple renewable, agriculturally derived raw materials, in combination with multiple processing methods, to provide the most profitable mix of higher value chemicals and energy products possible at a given location."

5.2.1
A Strategy Within a Strategy

An essential component of the structural shift from petroleum to biomass as the source of carbon is a "two-use" ethic. Everything that grows or is derived from organic sources (even plastics) should have at least two uses. MSW is collected and recycled to the biorefinery. Other organic materials, for example agricultural residues, used tires and plastics, and human and animal wastes, are converted into new chemicals or fuels in biorefineries. In this "two-use" ethic, carbon is recovered and recycled in much the same way that aluminum, iron, and lead are recycled today.

In contrast with the huge petrochemical complexes of today, biorefineries will probably be limited in total capacity to 1000 to 2000 tonnes of biomass per day.

This is because the distributed nature of agricultural production, forestry production, and municipal solid-waste management strategies limit the amount of material that can be economically assembled in one area, on a continuing basis, at an acceptable cost.

This means that biorefineries will be regional, and dispersed. This regionality not only means greater domestic security through dispersion and redundancy, but also wider distribution of new jobs and economic activity in rural areas.

5.2.2
Environmental Benefits

The use of biomass as a replacement for petroleum in the production of liquid fuels and industrial organic chemicals would have immediate and far-reaching environmental benefits.

- *First*, biomass resources are renewable. Most are annually renewable. This means that the carbon exhausted into the atmosphere as carbon dioxide when liquid fuels are burned would be recycled into new plant growth in the following years' crops. This factor alone will greatly improve air quality worldwide, and directly address the issue of global warming as a result of greenhouse gas emissions.
- *Second*, entire biomass resource needs are available domestically for many countries. No imports are needed. In the United States we *currently* have approximately 360 million tonnes per year of *non-fossil* carbon raw materials available to replace some, if not all, of the demand for petroleum for liquid fuels and industrial organic chemicals.
- *Third*, the assembly and refining of these resources will create a large number of jobs, primarily in rural areas.
- *Fourth*, the production and/or conversion of biomass resources to liquid fuels and organic chemicals involves processing steps that usually reduce the toxic burden associated with the petrochemical production of these products.
- *Fifth*, the required tonnage of carbon-rich biomass can be derived largely through the implementation of the "two uses" policy, i.e. the recycling of biomass. This provides a very economical input for the biorefinery.

5.2.3
The Business Structure

Because a major source of the biomass needed for this transition is "2nd use", this provides a unique opportunity for new business partnerships. Municipal solid wastes (MSW), agricultural crop residues, and forestry residues comprise the bulk of the 2nd-use sources.

The biomass input resources are the major component of the operating cost of production of liquid fuels and industrial organic chemicals for the biorefinery. Because these inputs are now considered to be of low or even negative value, the owners of these 2nd-use resources can very profitably move these biomass materials into the refining process, but delay taking their share of the profit until the final products are produced and sold. Thus, the 2nd-use producers would receive their fair share of the generated profits *after* the increased value has been added. This provides a considerably better return than the current negative, zero, or near zero waste value.

The 2nd-use strategy leads directly to the concept of a business partnership comprising the biorefinery owner(s) and the biomass production owner(s). For agricultural wastes and residues, assembly of these inputs could be achieved by use of already existing cooperatives and/or farmer organizations. Similarly, MSW inputs could be supplied through existing waste-management companies or municipal waste-management operations.

It is envisaged that the biomass suppliers would participate equally with the biorefinery companies in the direction and operation of the partnership. Essentially, the business model is one of vertical integration through a collaborative partnership or a joint venture business.

5.2.4
Cost Estimates

A biorefinery complex is not cheap. The approximate cost of a 1000 to 2000 tonnes per day multi-product plant is approximately $ 0.5 billion (US). In the United States, example, the biorefinery will draw raw materials from a radius of 150 to 300 km. This means, allowing for desert and inland waters, that from 300 to 500 biorefineries would eventually be built in the US. This represents an approximate $ 200 billion investment for the US. This is, however, approximately the same investment that will be required to replace approximately 200 petroleum refineries and petrochemical complexes that are now more than 30 years old and nearing the end of their useful lives.

5.3
Comparison of Petroleum and Biomass Chemistry

5.3.1
Petroleum Resources

Petroleum is a mixture of hundreds of hydrocarbon compounds. The dominant chemistry of petroleum is that of linear hydrocarbons, with relatively little unsaturation or branching. The chemical structure is polymers of the $-(CH_2)-$ mer, with the hydrocarbon chains typically from 4 to 30 units long. Lesser quantities of aromatic compounds (benzene derivatives), naphthenic compounds (benzene dimers), and anthracenes (benzene trimers) are present. Additional elements are incorporated into some molecules, for example oxygen, nitrogen, sulfur, or phosphorus, but the essential elements of petroleum are carbon and hydrogen.

Utilization of petroleum for the production of liquid fuels and organic chemicals involves both physical separation of the numerous different compounds and chemical synthesis. Fuels production is primarily a separation process, with additional synthesis needed for higher-quality products, for example reformulated gasoline, and for removal of sulfur and nitrogen. Crude petroleum is separated into different fractions according to molecular size by distillation. Distillation processes account for approximately three percent of the US total energy budget.

The largest-volume fuel produced from petroleum is gasoline. Gasoline is a mixture of smaller (four to eight carbon) straight-chain hydrocarbons recovered by distillation and synthetically created branched chain hydrocarbons with a similar number of carbon atoms. Diesel fuel consists of larger (nine to fifteen carbon) hydrocarbons that are recovered largely by distillation.

Nitrogen, sulfur, and phosphorus are elements that occur naturally in petroleum and must be removed from liquid fuels, largely because of the detrimental environmental effects of their combustion products. The removal processes typically involve catalytic reactions under extreme operating conditions.

Petrochemical products are, in general, based on chemical addition of organic functional groups such as hydroxyl, aldehyde, acid, ester, etc., or other elements, such as oxygen, nitrogen, and halides. Much of the synthetic chemistry used is based on addition of functional groups to olefin hydrocarbons such as ethylene, propylene, and butylenes. Ethylene, propylene, and butylene are derived by high-temperature processing of ethane, propane, and butane recovered from petroleum crude oil by distillation. Benzene occurs naturally in petroleum, but most of the benzene family of hydrocarbons is produced synthetically by catalytic reforming of hexane and/or alkylation reactions. A representation of the petrochemical products families is given in Fig. 5.1.

5.3.2
Biomass Resources

Although a tremendous variety of biomass resources is available, only four basic chemical structures present in biomass are of significance for production of fuels and industrial products:
- saccharides and polysaccharides (sugars, starches, cellulose, hemicellulose);
- lignins (polyphenols);
- triacylglycerides or lipids (vegetable oils and animal fats); and
- proteins (vegetable and animal polymers made up of amino acids).

In addition to these basic structural resources, there are hundreds of specific organic compounds of biomass origin that have commercial uses ranging from medicinal materials, nutrients and natural products, to industrial products.

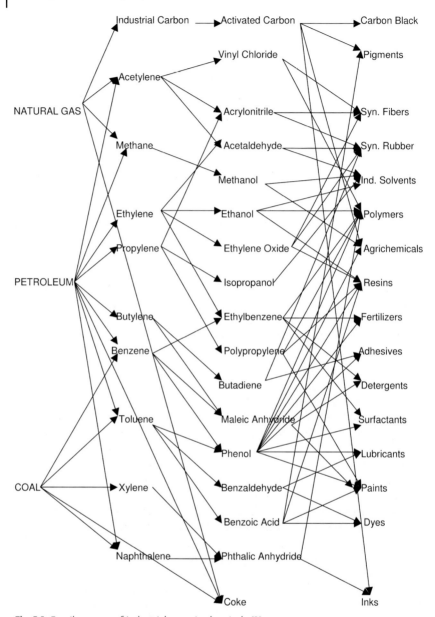

Fig. 5.1 Fossil sources of industrial organic chemicals [1].

5.3.3
Saccharides and Polysaccharides

Saccharides and polysaccharides may be characterized as hydroxycarbons because their basic chemical structure is CH_2O. Most hydroxycarbons occur naturally as either five- or six-membered ring structures. This ring structure may include only one or two connected rings (sugars) or they may be very long polymer chains (cellulose and hemicellulose).

The basic six-sided saccharide structure is exemplified by glucose. Long-chain polymers of glucose, or other hexoses, may be categorized as either a starch or a cellulose. The categorization depends on the configuration of the bonds formed across the oxygen molecule that joins two hexose units.

Starch is an energy-storage compound found in the seeds of many plants and is readily hydrolyzed enzymatically. Cellulose is found in association with two other polymers, hemicellulose and lignin, and is much more difficult to hydrolyze. Hemicellulose is a polysaccharide that has a large fraction of pentose sugars, with some hexoses, and is relatively easy to hydrolyze with acid.

Current industrial uses of starch and hexose sugars include the production of ethanol and other fermentation products, and the use of starch derivatives for polymers, absorbents, and adhesives. The pentose sugars from hemicellulose are a source of furfural and its derivatives and numerous xylose products.

5.3.4
Lignin

Lignin is a network polymer made up of multi-substituted, methoxy, arylpropane, and hydroxyphenol units. The resulting thermosetting polymer serves as the glue that holds the strands of cellulose and hemicellulose together in plant fibers to provide structure and strength. Together, the three polymers make up the largest biologically derived resource on earth – "lignocellulosics". The "lignocellulose" structure is the basis of the semi-rigid fibers found in all multi-cellular plants. The structural difference between a corn stalk, a tree, a flower stem, and a piece of waste paper is the difference between the relative amounts of hemicellulose, cellulose and lignin present and the shape and length of the fibers formed by the intertwined lignocellulosic chains.

The most significant current industrial uses for lignocellulosics are for construction materials and for pulp and paper products. The abundance of lignocellulosics is the basis for regarding them as the key input resources for the biorefinery strategy.

5.3.5
Triacylglycerides (or Triglycerides)

Triacylglycerides (or triglycerides) are the primary component of vegetable oils and animal fats. Irrespective of origin, these materials have identical chemical structures and very similar chemical compositions. The basic structure of a triglyceride looks like a comb with three long tines. The backbone of the comb is a three-carbon hydroxycarbon, dehydrated glycerol, with three medium to long-chain fatty acids attached. The fatty acid part of the molecule is a 7 to 31-carbon hydrocarbon chain with an organic acid group at one end. Triglycerides are relatively easily reacted with water or alcohols to form free fatty acids or fatty acid esters, respectively, with glycerol as co-product.

Vegetable oils and animal fats are an essential part of our diet. As such, they are available as recyclable materials in the form of recycled cooking oils and as the "float-grease" fraction recovered in municipal water treatment plants. In the United States an average of 10 kg of "waste" triglyceride materials is produced per person annually [2].

Derivatives of fats and oils have extensive use in non-food/feed applications. Current uses of triglyceride derivatives range from latex paints, high performance lubricants and polymers, to biodiesel fuel and personal care products.

The hydrocarbon structure of the fatty acid chain has facilitated the acceptance and use of triglycerides and their esters in conjunction with traditional petrochemical products. In fact, use of fats and oils for the production of industrial chemical products (oleochemical industry) is the largest contribution to the current industrial chemical industry made by biomass resources today.

5.3.6
Proteins

Proteins are long-chain polyamides based solely upon amino acid units. The –(NH)– (peptide) bonds characteristic of proteins are the same bonds found in industrial Nylons. The primary non-food/feed uses for proteins currently are as leather products, protein glues, and personal-care products. There are opportunities for the creation of "designer proteins", for example synthetic spider silk for light-weight, high strength cables or for polymer films and adhesives, but progress in this area has been somewhat slow.

5.4
The Chemistry of the Lignocellulosic Biorefinery

The production of liquid fuels and industrial chemicals from biomass will rely most heavily on the utilization of polysaccharide, lignocellulosic, and triacylglyceride feedstocks. These materials are available, easily assembled, and storable in the large quantities. In addition, these materials may be converted into products that are identical, or functionally equivalent, to current petroleum-based liquid fuels and industrial chemicals.

Petroleum is predominantly a liquid resource, with some gases and a small fraction of solid materials (waxes and asphalts). As such, every petroleum refinery begins with a massive distillation system to separate the crude oil into a large number of "cuts" that are further manipulated into the desired products.

Chemical manipulation in a petrochemical refinery usually can be characterized as the synthesis of structure – the conversion of linear hydrocarbons into more structured and substituted materials, or the creation of very large, synthetic polymer molecules.

Biomass materials are solids that include a sizable aqueous component. In general, initial treatment of biomass materials includes steps of drying and physical size reduction. The biomass materials already have a richly varied chemical structure. This means that the goal of biomass utilization is, in part, preservation of the intrinsic functional structures while depolymerizing the original material.

The process chemistries used in the depolymerization of biomass materials and their products are depicted in Fig. 5.2. These processes include:

- *Pyrolysis* – Treatment of biomass at moderate temperatures (300 to 600 °C) in the absence of oxygen to cause partial depolymerization of the material. Slow heating rates tend to favor production of volatile gases (CO, CO_2, hydrogen, methane, ethylene), organic acids and aldehydes, mixed phenols, and char. High heating rates tend to minimize liquid production and maximize gas production.

- *Gasification* – High-temperature (>700 °C) treatment of biomass in the absence of oxygen but with addition of steam, and possibly CO_2, to maximize the production of synthesis gas (syngas), a mixture of H_2, CO, CO_2, and CH_4. Syngas can be used directly as a fuel or as a chemical intermediate in the production of ammonia, methanol, and higher alcohols, organic acids and aldehydes, synthetic gasoline (using Fischer-Tropsch processing), and isobutene and isobutane.

- *Thermochemical Liquefaction* – Pyrolytic processing with addition of H_2, CO, CO_2, and selected catalysts to convert the biomass into hydrocarbons, mixed phenols (from the lignin fraction), and light gases. The key to commercial utilization of liquefaction processing is the separation and recovery of the multiple products created during the liquefaction process.

- *Hydrolytic Liquefaction* – This processing includes the use of acids, alkalis, or enzymes to depolymerize polysaccharides into their component sugars. These aqueous-phase reactions are used to provide basic polymers, for example cellulose and fermentable sugars for further processing, or hexose and/or pentose sugars for chemical conversion into other organic compounds.

- *Fermentation* – Biochemical processing uses microorganisms or/and enzymatic reactions to convert a fermentable substrate into recoverable products. Hexoses, particularly glucose, are the most frequently used fermentation substrates, but pentoses, glycerol, and other hydroxycarbons are also used. Fermentations are most commonly performed in aqueous solution, with the final products present in modest concentration.

- *Chemical Synthesis* – Cellulose recovered from a lignocellulosic matrix using hydrolytic liquefaction can be treated with several reagents to make materials such as cellulose acetate, nitrocellulose, and rayon. Xylose from the hydrolytic depolymerization of hemicellulose can be further reacted in the same process to

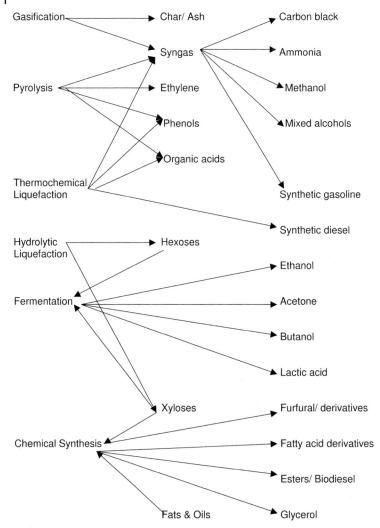

Fig. 5.2 Biomass-derived industrial organic chemicals.

make furfural. Furfural is the starting point for a large family of derivative chemical and polymer products. The adipic acid and the hexamethylene diamine used in the original synthesis of Nylon-6,6 were made by acid hydrolytic depolymerization of hemicellulose from oat hulls, followed by chemical synthesis of the monomers and condensation polymerization to form the Nylon-6,6.

There are several possible ways of using lignocellulosic and other categories of biomass for production of fuels and chemicals. Because the initial production steps involve solid materials, preparation and handling of the raw materials is more complicated and costly than using petroleum liquids. Also, as noted above, biomass materials are more disperse and less dense than petroleum. This means that assembly and storage of the raw materials is more complicated than for petroleum.

Finally, some of the biomass resources, notably crops and crop residues, are cyclical in production. This means that storage and integration with other resources are necessary in the design and management of a biorefinery complex.

5.5
Examples of Integrated Biorefinery Applications

5.5.1
Production of Ethanol and Furfural from Lignocellulosic Feedstocks

An approach to implementation of a biorefinery using lignocellulosic feedstocks (LCF) that has been given much attention in the United States, via USDOE-sponsored programs, is the use of chemical and enzyme treatments to depolymerize the LCF to produce fermentable sugars and lignin. The primary goal has been the production of ethanol. The basic process is:

Lignocellulosics + Water → Xyloses + Cellulose/Lignin (Acid Process)
Cellulose + Water → Glucose (Enzyme Process)
Glucose Fermentation → Ethanol + CO_2 + Biomass
Xylose Fermentation → Ethanol + CO_2 + Biomass
Lignin + Biomass → Heat + Steam

Unfortunately, with ethanol as the sole product, and no subsidies, this process facility does not make a profit. If, however, the xyloses are diverted from the fermentation process into the production of furfural, a highly versatile intermediate chemical, the overall operation can be highly profitable. Van Dyne et al. [3] showed that the optimum capacity for the integrated ethanol/furfural facility is 4360 tonnes per day of LCF. The discounted cash flow rate of return, after taxes, for this facility is approximately sixteen percent. At capacities below approximately 750 tonnes per day, the combined ethanol–furfural operation is not profitable, because the plant capital and operating costs are too large (economy of scale). On the other hand, the operation becomes increasingly less profitable for capacities above 4400 tonnes per day because the costs of assembling sufficient feedstock are too high.

5.5.2
Management of Municipal Solid Waste

Municipal solid wastes (MSW) are the largest single source of lignocellulosic materials available for utilization in modern society. Most localities have systems for collection and "disposal" of these materials. Too often the "disposal" consists of burial of the materials. Typically approximately 25% of the waste is either recyclable materials or inorganic materials such as stones, cement, and wallboard (gypsum) materials. The remaining 75% is non-recyclable organic solid waste materials (NROSW) that are available for production of a wide range of fuels and industrial chemicals.

There are numerous locations where the NROSW is burned, either to reduce the volume or, hopefully, to recover the energy value of the wastes. Using the biorefinery approach and the "Two-uses" paradigm, the following options should be considered for the NROSW:

A. Gasification $\rightarrow$ Syngas + Ash $\rightarrow$ Electrical power + CO_2
B. Gasification $\rightarrow$ Syngas + Ash $\rightarrow$ Chemical synthesis + CO_2
C. Gasification $\rightarrow$ Syngas + Ash $\rightarrow$ Fermentation $\rightarrow$ Ethanol
D. Liquefaction $\rightarrow$ Mixed organic liquids $\rightarrow$ Specialty chemicals and fuels

In many locations the use of the NROSW materials for gasification and the co-generation of electrical power is not competitive with other power sources, without special incentives. The production of a variety of specialty chemicals from syngas is commercial technology [4], although the easiest fuel source to use is often natural gas. Liquefaction processing of coal has long been commercially used for fuels and chemicals, with South Africa being the prime example.

Liquefaction of biomass is beginning to be used in commercial applications in some countries, including the US. The liquefaction strategy can be a very profitable alternative. As an example, a NROSW liquefaction plant handling 140 tonnes per day of MSW and 90 tonnes per day of waste tires costs about US $ 30 million. The facility produces a range of liquid fuels and a number of higher-value industrial organic chemicals. Using a 10 year project life, the facility produces a before-tax cumulative net profit of more than US $ 100 million.

5.5.3
Coupling MSW Management, Ethanol, and Biodiesel

Conventional ethanol production uses corn as the source of fermentable sugars to produce ethanol. The corn typically is dry milled and the entire milled kernel is added to the saccharification tank before fermentation. The process requires a sizable amount of process steam and electricity.

Biodiesel production requires modest amounts of energy, but requires an inexpensive source of fats or oils to be competitive. The oil can be, for example recycled restaurant grease, a virgin vegetable oil, or rendered animal fat. The corn that goes into the fermentation process contains approximately 3% by weight corn oil, which passes through the fermentation process as an inert material. Biodiesel also requires a source of alcohol to make the biodiesel from oil.

MSW, or other lignocellulosics, such as seed hulls, waste paper, etc., can be burned directly to provide steam and heat, but it is more compatible with the production of ethanol if the LCF is first converted to syngas to be used as a fuel gas. Also, the syngas can be converted into methanol – the most commonly used alcohol for making biodiesel.

The integrated process scheme for the biorefinery facility is:

Corn → Milling → Starch + Germ → Glucose → Ethanol
Germ → Corn oil + Defatted Germ Meal
Gasification + LCF → Syngas + Ash → Steam + Electricity
Syngas → Methanol
Corn Oil + Methanol → Biodiesel + Glycerol

In this process system, corn and LCF are the inputs and ethanol, biodiesel, defatted corn germ meal, and glycerol are the outputs. Economies of scale in the biodiesel plant may require additional sources of fats/oils, but this only makes the processes more profitable. The ethanol product is not used in the biodiesel because it is more valuable as an intermediate chemical or as a fuel on its own.

5.6
Summary

There is already significant use of renewable biomass resources for industrial chemicals [5, 6] and recognition of the opportunities for greatly expanded energy and fuel uses for biomass materials [7–11]. The biorefinery strategy advocated here is combining of the utility of multiple feedstocks with the utility of a wide array of conversion technologies to create a new, sustainable strategy to meet the world's needs for industrial chemicals and liquid fuels.

References

1 Morris, D. and I. Ahmed, The Carbohydrate Economy: Making Chemicals and Industrial Materials from Plant Matter, The Institute for Local Self Reliance, Washington, D.C., 1992.

2 Wiltsee, G., "Urban Waste Grease Resource Assessment," NREL/SR-570-26141, November, 1998.

3 Van Dyne, D. L., M. G. Blaise, and L. D. Clements, "A Strategy for Returning Agriculture and Rural America to Long-Term Full Employment Using Biomass Refineries," Perspectives on New Crops and New Uses, J. Janick, ed., ASHS Press, Alexandria, VA, 1999.

4 Spath, P. L. and D. C. Dayton, "Preliminary Screening – Technical and Economic Assessment of Synthesis Gas to Fuels and Chemicals with Emphasis on the Potential for Biomass-Derived Syngas," NREL/TP-510-34929, December, 2003.

5 Szmant, H. H., Industrial Utilization of Renewable Resources: An Introduction, Technomic Publishing Company, Lancaster, PA, 1986.

6 Johnson, R. W. and E. Fritz, Fatty Acids in Industry, Marcel Dekker, New York, 1989.

7 Donaldson, T. L. and O. L. Culberson, "Chemicals from Biomass: An Assessment of the Potential for Production of Chemical Feedstocks from Renewable Resources," ORNL/TM-8432, June, 1983.

8 Wise, D. L., Organic Chemicals from Biomass, The Benjamin/Cummings Publishing Company, Inc., Cambridge, MA, 1983.

9 Clements, L. D., S. R. Beck and C. Heintz, "Chemicals from Biomass Feedstocks," Chem. Engr. Prog., 79, 59–62 (1983).

10 Lowenstein, M. Z., Energy Applications of Biomass, Elsevier Applied Sciences Publishers, New York, 1985.

11 Thames, S., R. Kleiman and L. D. Clements, "How Crops Can Provide Raw Materials for the Chemical Industry," in New Crops, New Uses, New Markets – 1992 Yearbook of Agriculture, US Department of Agriculture, Washington, D.C., 1992.

6
Lignocellulosic Feedstock Biorefinery:
History and Plant Development for Biomass Hydrolysis

Raphael Katzen and Daniel J. Schell

6.1
Introduction

The current high level of interest in lignocellulosic biomass conversion technology is driven by the potential to produce fuels and chemicals to reduce dependence on petroleum, improve air quality, and reduce greenhouse gas emissions. Research and development efforts and attempts to commercialize biomass hydrolysis technology began in the early 1900s. This chapter discusses some of this early work which set the stage for current efforts to bring to fruition the lignocellulosic biorefinery. We highlight early efforts to pilot and commercialize lignocellulosic biomass conversion technology using acid hydrolysis processes and enzyme-based cellulose hydrolysis.

6.2
Hydrolysis of Biomass Materials

Producing ethanol from lignocellulosic biomass depends on converting the complex cellulosic and hemicellulosic carbohydrates into simple sugars which are then fermented to ethanol by a variety of microorganisms. This section briefly reviews both acid- and enzyme-based methods for hydrolyzing the polymeric carbohydrates into their constituent sugars.

6.2.1
Acid Conversion

Hydrolysis of cellulose and hemicellulose (primarily xylan) to sugars can be catalyzed by a variety of acids, including sulfuric, hydrochloric, hydrofluoric, and nitric acids. The hydrolysis process is represented by the following simple expressions:

Biorefineries – Industrial Processes and Products. Status Quo and Future Directions. Vol. 1
Edited by Birgit Kamm, Patrick R. Gruber, Michael Kamm
Copyright © 2006 WILEY-VCH Verlag GmbH & Co. KGaA, Weinheim
ISBN: 3-527-31027-4

cellulose → glucose → HMF → tars

xylan → xylose → furfural → tars

in which HMF is 5-hydroxymethylfurfural. If hydrolysis conditions are severe (e.g. high temperatures or acid concentrations) a large fraction of the sugars is degraded to other products, e.g. HMF, furfural, and tars.

Because dilute sulfuric acid is inexpensive, use of this acid is the most studied in acid conversion processes and these processes are most often used in plants based on acid conversion technology. Biomass is impregnated with a dilute sulfuric acid solution and treated with steam at temperatures ranging from 140–260 °C. At lower temperatures of 140–180 °C, xylan is rapidly hydrolyzed to xylose with little cellulose degradation. At higher temperatures, cellulose is also rapidly hydrolyzed to glucose and xylan is quickly converted to furfural and tars.

Concentrated acids are also used to hydrolyze cellulose and hemicellulose to sugars. Because low temperatures (100–120 °C) are typically used, high yields of sugars are obtained with little production of degradation products. The economic viability of this process depends, however, on the successful recovery of acid at low cost.

6.2.2
Enzymatic Conversion

Sugar yields are limited during acid hydrolysis because sugars are also converted to degradation products. Cellulase, a multi-component enzyme system, catalyzes cellulose hydrolysis and is 100% selective for conversion of cellulose to glucose; high yields are, therefore, possible. This enzyme is produced by a variety of microorganisms, most commonly, the fungus *Trichoderma reesei*.

Cellulose conversion rates are limited by the ability of the enzyme to access the cellulosic substrate. To increase accessibility, biomass is subjected to physical and chemical treatments that disrupt the biomass structure, usually by removing a fraction of the hemicellulose and/or lignin. Effective pretreatment is necessary to achieve good cellulose-to-glucose conversion yields.

6.3
Acid Hydrolysis Processes

6.3.1
Early Efforts to Produce Ethanol

Before World War II, research was conducted in the United States on hydrolysis of biomass to produce sugars for production of ethanol with emphasis on the use of forest and wood-processing wastes; no operation achieved true commercial success, however. Sherrard and Kressman [1] highlight developments in acid-based hydrolysis technology before World War II. In the early 1900s, a plant was built in Hattiesburg, MS, USA, to process wood waste using sulfurous acid, but never operated successfully [2]. A commercial operation was also set up in Georgetown, SC, USA in the 1910s to process wood waste using dilute sulfuric acid, but eventually failed because of low ethanol yields [3].

Process development was being investigated in Germany at the same time. One process used concentrated hydrochloric acid [4] to hydrolyze the carbohydrate fraction of wood waste. The treated material was then neutralized with caustic soda to yield a mixture of wood-based sugars and salt (sodium chloride), used primarily as cattle feed. In another process, a 7300 dry metric ton year^{-1} plant hydrolyzed wood chips in countercurrent diffusers by contact with 42% (*w/w*) HCl to produce a concentrated sugar solution [5]. After World War II the plant was extensively rebuilt to use a modified process known as the Udic–Rheinau process [6].

Work on sulfuric acid processes was also conducted in Germany at the same time, leading to the development of the Scholler process [7]. The Scholler process used a percolation reactor to hydrolyze wood waste, producing glucose as the primary product; this was then fermented to ethanol. Many such plants were built in Germany and Russia before World War II. The extensive use of water required for this process, however, produced a rather dilute (4%) sugar stream that was more costly to process.

In the late 1930s, a continuous wood-hydrolysis pilot plant was built in the United States to produce lignocellulosic plastics, and wood sugars, furfural, and acetic acid as by-products [3]. The plant was designed to hydrolyze wood slurries continuously with dilute sulfuric acid by pumping the mixture through heated hydrolysis tubes and then recovering the solid product. The plant produced 180–260 kg day^{-1} hydrolyzed product.

At the beginning of World War II molasses was fermented to ethanol as a raw material for synthesis of butanediol, which in turn was polymerized to produce synthetic rubber. Because German submarines were sinking transports from Cuba containing shipments of molasses and ethanol, the US government made the decision to develop technology for producing ethanol from wood waste for the synthetic rubber program. The Defense Plant Corporation, an organization of the US Government, awarded a contract to the Vulcan Copper and Supply Company (later known as Vulcan Cincinnati) to design and to construct a facility to produce ethanol. The author (Raphael Katzen) was involved as the senior process engineer and later as the project manager for design and construction of this facility in Springfield, OR, USA. The plant was designed to process 270 metric tons (dry basis) day^{-1} of softwood sawdust trucked from sawmills in the area, with the goal of producing 208 L/dry metric ton (50 gal/dry ton) ethanol.

This plant was based on modifications to the Scholler process, as a result of work at the Forest Products Laboratory (FPL) of the US Department of Agriculture in Madison, Wisconsin, USA. Based on early work by Ritter [8] and Sherrard [9], FPL built a pilot facility that improved upon the Scholler technology, yielding the Madison-Scholler process [10, 11].

Vulcan Cincinnati's design for their plant was based on the Madison-Scholler process and used information and data produced during test runs of the FPL pilot plant. Equipment was designed and fabricated at Vulcan's shops in Cincinnati, OH, USA, and construction was carried out in Springfield, OR, USA, with the assistance of contractors. Although construction was stopped at the end of World War II, the Defense Plant Corporation decided to complete the facility and test the technology.

Plant construction was completed in 1946 and the plant was started up under management of the Willamette Valley Wood Chemical Company, a group of individuals in the local forest products industry. Test runs were then initiated with Vulcan providing technical management under Raphael Katzen's supervision. Despite problems with tar formation and calcium sulfate deposits from neutralization of sulfuric acid used to hydrolyze the cellulose, the design production rate was achieved. The process proved too costly to compete with petroleum-derived synthetic ethanol which appeared on the scene at the end of World War II, however. Efforts were made to utilize the Springfield facility for production of waxy products, but it was not designed for this operation and the plant was shut down and dismantled.

With the prevalence of cheap petroleum-derived ethanol and other petrochemical products after World War II, there was little economic incentive to pursue cellulose hydrolysis technology further. In Germany many of the plants shut down and most of the Scholler process plants in Russia were converted to single-cell yeast production, because it was a more profitable product than ethanol. Research did continue, however, in various laboratories and pilot plants in different parts of the world. In the 1950s the Tennessee Valley Authority (TVA) built a dilute-sulfuric-acid-hydrolysis-based pilot plant using percolation reactors at Muscle Shoals, AL, USA [12]. The New Zealand Forest Products Laboratory built a similar plant in the 1980s [13]. Several pilot facilities were also built in the 1980s that performed continuous dilute-sulfuric-acid hydrolysis of cellulose and hemicellulose and were able to process 1–2 metric dry tons of biomass per day. Plug-flow reactor systems processing dilute biomass streams were constructed by the American Can Company [14] and at the Solar Energy Research Institute (SERI), now the National Renewable Energy Laboratory (NREL), in Golden, CO, USA [15]. Systems for processing high-solids biomass streams were constructed using twin-screw extruders at New York University [16] and in Canada by Bio-hol/St Lawrence Reactor [17], and TVA installed a new system using a modified pulp digester [18]. Except for the new reactor at TVA and a new but similar reactor recently installed at the NREL [19], none of these systems is currently operational.

In the mid-1980s researchers at the SERI proposed a "progressing batch reactor system" [20] that retained the simplicity of percolation reactors but achieved countercurrent flow of liquors to reduce sugar losses due to degradation reactions even further compared with percolation reactors. Further testing of the system, however, did not produce substantial sugar yield improvements [21]. In the late 1990s, the idea of a countercurrent shrinking bed reactor was also proposed for dilute-acid total cellulose hydrolysis [22], but operational difficulties limited the effectiveness of this system.

Several economic studies performed by engineering companies in the early 1980s to evaluate dilute-acid total hydrolysis processes for production of ethanol [23, 24] showed the economics to be favorable. The potential of enzymatic cellulose hydrolysis to achieve better yields was shifting emphasis away from acid hydrolysis to enzymatic-based processing, however [25].

Although there is no current active effort to build dilute-acid based cellulose plants, two companies are pursuing concentrated acid hydrolysis processing. Arkenol has examined the ability of using recombinant *Z. mobilis* to ferment acid hydrolysates produced by its concentrated-acid hydrolysis process [26] and is pursuing international opportunities to build a large-scale plant. Masada Resources Group plans to build a waste-handling facility in Middetown, NY, USA, that will use its patented OxyNol process to recycle or convert municipal solid waste. Profitable economics for both companies rely on achieving cost-effective recovery of the acid catalyst.

6.3.2
Other Products

Both glucose and xylose produced by acid-catalyzed hydrolysis of lignocellulosic biomass will, under the same conditions, further degrade to HMF and furfural, respectively. Furfural has been produced commercially from biomass but there has been no commercial interest in producing HMF. The Quaker Oats Company began production of furfural in the United States in the 1920s [27] and until recently was the major world producer of furfural from agricultural residues [28]. Furfural is produced from agricultural sources including corncobs, oat hulls, rice hulls, cereal grasses, and sugar cane bagasse. Early plants used batch production technology, but in 1965, at the recommendation of the Katzen Company [29], Quaker Oats agreed to pilot a continuous process in an existing leased pulping facility operated by Katzen. Successful results led to the design of the largest furfural plant in the world by the Katzen Company and the Black Clawson Company of Middletown, OH, USA. The plant is based on a highly modified Pandia digester system, originally used to pulp wood and agricultural residues.

The plant was constructed in Belle Glade, FL, USA and began operation in 1966. The feedstock for the plant was sugar cane bagasse from nearby sugar mills. When successful operation was demonstrated, the plant capacity was expanded to process 1800 dry metric tons day^{-1} bagasse to yield 137 metric tons day^{-1} furfural. By-product methanol and HMF were burned, with the lignocellulose residue, to provide steam and electrical energy for the plant. The plant was sited adjacent to a sugar mill operated by the Sugar Cane Growers Company of Florida, which provided transport and bulk storage of up to 227 000 metric tons (dry basis) of bagasse from nearby sugar mills, thereby enabling year-round operation. After 31 years of continuous operation this plant was shut down in 1997 because of the availability of lower cost crude furfural from China.

6.4
Enzymatic Hydrolysis Process

6.4.1
Early History

A new and exciting development in biomass conversion technology began when reports from US troops in the South Pacific during World War II described how "the green fungus among us" [30, 31] was destroying uniforms and other cotton gear. Reese, at the Natick Massachusetts Laboratory of the US Army Materials Command, analyzed samples of cotton items affected by this fungus in the 1950s [32]. He identified the fungus as *Trichoderma viride* and later named *T. reesei* QM 6a as the organism responsible for producing a cellulase complex that hydrolyzed cellulose to glucose. Serious studies of the use of this enzyme for biomass conversion began in the early 1970s with the pioneering work of Mandels and coworkers [33, 34]; this resulted in the development of improved *T. reesei* strain QM 9414.

In the late 1970s and early 1980s much research effort was devoted to mutating the wild *T. reesei* strains QM 6a or QM 9414 to enhance production of cellulase [34]. One such effort was conducted by researchers at several university laboratories in a cooperative program coordinated by Eveleigh at Rutgers University. This cooperative research program resulted in substantial improvement of the wild-type fungal strain and produced the widely known *T. reesei* strain RUT C30 [35]. Many other efforts from around the world have produced modified *T. reesei* strains.

6.4.2
Enzyme-Based Plant Development

In the late 1970s several industrial organizations became interested in enzymatic conversion of cellulose to sugars and ethanol. One of the first efforts to develop and pilot this technology was a collaboration between Gulf Oil Chemicals and Nippon Mining in a program carried out by the Bio-Research Corporation of Japan. This led to the building of a 900 kg day^{-1} pilot plant in Pittsburg, KS, USA. In addition to producing cellulase, the plant was the first to use a novel technology combining cellulase saccharification with glucose fermentation in the same reactor system, called simultaneous saccharification and fermentation (SSF) [36, 37]. The plant successfully processed paper mill waste, producing dilute beer streams containing 30–35 g L^{-1} ethanol, although problems with contamination in the SSF fermentors were reported [38, 39].

Although no commercial plants have been built for enzymatic cellulose conversion, several pilot-scale facilities were built in the 1980s throughout the world to test a variety of technology and feedstocks. For example, a pilot plant located in Soustons, France, utilized a Stake process [40] to pretreat biomass, followed by enzymatic saccharification. Ralph Katzen Associates International, with the

University of Arkansas and Procter and Gamble, erected a pilot plant at a pulp mill in Pennsylvania, USA, to process pulp mill waste through disc refiners followed by SSF in a 9500-L fermentor [30]. In 1987, a 3000 kg day^{-1} pilot plant that processed wheat straw through a batch digester (no catalyst) and used the washed pretreated solids to produce cellulase that was subsequently used to saccharify the remaining washed solids was constructed in the Voest-Alpine Biomass Technology Center [41]. Two pilot plants were also constructed in Japan. One operated from 1983 to 1987 and processed 500 kg day^{-1} bagasse or rice straw. It used mild alkaline pretreatment then enzymatic saccharification of the pretreated biomass with cellulase produced on Avicel as the carbon source, followed by sugar concentration using reverse osmosis and subsequent fermentation to produce ethanol [42]. The other plant operated from 1986 to 1990 and processed 1000 kg day^{-1} cedar wood or white birch chips. It used steam explosion to treat the wood that was then fermented with a strain of *Clostridium* [43].

In the early 1990s, the US Department of Energy (DOE) and NREL constructed a fully integrated 900 kg day^{-1} pilot plant to produce ethanol from a variety of lignocellulosic biomass sources [19] that used a modified pulp digester for pretreatment that has already been discussed. The plant includes unit operations for feedstock handling, pretreatment in a modified pulp digester, seed culture production, SSF in 9000-L fermentors, feed tanks for enzyme and nutrient addition, ethanol stripping in a sieve-tray distillation column, and solid–liquid separation. The plant has also extensive instrumentation for process control and data collection. The plant was operated on a corn fiber feedstock during a 15-day run [44] and was later operated continuously for up to six weeks [45].

The Iogen Company of Ottawa, Canada, recently built a 983,000-L-ethanol-per-year demonstration-scale plant processing nearly 5 metric tons day^{-1} agricultural residue. Because Iogen is a cellulase producer, they can supply the cellulase for the plant from an adjacent enzyme-production facility. Although little has been publicly disclosed about this facility and its performance, it has been reported to produce a 4% alcohol stream from conversion of lignocellulosic biomass [46].

6.4.3
Technology Development

The Biomass Research and Development Technical Advisory Committee, a group of biomass industry and academic experts, recently issued a "roadmap" document [47] outlining bioconversion research needs. The recommendations most relevant to enzyme-based processing are:
1. the need to improve physical and chemical pretreatments before fermentation;
2. the need for cost-effective chemical/enzymatic conversion; and
3. the need to overcome barriers associated with inhibitory substances in hydrolysate sugar streams.

Engineering catalyst and microorganisms to improve their tolerance are methods used to achieve the third goal.

Advances in all three areas will be required to achieve economic viability and thus success in the marketplace. The Consortium for Advanced Fundamentals and Innovation (CAFI), a group of independent academic researchers, is collaborating in an effort to identify and develop new pretreatment technology. The most promising technology is uncatalyzed steam explosion, liquid hot water, pH controlled hot water, flow-through liquid hot water, dilute acid, flow-through acid, lime, and ammonia-based processing [48].

Development of new and improved enzymes for biomass conversion has been a focus of the US DOE for the last few years. They have funded cost-shared efforts with the two largest cellulase producers, Genencor International and Novozymes, to produce cost-effective enzymes with a goal of achieving a tenfold cost reduction that would bring cost down to an estimated $ 0.50 gallon^{-1} ethanol. Both companies report success in reaching this goal, but further cost reduction is required and the DOE's goal is to achieve an effective enzyme cost of $ 0.10 gallon^{-1} ethanol.

Efficient conversion of all sugars derived from biomass to desired products is required for this technology to become economically viable. Development of genetically modified microorganisms able to utilize other sugars beside glucose has been an ongoing effort in many laboratories [49, 50]. As also emphasized by the last recommendation above, the ability to tolerate inhibitory substances is also a highly desirable characteristic. Currently, however, no microorganisms can tolerate inhibitory substances in dilute-acid pretreated biomass substrates without some type of conditioning process that removes inhibitors.

6.5
Conclusion

Early efforts to commercialize acid-based processes for producing products from cellulose hydrolysis were ultimately unsuccessful, because of competition from lower-cost petroleum-derived materials. These efforts, and ongoing work on enzyme-based processes, are, however, providing valuable knowledge and experience. The future is the multi-product biorefinery that can utilize all biomass components. We need to build upon past efforts and use new advances in technology to ensure the commercial success of the lignocellulosic feedstock biorefinery.

References

1 E. Sherrard, F. Kressman, *Ind. Eng. Chem.* **1945**, 37, 5.
2 Ruttan, *J. Soc. Chem. Ind.* **1909**, 28, 1291.
3 R. Katzen, D. Othmer, *Ind. Eng. Chem.* **1942**, 34, 314.
4 F. Bergius, *Trans. Inst. Chem. Engrs. (London)* **1933**, 11, 162.
5 F. Bergius, *Ind. Eng. Chem.* **1937**, 29, 247.
6 J. Wright, A. Power, P. Bergeron, *Evaluation of Concentrated Halogen Acid Hydrolysis Processes for Alcohol Fuel Production,*

Solar Energy Research Institute, SERI/TR-231-2074, Golden, CO **1984**.

7 H. Scholler, French Patent # 777,824, **1935**.

8 G. Ritter, *Ind. Eng. Chem. Anal. Ed.*, **1932**, 4, 202.

9 E. Sherrard, *Ind. Eng. Chem.* **1923**, 15, 1164.

10 E. Harris, E. Berlinger, G. Hajny, E. Sherrard, *Ind. Eng. Chem.* **1945**, 37, 12.

11 E. Harris, E. Berlinger, *Ind. Eng. Chem.* **1945**, 38, 890.

12 N. Gilbert, A. Hobbs, J. Levine, *Ind. Eng. Chem.* **1952**, 44, 1712.

13 R. Burton, *Proc. of the Royal Soc. of Canada Internat. Symp. on Ethanol from Biomass*, Royal Society of Canada, Ottawa, Canada, **1983**, 247.

14 J. Church, D. Wooldridge, *Ind. Eng. Chem. Res. Dev.* **1981**, 20, 371.

15 A. Brennen, W. Hoagland, D. Schell, *Biotechnol. Bioeng. Symp. No. 17*, John Wiley & Sons, New York, **1987**, 53.

16 B. Rugg, P. Armstrong, A. Dreiblatt, D. Wise, *Liquid Fuel Developments*, CRC Press, Baco Raton, FL, USA, **1983**, 139.

17 R. Lawford, R. Charley, R. Edamura, J. Fien, K. Hopkins, D. Potts, B. Zawadzki, H. Lawford, *Fifth Canadian Bioenergy R&D Seminar*, National Research Council of Canada, **1984**, 503.

18 M. Bulls, J. Watson, R. Lambert, J. Barrier, *Energy from Biomass and Waste XIV*, Institute of Gas Technology, Chicago, **1991**, 1167.

19 Q. Nguyen, J. Dickow, B. Duff, J. Farmer, D. Glassner, K. Ibsen, M. Ruth, D. Schell, I. Thompson, M. Tucker, *Bioresource Technol.* **1996**, 58, 189.

20 J. Wright, P. Bergeron, P. Werdene, *Ind. Eng. Chem. Res.* **1987**, 26, 699.

21 D. Schell, Personal Communication.

22 Y. Lee, W. Zhangwen, R. Torget, *Bioresource Technol.* **2000**, 71, 29.

23 Badger Engineers, Inc., SERI Subcontract Report No. ZX-3-03096-1, **1982**.

24 Stone & Webster Engineering Corp., SERI Subcontract Report No. ZX-3-03096-1, **1982**.

25 J. Wright, *Chem. Eng. Prog.* **1988**, 84, 62.

26 T. Yamada, M. Fitigati, M. Zhang, *App. Biochem. Biotechnol.* **2002**, 98-100, 899.

27 R. Kottke, *Kick-Othmer Encyclopedia of Chemical Technology, Supplement to 4th Ed.*, John Wiley & Sons, NY, **1998**, 155.

28 J. Levy, K. Yokose, *Chemical Economics Handbook*, Report 660.5000, SRI Consulting, Menlo Park, CA, USA, **2004**.

29 R. Katzen, Personal Communication.

30 R. Katzen, D. Monceaux, *App. Biochem. Biotechnol.* **1995**, 51/52, 585.

31 J. Sheehan, M. Himmel, *Biotechnol. Prog.* **1999**, 15, 817.

32 D. Ryu, M. Mandels, *Enzyme Microb. Technol.* **1980**, 2, 91.

33 M. Mandels, L. Hontz, J. Nystrom, *Biotechnol. Bioeng.* **1974**, 16, 1471.

34 I. Persson, F. Tjerneld, B. Hahn-Hagerdal, *Proc. Biochem.* **1991**, 26, 65.

35 B. Montenecourt, D. Eveleigh, *App. Environ. Microbiol.* **1977**, 34, 777.

36 F. Gauss, S. Suzuke, M. Takagi, US Patent 3 990 944, **1976**.

37 G. Huff, N. Yata, US Patent 3 990 945, **1976**.

38 D. Becker, P. Blotkamp, G. Emert, *Fuels from Biomass and Waste*, Ann Arbor Science Publishers, Ann Arbor, MI, USA, **1981**, 375.

39 K. Bevernitz, S. Gracheck, D. Rivers, D. Becker, K. Kaupisch, G. Emert, *Energy from Biomass and Waste XIV*, Institute of Gas Technology, Chicago, **1982**, 897.

40 J. Heard, W. Schabas, *Chem. Eng.* **1984**, 91 (6), 49.

41 M. Hayn, W. Steiner, R. Klinger, M. Sinner, H. Esterbauer, *Bioconversion of Forest and Agricultural Plant Residues*, CAB International, Oxon, U.K. **1993**, 33.

42 Y. Shirasaka, H. Ishibashi, H. Etoh, H. Michiki, H. Miyakawa, S. Moriyama, *Energy from Biomass and Waste XIII*, Institute of Gas Technology, Chicago, **1989**, 1311.

43 S. Matsui, *Conference on Alcohol and Biomass Energy Technologies*, NEDO-OS-9106, New Energy and Industrial Technology Development Organization, Tokyo, **1991**, 27.

44 D. Schell, C. Riley, N. Dowe, J. Farmer, K. Ibsen, M. Ruth, S. Toon, R. Lumpkin, *Bioresource Technol.* **2004**, 179.

45 D. Schell, Personal Communication.

46 B. Foody, From Presentation at the 27th Symposium on Biotechnology for Fuels

and Chemicals, Chattanooga, TN, USA, **2004**.

47 Biomass Research and Development Technical Advisory Committee, *Roadmap for Biomass Technologies in the United States*, **2002**, www.eere.energy.gov/biomass/progs/searchdb2.cgi?7219.

48 N. Mosier, C. Wyman, B. Dale, R. Elander, Y. Lee, M. Holtzapple, M. Ladisch, *Bioresource Technol.* **2005**, 96, 673.

49 R. Bothast, N. Nichols, B. Dien, *Biotechnol. Prog.* **1999**, 15, 867.

50 A. Aristidou, M. Penttila, *Current Opinions in Biotechnol.* **2000**, 11, 18.

7
The Biofine Process – Production of Levulinic Acid, Furfural, and Formic Acid from Lignocellulosic Feedstocks

Daniel J. Hayes, Steve Fitzpatrick, Michael H. B. Hayes, and Julian R. H. Ross

7.1
Introduction

The energy needs of the developed world are currently over-dependent on the utilization of finite mineral resources. Although renewable-power technologies, for example wind and photovoltaics, may, in the future, have major roles in the production of electricity, provision must still be made for the supply of industrial chemicals and motor fuels that are currently produced predominately from oil. In fact, of the approximately 170 chemical compounds produced annually in the US in volumes exceeding 4.5×10^6 kg, 98% are derived from oil and natural gas [1]. The vast majority of modern synthetic products are also derived from oil. Emerging biorefinery technologies offer a sustainable alternative by utilization of carbohydrates, the most abundant organic chemicals on the surface of the earth. This chapter will focus on the Biofine Process [2, 3], biorefinery technology that transforms carbohydrate feedstocks into products that include the platform chemicals levulinic acid, furfural, and formic acid in high yields. The process involves high-temperature acid-hydrolysis in two reactors and is one of the most advanced and commercially viable lignocellulosic-fractionating technologies currently available. The process involves the hydrolysis of polysaccharides to their monomeric constituents, and these are then in turn continuously converted into valuable platform chemicals.

7.2
Lignocellulosic Fractionation

The major polysaccharides of importance in biomass are the glucans and hemicelluloses. Of the glucans (carbohydrate homopolysaccharides consisting of repeating D-glucopyranose units), starch and cellulose are the most abundant. Technologies utilizing starchy feedstocks (e.g. maize) for production of ethanol, by fermentation of the liberated glucose monomers, are well-established and

Biorefineries – Industrial Processes and Products. Status Quo and Future Directions. Vol. 1
Edited by Birgit Kamm, Patrick R. Gruber, Michael Kamm
Copyright © 2006 WILEY-VCH Verlag GmbH & Co. KGaA, Weinheim
ISBN: 3-527-31027-4

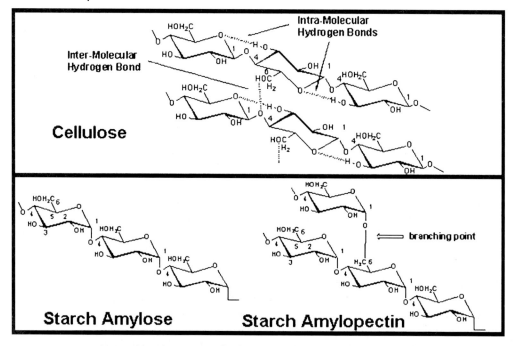

Fig. 7.1 Physical structures of cellulose and of starch amylose and amylopectin.

run at relatively high efficiencies. This is because of the comparative ease of starch hydrolysis, using mainly a-amylase and gluco-amylase enzymes [4]. In 1999 a total of 1.48 billion gallons (ca 5.3×10^9 L) of fuel ethanol was blended with gasoline for use in motor vehicles in the United States. About 94% of this was produced by fermentation from maize; most of the remainder was from other grain [5].

Cellulose is much more abundant in nature than is starch, and its annual production is estimated at 100×10^9 tonnes [6]. Furthermore, cellulosic feedstocks tend to be more productive and require less energy to produce than starch crops. Technologies for hydrolysis of the cellulosic feedstocks are currently not commercially developed at a scale approaching that for starch, however. This is because cellulose (Fig. 7.1) is of the order of 100 times more difficult to hydrolyze than starch [7]. The D-anhydroglucopyranose units in cellulose are linked through β-$(1 \rightarrow 4)$-glycosidic bonds, as opposed to the a-$(1 \rightarrow 4)$-linkages in the amylose component of starch and the a-$(1 \rightarrow 6)$ amylopectin branches in starch. The structure of cellulose enables intimate intermolecular associations that do not occur in starches, and this explains the relative resistance to degradation in cellulose fibrils and microfibrils compared with starch macromolecules.

7.2.1
Acid Hydrolysis of Polysaccharides

Cellulose is hydrolyzed in pure water by attack by the electrophilic hydrogen atoms of the H_2O molecule on the glycosidic oxygen (Fig. 7.2). This is a very slow reaction, because of the resistance of the cellulose to hydrolysis. The rate of the reaction can be increased by use of elevated temperatures and pressures or can be catalyzed by acids (concentrated or dilute), or by highly selective enzymes such as cellulases. The steps involved in the acid-catalyzed hydrolysis of cellulose are illustrated in Fig. 7.2. The H^+ ions equilibrate between the O atoms in the system, including those of water and the glycoside, with the consequence that there is an equilibrium concentration of protonated glycoside. This equilibrium tends towards the protonated form of the glycoside with increasing temperature. The protonated conjugate acid then slowly breaks down to the cyclic carbonium ion, which adopts a half chair conformation (while the other glucopyranose residue retains the OH at C-4). After rapid addition of water, free sugar is liberated. Because the sugar competes with the water, small amounts of disaccharides are formed as reversion products.

There is a time/temperature relationship whereby lower acid concentrations require more extreme conditions and longer times for cellulose degradation. The use of stronger acid may reduce the costs associated with higher-pressure vessels, but the costly effects of equipment corrosion and of acid loss may be excessive. Rates of cellulose hydrolysis may differ according to the degree of crystallinity of the cellulose (i.e. the proportions of crystalline and amorphous cellulose present), a factor which varies between feedstocks.

The mechanism of hydrolysis of hemicellulose polysaccharides is similar to that illustrated for cellulose in Fig. 7.2 and usually involves protonation of the glycosidic oxygen. Process conditions do not need to be as severe, however, given the lower degree of polymerization (formation of the carbonium ion occurs more rapidly at the end of a polysaccharide chain) and a tendency for the occurrence of less intermolecular bonding in most hemicelluloses. The rate of hydrolysis of hemicelluloses with a higher uronic acid content may be lower than for other hemicelluloses, however, as a result of the steric effects of the carboxyl groups.

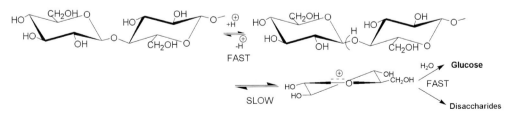

Fig. 7.2 Steps involved in the acid hydrolysis of cellulose [8].

The ash content of feedstocks is important because ash tends to lower the acidity of the mixture – the catalytic hydrogen ion is a function of the concentration of the acidic solution applied and the neutralizing power of the ash [9]. It is therefore useful to measure the titratable alkalinity of feedstocks to ascertain what acid levels may be necessary for their hydrolysis.

7.2.2
Production of Levulinic Acid, Formic Acid and Furfural

The Biofine Process involves the use of dilute sulfuric acid as a catalyst but differs from other dilute-acid lignocellulosic-fractionating technologies in that free monomeric sugars are not the product. Instead, the 6-carbon and 5-carbon monosaccharides undergo multiple acid-catalyzed reactions to give the platform chemicals levulinic acid ($C_5H_8O_3$) and furfural ($C_5H_4O_2$) as the final products.

Hydroxymethylfurfural (HMF) is an intermediate in the production of levulinic acid (4-oxopentanoic acid) from 6-carbon sugars in the Biofine Process. The series of consecutive reactions involved in its production are illustrated in Figs 7.3 and 7.4. These reactions have been established by numerous studies aimed at identification of intermediate products and analyses of pathways for their further transformation [10]. The enediol (1), obtained by enolization of D-glucose, D-mannose, or D-fructose, is the key compound in the formation of HMF. Further dehydration of the enediol (1) yields the product (2); which is

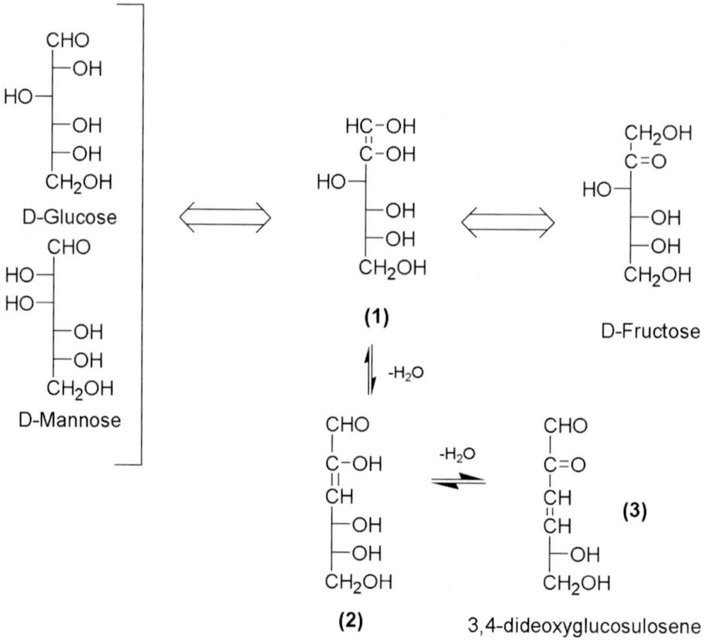

Fig. 7.3 Dehydration of the enediol (1) of D-glucose, D-mannose and D-fructose.

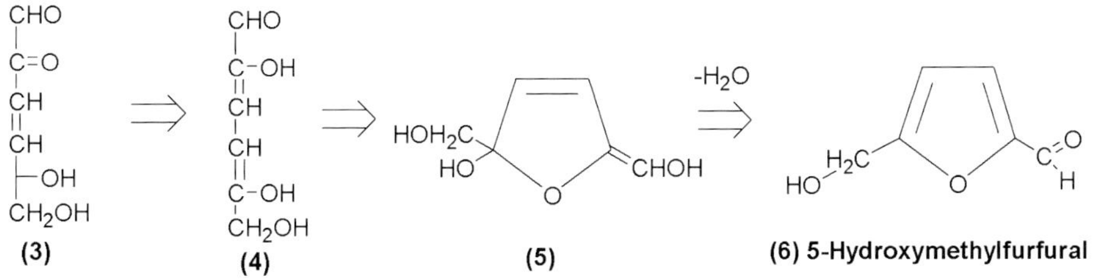

Fig. 7.4 Formation of hydroxymethylfurfural from 3,4-dideoxyglucosulosene-3.

further dehydrated to give 3,4-dideoxyglucosulosene-3 (**3**). 3,4-dideoxyglucosulo-sene-3 (**3**) is readily converted (Fig. 7.4) to the dienediol (**4**), which eventually results in the formation of 5-hydroxymethylfurfural (**6**) via the intermediate cyclic compound (**5**). Humic-type compounds can also be produced as side products in this reaction [11].

If the CH_2OH group of the hexoses is, instead, a hydrogen (as with the pentoses) a similar procedure occurs, but furfural is now the product.

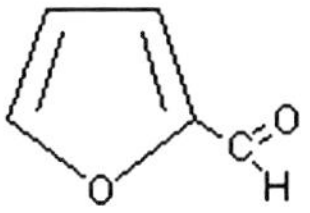

Furfural

Hydration of HMF, i.e. addition of a water molecule to the C-2–C-3 olefinic bond of the furan ring, leads to an unstable tricarbonyl intermediate (**7**) which decomposes to levulinic acid (LA) (**8**) and formic acid (HCOOH). A possible reaction process is shown in Fig. 7.5 [11]. The steps in the brackets in the mechanism below have not been proven and include several assumptions; these inter-

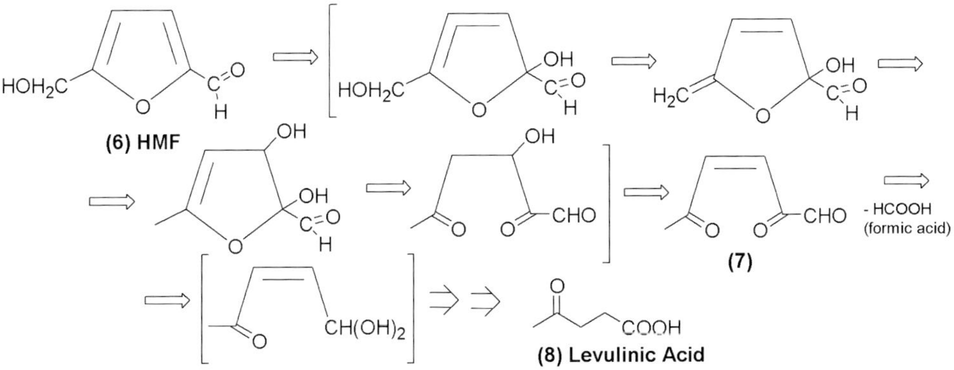

Fig. 7.5 A possible process for formation of LA from HMF [11].

mediates were proposed by Horvat et al. [12, 13] based on analysis of ^{13}C NMR spectra of the reaction mixture formed in the hydration of HMF.

7.3
The Biofine Process

Feedstock materials for a Biofine plant must be of appropriate particle size (ca 0.5 to 1 cm) to ensure efficient hydrolysis and optimum yields. The feedstock is therefore initially shredded before the biomass particulates are conveyed by high-pressure air injection system to a mixing tank. Here the feedstock is mixed with recycled dilute sulfuric acid (1.5–3%, depending on feedstock and titratable alkalinity). The Biofine Process then consists of two distinct acid-catalyzed stages (Fig. 7.6) that are operated to give optimum yields with a minimum of degradation products and tar formation.

The objective in the first reactor is the dominant, first-order, acid hydrolysis of the carbohydrate polysaccharides to their soluble intermediates (e.g. HMF). This reaction is favored by the use of a plug-flow reactor, at a temperature of 210–220 °C and a pressure of 25 bar. The rapid nature of the hydrolysis reaction means that a residence time of only 12 s is required. Given that the products are removed continuously, such a small residence time requires that the diameter of the reactor is kept small.

The completely mixed conditions of the second reactor favor the first-order reaction sequence leading to LA (Fig. 7.5) rather than higher-order tar-forming condensation reactions. Although the acid concentration remains the same as

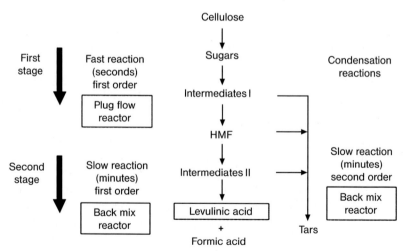

Fig. 7.6 Chemical conversion of cellulose to LA (major product), formic acid (byproduct), and tars (minor condensation products) in the two Biofine reactors.

in the first reactor, operating conditions are less severe (190–200 °C, 14 bar). This reactor is considerably larger than the first, however, because of the need for a residence time of approximately 20 min. Furfural and other volatile products tend to be removed at this stage while the tarry mixture of LA and residues are passed to a gravity separator. From here the insoluble mixture goes to a dehydration unit where the water and volatiles are boiled off. The heating of the mixture to boil off the LA is conducted under reduced pressure and results in the tarry material being "cracked", to give a bone-dry powdery substance ("char"). The crude 75% LA product can be purified up to a purity of 98%. The acid is recovered in the final recycle stage, enabling it to be re-used in the system.

In a complete Biofine plant, additional processing may then occur, depending on the final products required. For example, syngas production from the Biofine char (a dry, powdery material of calorific value comparable with that of bituminous coal, and composed of the residual materials in the Biofine Process which has value as a fuel and as a soil additive) can be conducted in a gasification unit or the LA can be esterified with ethanol to produce ethyl levulinate. The downstream conversions will be discussed further below.

7.3.1
Yields and Efficiencies of the Biofine Process

The maximum theoretical yield of LA from a hexose is 71.6% *w/w* and formic acid makes up the remainder [14]. How close to this theoretical yield is achieved in the conversion process will depend on the degradation reactions involved. In addition to cellulose and LA there are likely to be many intermediates other than those presented above. Some authors [12] have estimated there are over 100. These intermediates tend to cross-react and coalesce to form an acid-resistant tar which incorporates many insoluble residues such as humins. Previously developed technologies that attempted to produce LA from lignocellulosics were expensive because of low LA yields (approx. 3% by mass) and significant tar formation. The Biofine Process, because of its efficient reactor system and the use of polymerization inhibitors that reduce excessive char formation [2, 3], achieves from cellulose LA yields of 70–80% of the theoretical maximum. This translates to conversion of approximately 50% of the mass of 6-carbon sugars to LA, with 20% being converted to formic acid and 30% to tars. The mass yield of furfural from 5-carbon sugars is also approximately 70% of the theoretical value of 72.7%, equivalent to 50% of the mass, the remainder being incorporated in the Biofine char. These claims have been supported by process data from a pilot plant located in Glens Falls, New York State. This processes one dry tonne of feedstock per day and has been operational for several test-run periods since 1996. Its construction followed successful laboratory-scale demonstrations of the viability of the process at the National Renewable Energy Laboratory in Golden, Colorado. In the latter experiments, paper sludges from nearby paper mills were initially used as pilot plant feedstocks and gave LA yields ranging from 0.42 to

0.595 kg per kilo of cellulose (between 59 and 83% of the theoretical maximum yield).

The acid-insoluble ligneous and ash components of the feedstock become incorporated in the Biofine char with 100% mass conversion, although the properties of the resulting materials are likely to be altered under the "cracking" conditions of high-temperature and pressure. For most lignocellulosic feedstocks that may be processed in a Biofine unit, the dry mass balance of structural polysaccharides, lignin, and ash is likely to be close to 100%. Some feedstocks may have a relatively high proportion of extractives (extraneous components that may be separated from the insoluble cell wall material as a result of their solubility in water or neutral organic solvents). Bark, for example, may contain up to 25% by mass of extractives (predominately fats, waxes and terpenes) [15] whereas some grasses may contain a significant proportion (e.g. 20%) of water-soluble carbohydrates (WSC), depending on the time of year and environmental conditions. Although these WSC are also potential LA precursors, their fate in the Biofine process (as with other acid-hydrolysis schemes [16]) is likely to tend towards tar/residue formation because the process conditions are geared towards the conversion of cellulose and hence may be too strong to give LA as an end-product from WSC. Other extractive components are also likely to be incorporated in the Biofine char. That may be advantageous in instances where the char is to be combusted, given the relatively high heating values of these impurities [17].

7.3.2
Advantages over Conventional Lignocellulosic Technology

The Biofine Process is entirely chemical and does not rely on the use of any form of microorganism, as in enzymatic hydrolysis and in conventional dilute/concentrated acid hydrolysis technologies. The use of biological agents is often responsible for poor yields and a lower range of feasible feedstocks.

Most dilute acid hydrolysis technologies utilize microorganisms in the fermentation of the fully hydrolyzed monomers (e.g. *Saccharomyces cerevisiae* [18]). Some of the more recently developed schemes also utilize microorganisms in the hydrolysis of cellulose after hemicellulose extraction (simultaneous saccharification and fermentation, SSF). Even in the most advanced SSF technology the fermentation process takes a substantial time. After pretreatment, the cellulase enzyme and fermentation organisms require about 7 days to bring about the conversion to ethanol, compared with approximately 2 days for conversion of starch and approximately 30 min for conversion of cellulose to levulinic acid in the Biofine Process. Ethanol yields are also reduced as a result of the formation of sugar degradation products that inhibit the organisms/enzymes used for fermentation [19].

There are also significant problems associated with the fermentation of non-glucose sugars, particularly xylose. Although these sugars can be converted to ethanol by the genetically engineered yeasts that are currently available, for example *Pachysolen tannophilus* [20], ethanol yields are not sufficient to make the process economically attractive. It also remains to be seen whether the yeasts can be made "hardy" enough for production of ethanol on a commercial scale [21]. The inefficient utilization of nonglucose monosaccharide residues is a major disadvantage in fermentation schemes because these residues may be a significant proportion of the total polysaccharide mass (e.g. xylose makes up approximately 20% of the total dry mass in much woody and herbaceous biomass). The 50% (by mass) conversion of C5 sugars to furfural in the Biofine Process looks particularly attractive in such instances.

In avoiding the use of microorganisms, Biofine also enables use of a wider range of heterogeneous lignocellulosic feedstocks, including those (e.g. cellulosic municipal solid waste, sewage) that contain contaminants that might inhibit fermentation. The flexibility of the technology for a variety of feedstocks has been demonstrated over a four-month evaluation period during which the highly heterogeneous organic fraction of municipal solid waste (from the Bronx district of New York City) was successfully fractionated [22]. Furthermore, the lignin content of biomass has no inhibiting effect on the Biofine Process and this contrasts with enzymatic hydrolysis in which steric hindrance, caused by lignin–polysaccharide linkages, limits access of fibrolytic enzymes to specific carbohydrate moieties, this resulting in lower yields or the need for steam-explosion pretreatment [23].

7.3.3
Products of the Biofine Process

LA is a valuable platform chemical because of its particular chemistry – it has two highly reactive functional groups that enable many synthetic transformations. LA can react both as a carboxylic acid and as a ketone. The carbon atom of the carbonyl group is usually more susceptible to nucleophilic attack than that of the carboxyl group. Because of the spatial relationship of the carboxyl and keto groups, many of the reactions proceed with cyclization forming heterocyclic molecules (for example methyltetrahydrofuran). LA is readily soluble in water, alcohols, esters, ketones, and ethers. The worldwide market for pure LA at a price of $5 kg^{-1} has been estimated to be about only half a million kilograms. The key to an increased potential marketability for LA is the vast range of derivatives possible from this platform chemical (e.g. Refs. [24–26]) and its economical production via the Biofine Process. Figure 7.7 lists some of the sectors that offer markets for the products of the Biofine process. The following subsections will discuss some of the more promising products which potentially have the largest markets and hence the greatest potential for significantly replacing oil as a source of industrial chemicals and transport fuels.

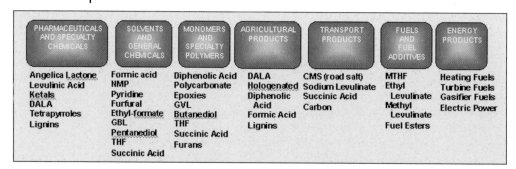

PHARMACEUTICALS AND SPECIALTY CHEMICALS	SOLVENTS AND GENERAL CHEMICALS	MONOMERS AND SPECIALTY POLYMERS	AGRICULTURAL PRODUCTS	TRANSPORT PRODUCTS	FUELS AND FUEL ADDITIVES	ENERGY PRODUCTS
Angelica Lactone	Formic acid	Diphenolic Acid	DALA	CMS (road salt)	MTHF	Heating Fuels
Levulinic Acid	NMP	Polycarbonate	Halogenated	Sodium Levulinate	Ethyl	Turbine Fuels
Ketals	Pyridine	Epoxies	Diphenolic	Succinic Acid	Levulinate	Gasifier Fuels
DALA	Furfural	GVL	Acid	Carbon	Methyl	Electric Power
Tetrapyrroles	Ethyl-formate	Butanediol	Formic Acid		Levulinate	
Lignins	GBL	THF	Lignins		Fuel Esters	
	Pentanediol	Succinic Acid				
	THF	Furans				
	Succinic Acid					

Fig. 7.7 Possible markets and saleable products from the Biofine process.

7.3.3.1 Diphenolic Acid

Diphenolic acid [4,4-bis-(4′-hydroxyphenyl)pentanoic acid] is prepared by reaction of levulinic acid with two molecules of phenol [27]. It may be a direct replacement for bisphenol A (BPA) in polycarbonates, epoxy resins, polyarylates, and other polymers. The acid also has numerous other uses including applications in lubricants, adhesives, and paints [28]. It can also copolymerize with BPA or can replace it in a variety of formulations. It contains a carboxyl group, absent from BPA, which confers additional functionality useful in polymer synthesis.

Diphenolic Acid   Bisphenol A

Diphenolic acid (DPA) was used commercially in various resin formulations before it was replaced by the petrochemically-derived BPA which could be supplied at a lower price. The reduced cost of LA production made possible with the Biofine Process may enable DPA to recapture some market share. Extensive research into near-term applications of DPA, particularly those that displace currently marketed BPA products, has been conducted at the Rensselaer Polytechnic Institute in New York State [29]. In the longer term DPA could be a viable alternative to oil in the production of plastics.

The cost of LA produced by other technologies is the principle reason for the high price of DPA (approx. $\phi 6 \text{ kg}^{-1}$). On the basis of Biofine estimates, the production of DPA from LA from the Biofine Process could result in a market price of $ 2.40 \text{ kg}^{-1}$. That price, based on Biofine estimates, could result in DPA capturing 20% of the US market ($2.5 \times 10^8 \text{ kg year}^{-1}$ for BPA). It may also result in DPA recapturing some of the $2.5 \times 10^6 \text{ kg year}^{-1}$ market it held for its old use as a coating material.

7.3.3.2
Succinic Acid and Derivatives

Oxidation of levulinic acid can lead to the production of succinic acid (Fig. 7.8). Currently, succinic acid is produced using a hydrocarbon-based process. A fermentation process using glucose derived from corn syrup can also produce succinic acid but this is not economically competitive. The most important uses of succinic acid are in food additives, soldering fluxes, and pharmaceutical products. The US market for succinic acid is approximately 4.50×10^8 kg year^{-1}, with a market price of approximately $ 2.8 kg^{-1}.

Succinic acid can be used to produce tetrahydrofuran (THF), 1,4-butanediol, and γ-butyrolactone (GBL). THF is formed by cyclization of succinic acid to give succinic anhydride which is then reduced and dehydrated to provide tetrahydrofuran. THF is a cyclic ether whose major use is as a monomer in the production of poly(tetramethylene ether glycol) (PTMEG), a component of, among other things, polyurethane stretch fibers (Spandex). A smaller amount of THF is used as a solvent in poly(vinyl chloride) (PVC) cements, pharmaceuticals, and coatings and as a reaction solvent. The Western European market for tetrahydrofuran is estimated to be approximately 7.5×10^7 kg, valued at $ 2.6 kg^{-1}. Almost 80% of production is used captively, mostly for PTMEG [30].

γ-Butyrolactone ($C_4H_6O_2$) is used as a chemical intermediate in the manufacture of the pyrrolidone solvents. It can be used in the production of pesticides, herbicides, and plant-growth regulators. Mechanisms for the production of GBL are currently being refined – catalysts have been identified for the selective reduction of succinic acid to GBL in the presence of acetic acid [31]. Although high GBL yields have been successfully demonstrated, catalyst productivities are currently still below commercially attractive rates [31]. The market price for 1,4-butanediol, another possible derivative of succinic acid, is approximately $2.30 kg^{-1} [30].

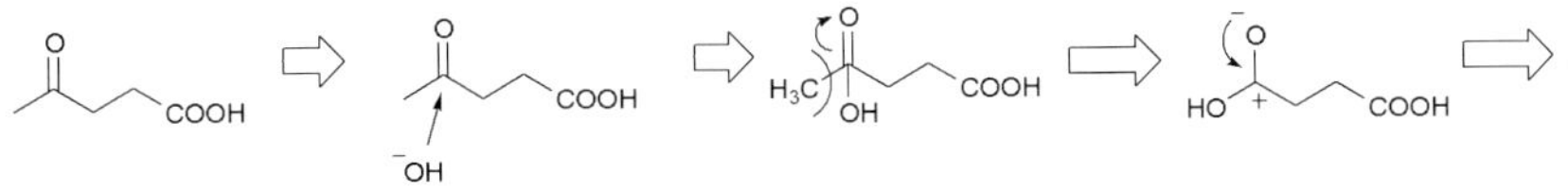

Fig. 7.8 The production of succinic acid in base (e.g. NaOH).

7.3.3.3 **Delta-aminolevulinic Acid**
δ-Aminolevulinic acid (DALA) is a naturally occurring substance present in all plant and animal cells [32–34]. It is the active ingredient in a range of environmentally benign, highly selective, broad-spectrum herbicides. It has high activity against dicotyledonous weeds and little activity against monocotyledonous crops such as corn (maize), wheat, or barley [35]. DALA also has use as an insecticide [36] and in cancer treatment [37].

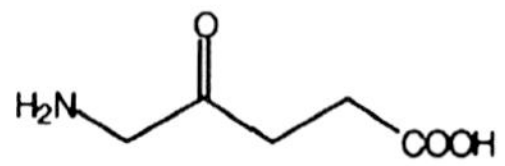

DALA

Difficulties experienced in production of DALA from LA involve the selective introduction of an amino group at the C5-position. The most common approach for activating the C5 position toward amination is bromination of LA in an alcohol medium to give mixtures of 5-bromo- and 3-bromoesters that are separated by distillation [38]. The 5-bromolevulinate is then aminated using a nucleophilic nitrogen species [39]. These conventional mechanisms give low yields at very high cost. The National Renewable Energy Laboratory (NREL) process (Fig. 7.9), significantly improves yields and reduces costs. It also results in the production of two moles of formic acid per mole of DALA, the resulting DALA being obtained at a purity of greater than 90%. During initial testing in a greenhouse environment, NREL found that this crude DALA was active as a herbicide.

A significant amount of research is still being conducted on the formation of DALA from LA. The complexity and low yields of conventional DALA synthesis techniques mean that it is currently a very expensive product, being used only for highly selective herbicidal treatment and some cancer therapies. There is a large potential in the agricultural and horticultural sector for lower-cost Biofine-derived DALA; however, quantification of this area is not possible at present because specific commercial formulations must be developed.

7.3.3.4 Methyltetrahydrofuran

The production of fuel additives via renewable feedstocks offers perhaps the greatest potential for mass-market penetration of LA. Methyltetrahydrofuran (MTHF) can be added to petroleum in amounts up to 30% by volume with no adverse effects on performance, and engine modifications are not required. Some important properties of MTHF are listed in Table 7.1. Although it has a

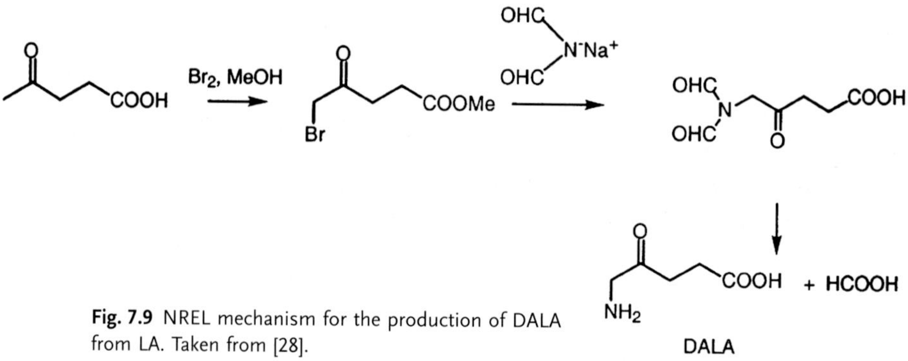

Fig. 7.9 NREL mechanism for the production of DALA from LA. Taken from [28].

Table 7.1 Selected properties of MTHF and ethyl levulinate [42–44].

	MTHF	Ethyl levulinate
Boiling point (102 mmHg), °C	20	93
Boiling point (Atm.), °C	80	206.2
Flash point, °C	11	195
Reid vapor pressure, psig	5.7	<0.01
Lower heating value, kJ kg^{-1}	32000	24300
Specific gravity	0.813	1.016
Octane rating	80	
Cetane number	–	<10
Lubricity (HFRR micros)	–	287

lower heating value than regular petroleum, it has a higher specific gravity and hence mileage from MTHF blended fuel would be competitive. MTHF substantially reduces the vapor pressure of ethanol when coblended in gasoline. This has led to the development of "P-Series" fuels, i.e. fuels miscible with petroleum designed for vehicles with flexible-fuel engines and containing "pentanes-plus" hydrocarbons from natural gas, ethanol (preferably from biomass), and methyltetrahydrofuran as a co-solvent for ethyl alcohol (high-octane) [40]. P-Series fuels can be used alone or may be mixed in any proportions with petroleum. Vehicle tailpipe and evaporative emissions tests have been conducted on three P-Series formulations by the Environmental Protection Agency [41] and the results have been compared with those obtained from reformulated gasoline (RFG). It was found that the formulations had a reduced ozone-forming potential (OFP) and resulted in reduced emissions of nonmethane hydrocarbons and total hydrocarbons – approximately a third of that formed with Phase 2 RFG. It has been estimated that when the MTHF and ethanol are derived from biological materials, the full fuel-cycle greenhouse gas emissions will be between 45 and 50% below those of reformulated gasoline [41]. These successful emission and performance tests have recently resulted in the P-Series formulations being approved by the US Department of Energy as an alternative gasoline, meeting the requirements of the Energy Policy Act for automobile fleet usage. It should be noted, however, that P-Series fuels can only be used in "flexible fuel engines" and have to be distributed at gasoline stations supplied with pumps specially modified for alcohol-based fuels. Their short-term markets may therefore be limited to captive fleets (e.g. city buses).

Direct conversion of LA to MTHF occurs in low yield, hence indirect routes are utilized (Fig. 7.10). One possible mechanism involves the catalytic hydrogenation of LA to γ-valerolactone (GVL) which, on further hydrogenation, yields 1,4-pentanediol and, finally, MTHF [28]. An efficient application of this mechanism was devised by scientists at the Pacific Northwest Laboratory (PNL) in the US [45]. The process is conducted at elevated temperatures and pressures using a continuous-flow catalytic reactor. Levulinic acid is pumped into a tube where it is warmed to approximately 40 °C, then mixed with hydrogen. Both com-

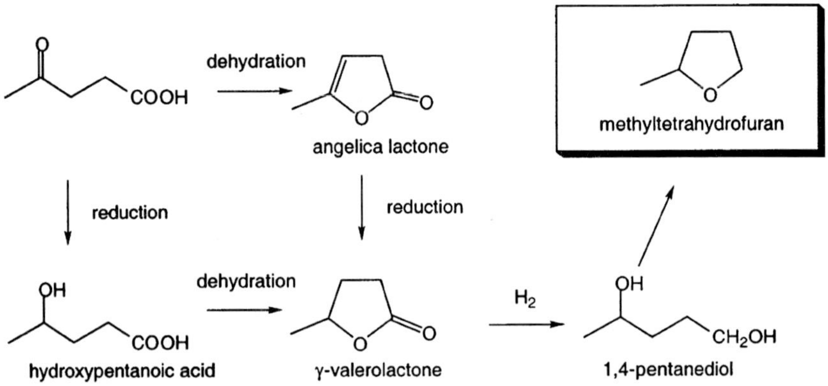

Fig. 7.10 Possible mechanisms for formation of MTHF from LA [28].

pounds are then pumped through a reactor filled with a catalyst in which a series of chemical reactions occurs at approximately 240 °C and 100 atmospheres pressure to create MTHF. The procedure requires three moles of hydrogen per mole LA. Laboratory tests indicated the yield was 83% on a theoretical (molar) basis [45]. This would be equivalent to a yield of approximately 63 kg (71 L) MTHF for every 100 kg of LA, or 81 L of MTHF for every 100 L of LA. The yield of the PNL process is significantly greater than that of other processes. These usually used mechanisms in which MTHF was a merely a byproduct, with final yields of approximately only 3%.

The extra costs involved in producing MTHF from LA are minimal – for a Biofine plant processing 1000 dry tonnes of biomass per day, the estimated extra capital cost for an MTHF production facility would be $ 10 Mio. The required 6 kg of hydrogen for every 100 kg of LA could be supplied from the residual process char (via a syngas production unit, see below) with an estimated cost of hydrogen production of 5 c kg^{-1}.

In addition to transport, MTHF has value in other markets – it is, for example, an excellent general solvent that is, in many regards, superior to tetrahydrofuran. It should also be noted that catalytic production of MTHF from furfuryl alcohol is possible, as is the production of dimethyltetrahydrofuran (DMTHF) from hydroxymethylfurfural (the product of the first Biofine reactor). It is hypothesized that the additional methyl group in DMTHF may afford superior performance and mileage over MTHF, although vehicle tests have yet to be carried out.

7.3.3.5 Ethyl Levulinate

Esters of LA produced from either methanol or ethanol have significant potential as blend components in diesel formulations. LA esters are similar to the biodiesel fatty acid methyl esters (FAME) that are used in some low-sulfur diesel formulations but they do not have their principal drawbacks (cold flow properties and gum formation [46]). Addition of ethyl or methyl levulinate to FAME would be expected to alleviate both these problems.

The most studied of the LA esters is a low-smoke diesel formulation developed by Biofine and Texaco that uses ethyl levulinate (made by esterifying LA with fuel-grade ethanol) as an oxygenate additive. The 21:79 formulation consists of 20% ethyl levulinate, 1% co-additive, and 79% diesel and can be used in regular diesel engines. The oxygen content of ethyl levulinate (EL) is 33%, w/w, giving a 6.9%, w/w, oxygen content in the blend, resulting in a significantly cleaner burning diesel fuel [44].

The ethyl levulinate blend gives lower sulfur emissions than does regular diesel. This is because ethyl levulinate contains no sulfur. Lower sulfur emissions can also be attributed to the high lubricity of EL blends. Fuel lubricity is used to determine the amount of wear that occurs between two metal parts covered with the fuel as they come into contact. Fuels of higher lubricity result in less wear and prolong engine component life. The sulfur level of diesel is reduced in the refinery using a hydro-treating process; this results in undesirable removal of some of the lubricity components from the fuel and hence a decrease in diesel lubricity. Addition of EL, with high lubricity, will therefore mean that diesel blend-stocks of low lubricity, and hence lower S content, can be used without reducing the all-over lubricity of the end product. In Europe lubricity is measured by use of the high frequency reciprocating rig (HFRR) test with lower values indicating higher fuel lubricity. Biofine has shown that addition of 20% EL to a standard No 2 base fuel improves the HFRR from 410 to 275 [44]. Importantly, the significant losses of engine efficiency (a decrease of up to 15% in the distance driven per unit volume is found with other diesel oxygenates, for example ethanol) do not occur with ethyl levulinate. This is because of the high energy content of the 21:79 formulation (selected properties of EL are listed in Table 7.1).

The levulinate esters also have potential as replacements of kerosene as a home heating oil and as a fuel for the direct firing of gas turbines for electrical generation [47]. The production of levulinic acid esters from LA formed in the Biofine Process has the added advantage over conventional bioesters that there is no coproduction of glycerol which would have to be disposed of.

7.3.3.6 Formic Acid

Formic acid (HCOOH) is a byproduct in the production of levulinic acid from cellulose. It can be purified by distillation and sold directly as a commodity chemical. It is conventionally produced, usually as a byproduct of acetic acid production, by liquid phase oxidation of hydrocarbons. It is used extensively as a decalcifier, as an acidulating agent in textile dying and finishing, and in leather tanning [48]. It is also used in the preparation of organic esters and in the manufacture of drugs, dyes, insecticides, and refrigerants. Formic acid can also be converted into calcium magnesium formate for use as a road salt. In Europe, the largest single use of formic acid is as a silage additive. For example, the AMASIL additive produced by BASF Ireland contains 85% formic acid which is bought at a price of € 1.35 per liter.

The catalyst-preparation sector is a very large potential future market for formic acid. As well as being used in the manufacture of many catalysts, formic acid is also used in the regeneration of catalyst metals poisoned with sulfur. The increasing demand for low-sulfur fuels will result in increased demand for the catalysts produced using the formates and, consequently, will require formic acid. Additionally, esters of formic acid (e.g. methyl and ethyl formate) may also have value as fuel components and as platform chemicals.

In 2000, world consumption of formic acid amounted to approximately 4.15×10^8 kg [48], roughly half of which was consumed in Europe. A Biofine plant processing 300 dry tonnes of feedstock per day would produce approximately 9×10^6 kg formic acid per year (assuming a cellulose content of 40%). Where supply of formic acid exceeds demand for its conventional uses, the merchant market price may fall to around $ 0.16 per liter, which is the price needed to open up other markets such as its use as a road salt or for formaldehyde production [49]. If even these markets are not available, the formic acid byproduct still has value, because it can provide energy via gasification or anaerobic digestion.

7.3.3.7 Furfural

Furfural is produced from the hemicellulosic pentose fractions of biomass. Xylose is the predominant pentose in most feedstocks, with hemicellulosic arabinose found to a lesser extent. Furfural can be sold as a solvent or used in the production of furfuryl alcohol, tetrahydrofuran (THF), and LA. Furfuryl alcohol (Fig. 7.11) is a monomer for furan resins, these being used mainly as foundry binders. It is prepared by hydrogenation of furfural. THF is produced by decarbonylation of furfural to furan, then catalytic hydrogenation [50]. LA is produced by first converting furfural to furfuryl alcohol. Figure 7.11 shows the mechanism involved – furfuryl alcohol, when boiled in ethyl methyl ketone in the presence of HCl, gives rise to 90–93% levulinic acid, the reaction occurring via hydroxy derivatives [11].

Global production of furfural in 2001 amounted to 22.5×10^7 kg year^{-1} [51]. Approximately 4×10^7 kg furfural was consumed in Europe in 2000, furfuryl alcohol being the major market. Most furfural is now produced in China, whose total capacity is 15–20×10^7 kg year^{-1} [51]. Low labor and feedstock prices in Chi-

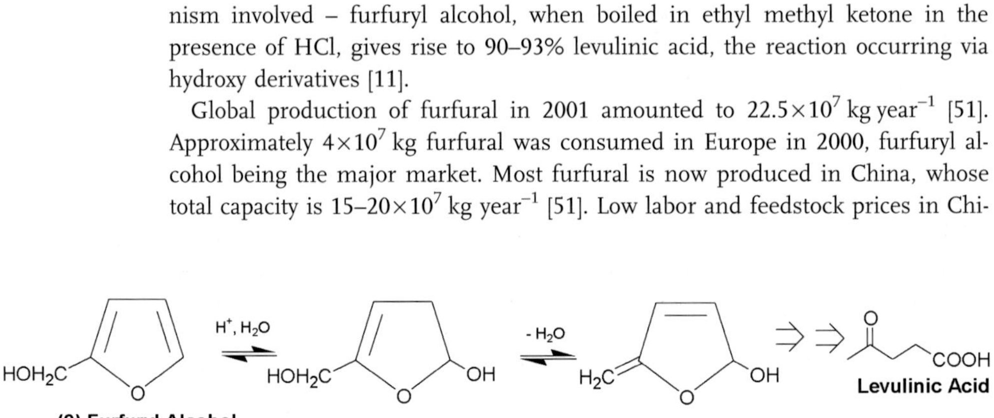

(9) Furfuryl Alcohol

Fig. 7.11 Production of LA from furfuryl alcohol.

na, coupled with increasing Chinese capacity, have resulted in prices falling over the last decade – the current market price of furfural is approximately $ 1 kg^{-1} compared with prices in 1990 of $ 1.74 kg^{-1} for furfural and $ 1.76 kg^{-1} for furfuryl alcohol [50]. EU and US import tariffs are placed on furfural from China, these being designed to lessen this effect of this price differential, but market prices are still highly dependent on Chinese supply. (A significant rise in price between 1995 and 1998 was attributed to a drought in China during that period).

A Biofine plant processing 300 dry tonnes of feedstock per day would produce, from hemicelluloses, approximately 1.3×10^7 kg furfural per year (assuming 25% pentosans by mass). This represents 32.5% of the total consumption of furfural/furfuryl alcohol in Europe in 2000. Furfural conversion products, whether THF or LA and their subsequent downstream products, may therefore be more marketable final products than furfural itself in large biorefinery schemes, especially if the fuel additive market is explored.

7.3.4
Biofine Char

The quantity of residual char from the Biofine process and its calorific value will depend on the acid-insoluble lignin content of the biomass, the ash content, any insoluble proteins present, and the amount of degradation and reversion products formed from the cellulose and hemicellulose fractions. The boiling off from the char of volatiles and LA gives rise to a "cracking" of the char. It is, therefore, difficult to predict the final composition of the char from the mass compositions of virgin biomass. The composition would be predictable with greater certainty if each potential feedstock was tested in the Biofine Process.

Biofine char has much promise as a fuel. Residual char from the processing of paper sludge in the Biofine pilot plant was found to have a heating value of approximately 25.6 MJ kg^{-1} (with 15% ash content), a value that was significantly larger than that of the original feedstock (18.6 MJ kg^{-1}). It was found that combustion of the dry Biofine char (the mass of which was 15% of that of the original paper sludge) yielded more energy than combustion of the entire feedstock (at its initial 50% moisture content).

It has been estimated that the energy provided by the residual char is greater than that needed to completely fuel the steam and electric power needs of the biorefinery when the scale of operation is equal to or greater than approximately 270 dry tonnes of feedstock per day (assuming a feedstock lignin content of approximately 25%). Appropriately sized plants may therefore expect to gain significant revenue from the marketing of surplus electricity.

Research is ongoing for alternative uses and markets for Biofine char. It is believed it may have value as a soil conditioner. Figure 7.12 compares the FTIR spectra of lignin with those of chars obtained from paper sludge and straw feedstocks. It can be seen that straw char retains many of the functionalities of lignin, characterized by absorbance in the 1000–1800 cm^{-1} region of the spectrum.

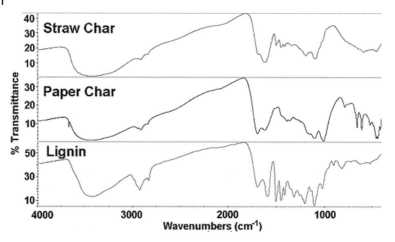

Fig. 7.12 FTIR spectra for lignin and Biofine chars from paper sludge and straw feedstocks.

The chars from straw and from paper have significant carbonyl/carboxyl functionality and the presence of significant acidic functionality was confirmed by titration data. Solid-state NMR will indicate the nature of the aromatic functionality and whether or not the Biofine chars have the fused aromatic structures characteristic of charcoals.

We have performed thermogravimetric analyses on several feedstocks and on the chars from straw and paper. In thermogravimetry, sample weight loss is monitored as a function of increasing temperature. Thermograms, and their first derivatives (rate of weight loss with respect to temperature) for the renewable energy crop Miscanthus, for a lignin extract, and for the Biofine chars from paper sludge, and straw feedstocks are shown in Fig. 7.13. Weight loss in the range 50–120 °C is associated with volatilization of water whereas that resulting from loss of low-molecular-weight compounds and other volatile organic compounds (extractives in woods/grasses) occurs from 120–250 °C; degradation of hemicelluloses occurs in the 250–300 °C range, and cellulose degrades very sharp at approximately 300–340 °C in air (higher in nitrogen). The thermogram for Miscanthus is strong evidence for hemicellulose, cellulose, and lignin components. The two thermograms for the chars are similar and clearly show that the hemicellulose and cellulose components are greatly diminished – indicated by a significant shift of the peaks to the right compared with the Miscanthus thermogram. This shift reflects a predominance of the ligneous type components, this being indicated by a similarity between the char thermograms and those of the lignin extract.

Another possible use of the char is steam gasification (thermochemical production of hydrogen from a feedstock, for example biomass materials, or, in this context, Biofine char) followed by upgrading of the synthesis gas produced. Although little work has yet been done along these lines using the Biofine char,

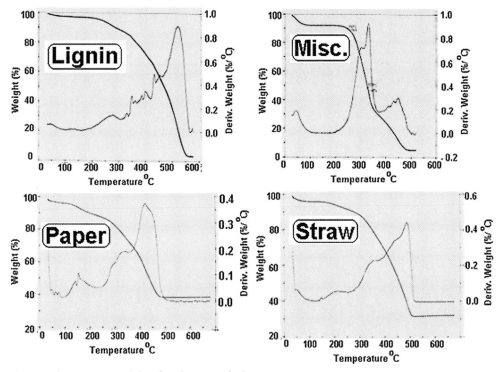

Fig. 7.13 Thermograms and their first derivatives for lignin, Miscanthus, and Biofine chars from paper and straw feedstocks.

there has been much work over the years on the gasification of equivalent materials, for example peat or coal [52, 53]. Coal gasification was originally used for the production of syngas for use in, for example, the Fischer-Tropsch Process. More recently, interest in connection with that process has shifted to the reforming of natural gas as a source of the syngas for the process (e.g. Ref. [54] and other articles in the same volume). The steam gasification of carbon can be represented simply by a combination of the gasification reaction:

$$C + H_2O \rightarrow CO + H_2$$

followed by the water-gas shift reaction:

$$CO + H_2O = CO_2 + H_2$$

The exothermic water-gas shift reaction is favored by operation at low temperatures whereas high temperatures favor the reverse reaction. Hence, a product gas containing largely hydrogen is produced if the temperature is low and a syngas with a CO/H_2 ratio of 1 is obtained if the temperature is high. The syngas can be used as a fuel (e.g. to give the energy needed for the Biofine process) but it can also be used in a variety of reactions such as methanol synthesis:

$$CO + 2H_2 \rightarrow CH_3OH$$

Alternatively, it can be used in the Fischer–Tropsch process mentioned above; this can be depicted simplistically as:

$$nCO + mH_2 \quad CnH_2m$$

in which the product hydrocarbons are usually aliphatic in nature and can be used as diesel substitutes. Much work has recently been performed on so-called GTL technology (GTL=Gas to Liquids – technology that converts synthesis gas (from gasification of biomass or biorefinery process chars, for example) into liquid fuels), and many of these developments have been summarized recently [55].

7.3.5
Economics of the Biofine Process

The Biofine technology is commercially viable. A commercial plant (Fig. 7.14) processing 50 dry tonnes of feedstock per day has been constructed in Caserta, Italy (with joint funding from the EU and private investment) and is expected to be operational in 2005. The primary feedstocks will be paper sludge, agricultural residue, and waste paper with the major products being LA and EL (for use as a fuel). The process char will be gasified to produce a fuel gas for the process boilers. The modular nature of the technology means that the capacity can easily be upgraded, and there are plans for a supplemental 250 tonne per day reactor system to be installed eventually – bringing the total capacity to 300

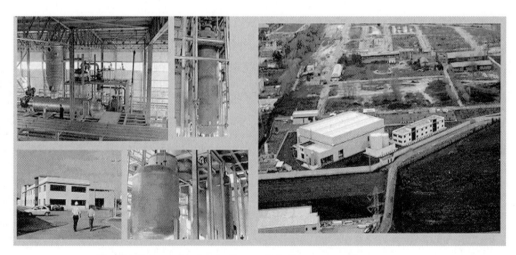

Fig. 7.14 Commercial plant in Caserta, Italy. Recovery vessels
(top); outside of building (bottom left); mixing tank
(top middle); second reactor (bottom middle);
arial view (right).

tonnes per day. Indeed, the Biofine process is extremely compact – a feasibility study conducted by a marine architectural company concluded that a self-contained 1000 tonne per day facility could be accommodated on an ocean-going "Panamax" barge [56].

Significant economies of scale can accrue with increasing plant size, as shown in Fig. 7.15 a and b. Figure 7.15 c shows, for various plant sizes, the trend in the cost of ethyl levulinate production with feedstock cost. Table 7.2 shows a detailed breakdown of these costs and of byproduct revenues for a plant processing 1000 dry tonnes of feedstock per day. It is assumed that the feedstock is of composition, by mass, 50% cellulose, 20% hemicellulose, 20% lignin, and 5% ash (comparable with many woody and herbaceous energy crops). It is also assumed that the plant is operational for 350 days per year, that all of the furfural

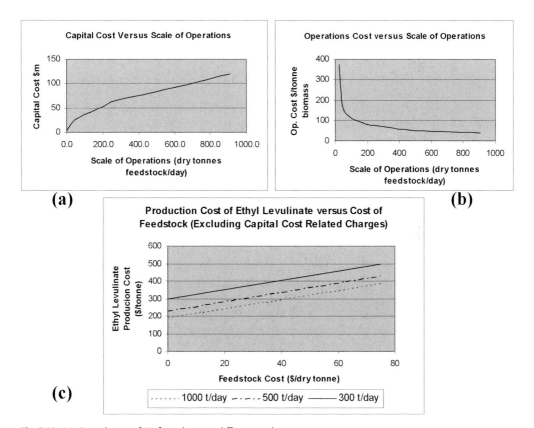

Fig. 7.15 (a) Capital cost of Biofine plants at different scales of operation; (b) Operating cost ($ per dry tonne of feedstock processed) at different scales of operation; (c) Production cost of ethyl levulinate with three plant sizes (1000, 500 and 300 dry tonnes of feedstock processed per day) and varying feedstock cost.

Table 7.2 Data provided by Biofine on estimated operating costs and byproduct revenues from a plant processing 1000 dry tonnes of feedstock per day for the production of ethyl levulinate.

Scale of Operation – 1000 dry tonnes per day (350 000 dry tonnes/year)
Capital Cost – $ 150 million (Grassroots, fully self-contained and integrated)
Production Output – 133 000 tonnes per year ethyl levulinate

Raw materials:			
Feedstock	350,000 dt/y	@$ 40/t	$ 14,000,000/y
Sulfuric acid	3,500 t/y	@$ 100/t	$ 350,000/y
Caustic soda	500 t/y	@$ 120/t	$ 60,000/y
Ethanol	35,000 t/y	@$ 350/t	$ 12,250,000/y
Hydrogen	120 t/y	@$ 1,500/t	$ 180,000/y
Others	allow.		$ 160,000/y
Subtotal			$ 27,000,000/r
Utilities:			
Steam	250,000 lb/h	gen. on-site	0
Electric	14.4 MW	gen. on-site	0
Electric usage	11.3 MW		0
Electric sold	3.1 MW		
Water	250 gpm		$ 500,000/y
Gas (boiler)	294 m BTU/h	gen. on-site	0
Subtotal			$ 500,000/y
Labor and Maintenance:			
Operators	17 per shift	@$ 20 per hr	$ 2,800,000/y
Supervision	2 per shift	@$ 24 per hr	$ 400,000/y
Maintenance		@4% of cap cost/yr	$ 6,000,000/y
Subtotal			$ 9,200,000/y
Overheads			
Direct	@30% of labor		$ 1,000,000/y
General	@25% of Lab. & Maintenance		$ 2,300,000/y
Taxes and Insurance	allow.		$ 3,700,000/y
Subtotal			$ 7,000,000/y
Disposal Costs:			
Ash:	17,500 t/y	@$ 35/t	$ 600,000/y
Subtotal			$ 600,000
Gross Production costs			**$ 44,300,000**
Byproducts: Formic acid	38,500 t/y	@$ 110/t	$ 4,200,000
Electric sold	26,000 MWhr/y	@$ 60/MWhr	$ 1,500,000
Subtotal			$ 5,700,000
NET PRODUCTION COST			**$ 38,600,000**
Production cost per to Ethyl Levulinate (no capital charges)			*$ 291 per tonne*
Equivalent Energy price			*12 per GJ*

is converted to LA, and that formic acid is sold for 10 c kg^{-1} and electrical power for 6 c kw h^{-1}. It can be seen that ash is the only waste product, incurring a disposal charge (\$ 35/tonne). Disposal need not be a problem, however. The Caserta plant will supply an adjacent tile factory with the ash, avoiding such costs. The ash can also be used as a fertilizer on agricultural land. The ethyl levulinate production cost of \$ 291 tonne^{-1} is equivalent to a price of \$ 12 GJ^{-1}, competitive with the \$ 16 GJ^{-1} of gasoline at \$ 2 gallon^{-1} or \$ 10 GJ^{-1} for crude oil at \$ 50 per barrel.

7.4
Conclusion

Lignocellulosic fractionating technology offers the potential for inexpensive production of a range of chemicals and fuels that are currently competitive only from petrochemical reserves. The Biofine Process is among the most advanced of this technology and provides high yields of levulinic acid (LA), furfural, and formic acid. Furthermore, unlike most other processes aimed at harvesting added value from carbohydrate feedstocks, the Biofine process is continuous, compact, easily expandable and entirely chemically based. Feedstocks that contain reasonable concentrations of carbohydrates can be utilized. Thus heterogeneous biomass reserves such as cellulosic municipal solid waste and animal manures may be processed as well as the more conventional lignocellulosic feedstocks such as sugar cane bagasse and high-yielding energy crops. Maximum value is targeted from the diverse chemical constituents of biomass – the moist nature of the biomass is exploited in the acid hydrolysis of polysaccharides to provide platform chemicals such as LA (unlike in combustion/gasification schemes where moisture is a barrier). The dry char residue has a significantly higher fuel calorific value than the feedstock and it has potential for syngas production and as a soil conditioner. The technology offers a potentially sustainable "bio-recycling" solution in a world where rising and erratic oil prices and unpredictable oil supplies are coupled with growing levels of waste production. The extent to which this potential is realized will depend on the size of the market for LA, furfural, and their derivatives. Mechanisms already exist for the production of numerous saleable industrial chemicals from these, and promising research indicates avenues for expansion into the potentially huge transport, agricultural, and plastics sectors. It is therefore feasible that such a technology can stimulate a transition from a hydrocarbon to a carbohydrate-based economy (i.e. economy in which chemical, energy, fuel, and consumables requirements are provided by carbohydrate rather than hydrocarbon feedstocks) where local self-sustainability is possible. This concept is supported by the range of commercial-scale Biofine plants planned for Ireland, the UK, and the US.

References

1 Szmant, H. H. (1989), *Organic Building Blocks of the Chemical Industry.* Wiley & Sons, New York.

2 Fitzpatrick, S. W. (1990), *Lignocellulose degradation to furfural and levulinic acid: U.S. Patent 4,897,497*

3 Fitzpatrick, S. W. (1997), *Production of levulinic acid from carbohydrate-containing materials: U.S. Patent 5,608,105*

4 McAloon, A., Taylor, F., Yee, W., Ibsen, K. and Wooley, R. (2000), *Determining the Cost of Producing Ethanol from Corn Starch and Lignocellulosic Feedstocks,* NREL/TP-580-28893. NREL, Golden, CO.

5 Broder, J. D., Harris, R. A. and Ranney, J. T. (2001), Using MSW and industrial residues as ethanol feedstocks. *Bi°Cycle* 42(10): 23–26.

6 Bozell, J. J. (2001), *Chemicals and Materials from Renewable Resources.* American Chemical Society, Washington DC.

7 Klass, D. L. (1981), *Biomass as a nonfossil fuel source.* American Chemical Society, Washington DC.

8 Sjostrom, E. (1981), *Wood Chemistry: Fundamentals and Applications.* Academic Press, Inc., London, UK.

9 Zerbe, J. I. and Baker, A. J. (1987), Investigation of fundamentals of two-stage, dilute sulphuric acid hydrolysis of wood. In: D. L. Klass (eds), *Energy from Biomass and Wastes X.* Institute of Gas Technology, Chicago, 927–947.

10 Kooherkov, N. A., Bochkov, A. F., Dimitriev, B. A., Usov, A. I., Chizbov, O. S. and Shibaev, Y. N. (1967), *Khimiya Uglevodov (The Chemistry of Carbohydrates).* Khimiya, Moscow.

11 Timokhin, B. V., Baransky, V. A. and Eliseeva, G. D. (1999), Levulinic acid in organic synthesis. *Russian Chemical Reviews* 68(1): 73–84.

12 Horvat, J., Klaic, B., Metelko, B. and Sunjic, V. (1985), Mechanism of levulinic acid formation. *Tetrahedron* 26: 2111–2214.

13 Horvat, J., Klaic, B., Metelko, B. and Sunjic, V. (1986), Mechanism of levulinic acid formation in acid-catalyzed hydrolysis of 2-hydroxymethylfuran and 5-hydroxymethylfuran-2-carbaldehyde. *Croat. Chem. Acta* 59: 429–438.

14 Leonard, R. H. (1956), Levulinic acid as a basic chemical raw materials. *Ind. Eng. Chem.* 48(8): 1331–1341.

15 USDA (1971), *Bark and its Possible Uses.* US Department of Agriculture, Madison, WI.

16 Wiselogel, A. E., Agblevor, F. A., Johnson, D. K., Deutch, S., Fennell, J. A. and Sanderson, M. A. (1996), Compositional changes during storage of large round switchgrass bales. *Bioresource Technology* 56(1): 103–109.

17 Susott, R. A., DeGroot, W. F. and Shafizadeh, F. (1975), Heat content of natural fuels. *J. Fire and Flammability* 6: 311–325.

18 Nguyen, Q. (1998), *Milestone Completion Report: Evaluation of a Two-Stage Dilute Sulfuric Acid Hydrolysis Process. Internal Report.* National Renewable Energy Laboratory, Golden, Colorado.

19 Gregg, D. and Saddler, J. N. (1996), A techno-economic assessment of the pretreatment and fractionation steps of a biomass-to-ethanol process. *Appl. Biochem. Biotech.* 57/58: 711–726.

20 Beck, M. J. and Strickland, R. C. (1984), Production of ethanol by bioconversion of wood sugars derived from two-stage dilute acid hydrolysis of hardwood. *Biomass and Bioenergy* 6: 101–110.

21 Cooper (1999), A Renewed Boost for Ethanol. *Chemical Engineering* 106(2): 35.

22 BioMetics Inc. (1996), *Municipal Solid Waste Conversion Project, Final Report,* Contract No: 4204-ERTER-ER-96. Biometics Inc., Boston, MA.

23 Donaldson, L. A., Wong, K. K. Y. and Mackie, K. L. (1988), Ultrastructure of steam-exploded wood. *Wood Science and Technology* 22: 103–114.

24 Oono, T., Saito, S., Shinohara, S. and Takakuwa, K. (1996), *Fluxes for electric circuit board soldering and electric circuit boards: Japanese patent 08243787*

25 Shimizu, A., Nishio, S., Wada, Y. and Metoki, I. (1996), *Photographic processing method for processing silver halide photo-*

graphic light-sensitive material: European patent 704756

26 Adams, P.E., Lange, R.M., Yodice, R., Baker, M.R. and Dietz, J.G. (1998), *Intermediates useful for preparing dispersant-viscosity improvers for lubricating oils: European patent 882745*

27 Isoda, Y. and Azuma, M. (1996), *Preparation of bis(hydroxyaryl)pentanoic acids: Japanese patent 08053390 to Honshu Chemical Ind.*

28 Bozell, J.J., Moens, L., Elliott, D.C., Wang, Y., Neuenschwander, G.G., Fitzpatrick, S.W., Bilski, R.J. and Jarnefeld, J.L. (2000), Production of levulinic acid and use as a platform chemical for derived products. *Resources, Conservation and Recycling* 28: 227–239.

29 Moore, J.A. and Tannahill, T. (2000), Homo- and co-polycarbonates and blends derived from diphenolic acid. *High Performance Polymers* 13: 305–316.

30 Ring, K.-L., Kaelin, T. and Yoneyama, M. (2001), *CEH Report: Tetrahydrofuran.* SRI, Menlo Park, CA.

31 Nghiem, N., Davison, B.H., Donnelly, M.I., Tsai, S.-P. and Frye, J.G. (2001), An integrated process for the production of chemicals from biologically derived succinic acid. In: J.J. Bozell (eds), *Chemicals and Materials from Renewable Resources.* American Chemical Society, Washington DC, 160–173.

32 Gibson, H.D., Laver, W.G. and Neuberger, A. (1958), Initial stages in the biosynthesis of porphyrins. II. The formation of 5-aminolevulinic acid from glycine and succinyl-CoA by particles from chicken erythrocytes. *Biochem. J.* 70: 71–81.

33 Beale, S.I. and Castelfranco, P.A. (1974), The biosynthesis of delta-aminolevulinic acid in higher plants. II. Formation of ^{14}C-delta-aminolevulinic acid from labelled precursors in greening plant tissues. *Plant Physiol.* 53: 297.

34 Chen, J., Miller, G.W. and Takemoto, J.Y. (1981), Biosynthesis of δ-aminolevulinic acid in *Rhodopseudomonas spaeroides. Arch. Biochem. Biophys.* 208: 221–228.

35 Rebeiz, C.A., Montazer-Zouhoor, A., Hopen, H.J. and Wu, S.M. (1984), Photodynamic herbicides: Concept and phenomenology. *Enzyme and Microbial Technology* 6: 390–401.

36 Rebeiz, C.A., Gut, L.J., Lee, K., Juvik, J.A., Rebeiz, C.C. and Bouton, C.E. (1995), Photodynamics of porphyric insecticides. *Crit. Rev. Plant Sci.* 14: 329–366.

37 Bedwell, J., McRoberts, A.J., Phillips, D. and Brown, S.G. (1992), Fluorescence distribution and photodynamic effect of ALA-induced PP IX in the DMF rat colonic tumor model. *Br. J. Cancer* 65: 818–824.

38 MacDonald, S.F. (1974), Methyl 5-bromolevulinate. *Can. J. Chem.* 52: 3257–3258.

39 Ha, H.-J., Lee, S.-K., Ha, Y.-J. and Park, J.-W. (1994), Selective bromination of ketones. A convenient synthesis of 5-aminolevulinic acid. *Synth. Commun.* 24: 2557–2562.

40 Lucas, S.V., Loehr, D.A., Meyer, M.aE. and Thomas, J.J. (1993), *Exhaust emissions and field trial results of a new, oxygenated, non-petroleum-based, waste-derived, gasoline blending component, 2-methyltetrahydrofuran.* Soc. Auto. Eng. Fuels and Lubricants Sect. Mtg., Philadelphia, PA.

41 DoE (1999), *10 CFR Part 490: Alternative Fuel Transportation Program; P-Series Fuels; Final Rule.* Office of Energy Efficiency and Renewable Energy, Department of Energy (DOE).

42 Bayan, S. and Beati, E. (1941), *Chemica e Industria* 23: 432–434.

43 Thomas, J.J. (1986), *Biomass Derived Levulinic Acid Derivatives and Their Use as Liquid Fuel Extenders.* Biomass Energy Dev. [Proc. South Biomass Energy Res. Conf.], Plenum.

44 Texaco/NYSERDA/Biofine (2000), *Ethyl Levulinate D-975 Diesel Additive Test Program,* Glenham, NY.

45 Elliott, D.C. (1999), *U.S. Patent 5,883,266*

46 Huang, C. and Wilson, D. (2000), *91st AOCS Annual Mtg., April 26th, 2000.*

47 Erner, W.E. (1982), *U.S. Patent 4,364,743*

48 Bizzari, S. and Ishikawa, Y. (2001), *CEH Report: Formic acid.* SRI, Menlo Park, CA.

49 Idriss, H., Lusvardi, V. S. and Barteau, M. A. (1996), Two routes to formaldehyde from formic acid on TiO$_2$(001) surface. *Surface Science* 348(1/2): 39–48.

50 Gravitis, J., Vedernikov, N., Zandersons, J. and Kokorevics, A. (2001), Furfural and levoglucosan production from deciduous wood and agricultural wastes. In: J. J. Bozell (eds), *Chemicals and Materials from Renewable Resources.* American Chemical Society, Washington DC, 110–122.

51 Levy, J. and Sakuma, Y. (2001), *CEH Report: Furfural.* SRI, Menlo Park, CA.

52 Rieche, A. (1964), *Outline of Industrial Organic Chemistry.* Butterworths, London.

53 Sutton, D., Kelleher, B. P. and Ross, J. R. H. (2001), Review of Literature on Catalysts for Biomass Gasification. *Fuel Processing Technology* 73(3): 155–173.

54 Bakkerud, P. K., Gol, J. N., Aasberg-Petersen, K. and Dybkjaer, I. (2004), Preferred Synthesis Gas Production Routes for GTL. (eds), *Studies in Surface Science and Catalysis.* Elsevier, New York, 147: 13–18.

55 Bao, X. and Xu, Y. (2004), *Natural Gas Conversion VII*, Studies in Surface Science and Catalysis, 147. Elsevier, New York.

56 Seaworthy Systems Inc. (1997), SSI Report #403-01-01.

Whole Crop Biorefinery

8
A Whole Crop Biorefinery System:
A Closed System for the Manufacture of Non-food Products from Cereals

Apostolis A. Koutinas, Rouhang Wang, Grant M. Campbell, and Colin Webb

8.1
Introduction

Selection of the appropriate renewable raw material to supply sustainable processes is dependent on infrastructural, economical and technological factors (e.g. availability, skilled workforce, pretreatment technology and costs, transportation). Cereals meet most of these prerequisites and have the potential to be used for the production of not only traditional foods but also novel functional foods and non-food products (e.g. biodegradable plastics, chemicals, fuels). However, cereal-based processes are currently more expensive than petroleum-based ones. The reduction of processing costs is strongly dependent on restructuring, integrating and optimizing current processes. To achieve this, the introduction of contemporary low-cost unit operations, the reduction of utilities costs and capital investment, and the creation of added-value byproducts in line with core end-products is imperative. The starting point would be to evaluate current cereal fractionation processes as the basis for a biorefinery and to identify focus areas for optimization, operating/capital cost reduction and end-product/byproduct production.

The concept of the whole crop biorefinery is inextricably linked to cereals as one of the most energy intense and chemically rich groups of agricultural crops. Cereals are also amongst the most developed crops having been progressively 'improved' throughout the past 10 000 years. They have been continuously optimized in terms of yield, with many now exceeding 10 tonnes per hectare. However, it is still the case that for every tonne of readily processable, starch-rich cer-

Biorefineries – Industrial Processes and Products. Status Quo and Future Directions. Vol. 1
Edited by Birgit Kamm, Patrick R. Gruber, Michael Kamm
Copyright © 2006 WILEY-VCH Verlag GmbH & Co. KGaA, Weinheim
ISBN: 3-527-31027-4

eal grain there is approximately another tonne of rather less accessible lignocel-lulosic material such as straw and other residues. How to deal with this material is one of the prime challenges of the whole crop biorefinery. Not only is there less to be had from the straw component of the crop than from the grain but it is also more difficult to get at; requiring tedious and often costly preprocessing. In addition, there is a major impediment to transportation of this fraction of the crop because it has a bulk density of only about a fifteenth of that of the grain, thereby requiring vastly more voluminous vehicles to move it around.

Ideally, of course, the whole crop biorefinery would involve harvesting the whole of the crop and transporting it directly to the refinery where fractionation would begin. Unfortunately, this is unlikely to be the reality and the more prag-matic approach of separation in the field followed by utilization of the straw as a primary energy source, through combustion, or incorporation into building composites, is more likely to prevail for some time to come. It must also be conceded that traditional outlets for straw such as re-incorporation into the soil, animal feed, and animal bedding, will continue to be "first call" uses in the fore-seeable future [1]. Thus one of the principal conclusions of a European study to determine the profitability of a wholecrop biorefinery [2] was that "*Combine har-vesting with grain processing in a biorefinery is more profitable than wholecrop.*" In view of these observations, this chapter will consider the biorefinery concept as one in which on-site separation of grain is carried out prior to fractionation and conversion of the whole grains at a remote site. Should it become feasible to process straw and other residues alongside the grain, such processing could readily be integrated within the biorefinery.

Current cereal fractionation processes (CFP) break down the grain into macro and micro components that are used either as end-products (e.g. gluten, oil) or as raw materials (e.g. starch) for secondary processing in many industries (e.g. food, pharmaceuticals, textiles, cosmetics, fermentation). The term macro com-ponent incorporates any high molecular weight compound (e.g. starch, protein, cellulose, hemicellulose, oil, gums), while micro components are defined as rel-atively low molecular weight molecules (e.g. lipids, vitamins, minerals). Tradi-tional CFP can be categorized into dry and wet milling operations. Dry milling involves the use of successive grinding and sieving steps aiming at the maxi-mum economic separation of bran from endosperm. Dry milling operations are relatively inexpensive and result in incomplete macro component separation. Wet CFP can be generally categorized into wet–aqueous and wet–nonaqueous processes resulting in selective separation of one or more cereal components. Wet fractionation processes could be applied to the end-products of a primary dry milling operation.

Traditional CFP have been developed to suit the needs of the food industry and do not exploit the potential of cereal grains for non-food applications. The development of viable whole-crop biorefineries depends on the constructive inte-gration of physical, chemical, thermal and biological processing resulting in var-ious products, such as functional proteins, oils, antioxidants, polysaccharides, fine and bulk chemicals, biofuels and biodegradable plastics. Novel cereal fractionation plants could be of three kinds depending on their production capacity:

- Small-scale plants that will not focus directly on the market outlets of the traditional cereal processing plants but will target specialty industries (e.g. cosmetics, pharmaceuticals) by extracting value-added minor constituents (e.g. antioxidants). Such plants will utilize only one cereal grain and will leave the majority of the raw material unprocessed, creating the need to find market outlets for this bulk quantity of material. The use of the remaining material for the production of fine or platform chemicals through microbial bioconversion would be an attractive option.
- Intermediate-scale plants may have wider flexibility in terms of the cereal grains that they can process. They will be able to market more end-products. Their commercial survival though will be dependent on continuous research and development and process improvements.
- Large-scale plants would be able to utilize any cereal grain for the simultaneous commercialization of traditional end-products, value-added minor components as well as biofuels and biodegradable plastics. Extensive technical and market research should certify high efficiency, cost-competitiveness and customer demand for all the end-products.

In this chapter, potential whole-crop biorefineries based on wheat and oats are presented. Future biorefineries based on cereals should aim to exploit the vast complexity of cereal grains by extracting valuable macro and micro components and converting the starch fraction into platform chemicals, biodegradable plastics and biofuels via microbial bioconversions. This approach targets waste and cost reductions and the creation of more market outlets.

8.2
Biorefineries Based on Wheat

8.2.1
Wheat Structure and Composition

The structure of the wheat grain consists of several layers with varying composition and functions (Fig. 8.1 and Table 8.1). The two main parts of the kernel are the pericarp and the seed. The pericarp covers the entire wheat kernel and is divided into the outer and the inner pericarp. Beneath the inner pericarp, the seed coat and the pigment strand provide a complete covering around the seed. The nucellar epidermis and the nucellar projection are located underneath the seed coat and surround the endosperm and embryo. One of the most nutritionally important wheat layers, the aleurone layer, is situated below the nucellar tissues. This is a one-cell-thick layer that encompasses the entire endosperm and part of the embryo. The embryo lies on the lower dorsal side of the wheat kernel and its two major components are the embryonic axis and the scutellum.

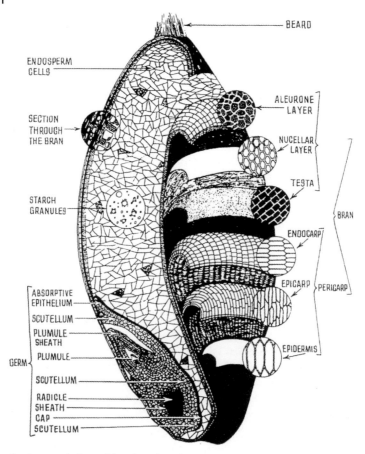

Fig. 8.1 Morphology of the wheat kernel [3].

Table 8.1 Wheat nutrients and their location in the kernel.

Constituent		Function	Mass[a)]	Composition
Pericarp			5	
Seed coat, pigment strand and nucellus	Bran	Protect the grain	3	Fiber, K, P, Mg, Ca
Aleurone layer		Encases endosperm	7	Niacin, phytic acid, minerals (especially P)
Endosperm		Stores food	82	Starch, protein, pantothenic acid, B_2, minerals
Embryo		Root and shoot	1	Fats, lipids, sugars
Scutellum		Stores food	2	P, B vitamins (especially thiamine)

a) Mass fraction of the constituent within the kernel as % on a dry basis (db)

The scutellum is a storage organ that is considered a cotyledon. The embryo, known as germ to a miller, when separated by traditional milling processes, consists principally of the embryonic axis.

A detailed analysis of the chemical composition of wheat grain is given by Pomeranz [4] and MacMasters et al. [5]. Each wheat layer has a unique composition in certain micro and/or macro components. In addition, wheat chemical composition and distribution in grain varies between varieties. The average chemical composition of pericarp is crude fiber (20–21%), cellulose (23.5–24%), and arabinoxylan (25–28%). Small amounts of protein (2.5–4%) and fat (<1%) are also present. In comparison with the pericarp, the seed coat contains much more protein (10–17%), less arabinoxylan (12–13.5%), much less crude fiber (ca. 1.0%), and no cellulose. The aleurone layer contains high levels of total phosphorus (2.7%), phytate phosphorus (2.4%), and niacin (B3) (530–640 $\mu g\ g^{-1}$). The niacin in the aleurone layer represents about 80% of the total amount in the entire grain. Pyridoxine (B_2) occurs in a pattern similar to that of niacin, with over 60% of all pyridoxine in the aleurone layer (30 $\mu g\ g^{-1}$). The aleurone layer is also an important contributor of pantothenic acid (B_5), containing more than 40% of the total in the wheat grain (40 $\mu g\ g^{-1}$) [6]. Total free sugar accounts for 10% of the aleurone materials, including sucrose 42%, raffinose 31%, neokestose 20%, and fructosyl raffinose 6% [7]. Monosaccharides, disaccharides (maltose) and higher oligosaccharides which occur in other parts of the grain are absent from the aleurone cells. The content of total lipids in aleurone cells accounts for between 8 and 11% [8], of which 70–80% are nonpolar.

Endosperm contains mainly starch (55–65%) and protein (7–11%). Peripheral cells have the lowest starch content and the highest protein content. Values as high as 54% protein have been found in subaleurone cells [9]. The main constituents of endosperm cell walls include polysaccharides (75%) and protein (15%). Arabinoxylan contributes 85% of the total polysaccharide content in endosperm cell walls and β-glucan and β-glucomannan account for the remainder in equal amounts [10]. Non-starch lipids and starch lipids contribute nearly evenly to the 1.5–2.5% total lipids in wheat endosperm. Wheat germ is rich in lipids (25–30%), protein (21–23%), phosphorus (3%) and B vitamins including B1, B2, B3, B5, B6. Sucrose (10%) and raffinose (7%) are the two sugars abundant in wheat germ and no substantial amount of the other oligosaccharides has been located.

8.2.2
Secondary Processing of Wheat Flour Milling Byproducts

In the traditional wheat flour milling process, wheat is milled into various flour fractions involving a large number of milling and sifting operations developed originally to serve the needs of the food industry. In particular, wheat grains are initially cleaned from impurities and tempered with water for an average of 12 hours to detach the outer bran layers from the endosperm, facilitating their separation. The tempered grains are subsequently processed through a series of break and reduction roller mills and sifting stages. The main aim of the conventional dry milling process is to produce flour fractions with the lowest possible bran impurities. However, the nature of this process will never produce any flour fraction 100% free from germ and bran. Current wheat flour mills operate at 70–80% grain to flour conversion efficiency where the remaining 20–30% constitutes various byproduct streams that contain predominantly bran as well as lower amounts of germ and flour. The byproduct streams are mixtures of all coarse streams from each break and reduction roll and are usually used as animal feeds or commercial bran.

As a whole, the dry milling process of wheat produces many flour streams of varying particle sizes and compositions in endosperm, bran and germ. This means that the separation of certain wheat layers enriched in specific value-added chemical components is not possible. This way of processing results in high capital investment, high operating costs for milling, conveying and sifting, and products of low purity. Thus, traditional dry milling of wheat cannot be considered as the basis for the development of a viable biorefinery for non-food applications.

The most realistic option to use traditional mills for non-food applications is through bioconversion of the significant amounts of byproduct produced. In 1999/2000, 5624×10^3 tonnes of wheat (83% of which was home grown) was processed by UK flour millers resulting in 4481×10^3 tonnes of flour and 1148×10^3 tonnes of byproducts. The majority of this byproduct stream, known as wheatfeed or middlings, contains 15–19% protein (75% of which is degradable), 20–35% starch and around 1% phosphorus. However, the high crude fiber content (7–11%), low essential amino acid content (0.6% Lys, 0.5% Thr, 0.2% Try, 0.4% Met) and the presence of phytic acid (containing about 60–80% of the total phosphorus) reduce its nutritional value. Consequently, its use as animal feed is restricted only to pigs and cattle. Phytic acid, in particular, has been identified as a certain antinutritional compound that forms complexes with iron and zinc ions and makes these metal ions less accessible for assimilation by humans and other monogastric animals [11]. Nonruminants excrete most of it as they do not have an efficient system for making phosphate available from phytate. This forces producers to add inorganic phosphate to animal feed as a supplement, leading to excessive phosphate excretion, which worsens water pollution and eutrophication [12]. The addition of enzyme preparations such as phytase, xylanase and protease could increase the overall digestibility of flour milling byproducts, allowing animals to consume phosphorus from the phytic acid and better assimilate the iron and zinc ions. For this reason, the animal feed industry is currently developing large-scale enzyme applications [12].

The development of an integrated biorefinery that leads to the production of high quality wheat flour and upgrades the byproduct stream into a nutrient-enriched animal feed and value-added chemicals through microbial bioconversions is an attractive option. Figure 8.2 shows such a process based around the bioproduction of succinic acid as a major potential platform chemical. The byproducts from a traditional wheat flour mill could be treated with successive washing and screening stages to separate the majority of starch and some of the pro-

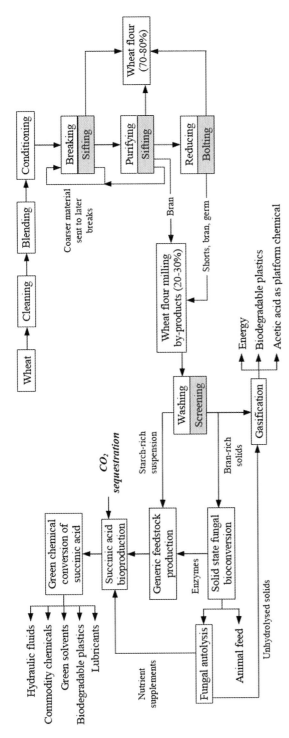

Fig. 8.2 Schematic diagram of a possible biorefinery utilizing traditional wheat flour milling byproducts.

tein, as well as other soluble nutrients. The starch-rich suspension would be used for production of the bioconversion feedstock, while bran will be used in fungal solid state bioprocessing (SSB) for enzyme production. The crude enzymatic mixture produced by SSB would be used to hydrolyze wheat macromolecules (e.g. starch, protein) contained in the starch-rich suspension. In-situ production of enzymes through SSB would reduce operating costs by eliminating the purchase of unnecessarily purified commercial enzymatic solutions. SSB would also provide a potential use for residual solids as a value-added animal feed, enhanced by the presence of enzymes that increase digestibility and fungal cells that contain high levels of essential amino acids (3.3% Lys, 2.82% Thr, 1.18% Try, 1.46% Met) [13, 14]. The solids could also be used for the production of nutrient supplements similar to yeast extracts by exploiting the natural degradation of fungal hyphae via the excretion of autolytic enzymes under oxygen limiting conditions [15]. Optimization of bran utilization for enzyme production could lead to the exploitation of the excess bran as raw material for gasification. The synthesis gas produced in this way could be used either for energy production to minimize the non-renewable energy requirements for the whole process or as crude feedstock for the production of value-added chemicals via microbial bioconversion or chemical synthesis.

The generic nature of the microbial feedstock produced from wheat flour milling byproducts can be used in various microbial bioconversions for the production of value-added chemicals. This specific biorefinery should target the production of low-to-medium volume and medium-to-high value chemicals because of the relatively small amount of raw materials (milling byproducts contain 20–35% starch) available for microbial bioconversion. It should be taken into consideration that the main activity of this biorefinery is the production of wheat flour, while only an average of 25% of the initial grain will be used for non-food applications. In the case of high-volume, low-value chemicals, fuels and plastics, economies of scale apply and small plants are not profitable. However, an economic analysis is necessary as the revenue derived from the primary market outlet may lead to the creation of an overall viable biorefinery even for commodity materials.

For this biorefinery, a potential market opportunity could be the production of succinic acid, which has the potential to be a future intermediate molecule for the production of a wide variety of commodities and specialties [16]. Succinic acid is currently produced petrochemically; maleic anhydride produced via butane oxidation is hydrated to maleic acid and then hydrogenated to succinic acid. Global production via this route exceeds 15,000 tonnes per annum. At a selling price between \$ 6–8.8 kg^{-1}, succinic acid is a valuable commodity, but is too expensive to be considered a feasible bulk chemical [16]. A preliminary material balance based on reaction stoichiometries (eqs 1–3) demonstrates the potential commercial and environmental impact of using wheat flour milling byproducts as the raw material for succinic acid production:

$$[C_6H_{10}O_5]_n + nH_2O \ \rightarrow \ nC_6H_{12}O_6 \tag{1}$$

$$C_6H_{12}O_6 + 2CO_2 + 4[H] \ \rightarrow \ 2C_4H_6O_4 + 2H_2O \tag{2}$$

$$C_6H_{12}O_6 \ \rightarrow \ 2C_2H_5OH + 2CO_2 \tag{3}$$

The total amount of wheat flour milling byproducts (1.1×10^6 tonnes) available per annum in the UK contains on average 30% starch, i.e. equivalent to 3.66×10^5 tonnes of glucose (eq. 1). The theoretical yield from glucose to succinic acid is 1.31 kg acid kg^{-1} glucose (eq. 2), giving a theoretical maximum of 4.8×10^5 tonnes succinic acid per annum for the UK. This is far greater than the current world production of 1.5×10^4 tonnes. At the same time, succinic acid production would result in 1.8×10^5 tonnes per annum CO_2 sequestration (eq. 2) because mass production of the acid requires CO_2 fixation in the metabolism of the microorganism involved. This is equivalent to the CO_2 released from the production of 2.4×10^5 tonnes of bioethanol (eq. 3). In addition, current bioprocessing practices could reduce the succinic acid production cost to lower than $ 0.6 kg^{-1} [17]. Thus, by utilizing a low-cost agro-industrial raw material succinic acid could be transformed into a low-cost platform intermediate. Such alternative use of wheat flour milling byproducts would also give flexibility to farmers and industrialists in exploring new market opportunities.

8.2.3
Advanced Wheat Separation Processes for Food and Non-food Applications

Traditional wheat processing for food (excluding breadmaking) and non-food applications concentrates mainly on the extraction of the bulk macromolecules, starch and gluten. However, the extraction of a number of value-added components from individual wheat layers could upgrade wheat processing into a novel whole-crop biorefinery producing both low-volume, high-value and high-volume, low-value products. In recent years, there has been a growing interest in the utilization of advanced cereal fractionation technologies to reduce operating/capital costs and to separate/purify value-added macro and micro components from cereal grains. The desired functional component may be concentrated in a particular layer in the cereal grain (e.g. aleurone layer, pericarp, germ). For this reason, novel CFP involve the selective separation of the outer bran layers including the aleurone layer and the germ.

8.2.3.1 Pearling as an Advanced Cereal Fractionation Technology
In the 1990s, a new technology was commercialized for wheat dry milling, which involves gradual removal of the outer layers (e.g. pericarp, aleurone cells) of the wheat kernel as a means to increase wheat milling efficiency [18]. In this process, the wheat bran layers are removed sequentially by friction and abrasion operations, while the byproducts of pearling hold great promise as novel food

ingredients with physicochemical and nutritional properties that differ from those of previously available cereal products [18, 19]. There are a number of pearling devices for sequential removal of cereal outer layers [20–22]. Wheat pearling can be used as a preprocessing stage before conventional dry milling or non-food applications.

The Tkac and the PeriTec model Satake VBW5A pearling systems have been presented in a previous publication [18]. The fourth generation Satake pearling system VCW5A is presented in Fig. 8.3 [23]. Wheat is fed to the top of the pearling equipment into the abrasion chamber where the wheat kernels are evenly distributed by a rotating scroll. The abrasion chamber contains abrasive wheels, a slotted screen and four vertically adjusted resistance bars. The wheat kernels are rubbed between the abrasive wheels and the resistance bars resulting in the removal of the outer kernel layers. The bran is collected through the slotted screen by an air stream that is blown through the holes of a hollow central shaft. The degree of debranning in the abrasion chamber is set by a weighted flap on the outlet of the chamber. The partly pearled wheat kernels are transferred through a screw conveyor into the friction chamber. This section contains a cast steel cylinder with two vertical agitator bars on it, which rotates around a slotted screen. The wheat kernels are further debranned by rubbing against the slotted screen. The friction stage is efficient only when the tough and oily testa

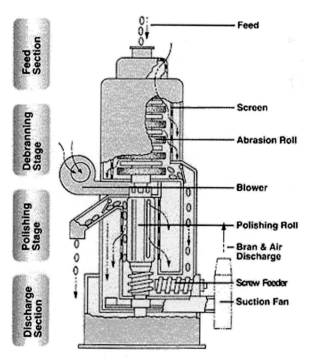

Fig. 8.3 The Satake VCW5A debranning apparatus.

layer has been disrupted during the abrasion stage. The bran separated during the friction stage is removed through the screen by an air stream blown into the center of the chamber via a perforated main shaft.

Research and commercial implementation of pearling has revealed the numerous potential uses of this advanced CFP. When pearling is used prior to conventional milling, it can improve flour quality and reduce operating costs [24]. The application of pearling can lead to the production of bran-rich streams that can be used as food ingredients. Cui et al. [19] reported that non-starch polysaccharides (NSP) from a wheat bran fraction produced by the Tkac and Timm pearling technology exhibited novel rheological properties. The NSP extracted from a pearling fraction that contained 13.4% starch, 29.2% insoluble dietary fiber, 8.5% soluble dietary fiber and 2.6% β-glucan, exhibited shear-thinning flow behavior at low concentrations in water (0.5%, 25 °C) and formed a thermally reversible gel upon cooling at 4 °C [19].

The bran-rich fractions produced by pearling are also rich in value-added components (e.g. antioxidants, β-glucan) in comparison to the bran-rich fractions produced from conventional milling operations. This occurs because the latter contain higher quantities of starchy endosperm, diluting the overall amounts of added-value components [25]. In the case of wheat, Dexter and Wood [18] used the Tkac debranning system, which produced friction fractions rich in pericarp and enriched in dietary fiber, while the abrasion fractions were rich in aleurone cells and enriched in protein, β-glucan and soluble fiber in comparison to whole wheat. Marconi et al. [26] used barley pearlings enriched in β-glucan and dietary fiber for the production of functional pastas with the aim of meeting the Food and Drug Administration (FDA) requirements of 5 g of dietary fiber and 0.75 g of β-glucan per serving (56 g in the US and 80 g in Italy). It has been reported that pearling fractions from oats may contain significant quantities of specific antioxidants [27]. It has also been reported that by-products that are produced from the pearling stage prior to dry milling of barley are enriched in β-glucans, tocopherols, and tocotrienols [28]. Cereal constituents with antioxidant properties can be used in pharmaceutical and cosmetic applications.

Using pearling before wheat milling could also lead to increased gluten extraction yield from pearled wheat grains [29]. The gluten extraction yield from ground, pearled wheat (11.4% of bran and germ was removed during pearling) was 20–25% higher than from conventionally milled flour in a process achieving 70% extraction of flour from wheat.

Apart from milling operations that produce flour streams for food, pharmaceutical and cosmetic purposes, the usefulness of pearling has also been recognized in the case of non-food applications. Wang et al. [30] used whole grain flour and pearled grain flour as fermentation medium for bioethanol production and the latter increased ethanol yields by 6.5–22.5%. This occurred because the use of pearling reduced the bran content in the fermentation feedstock, while at the same time the starch throughput per batch increased by an average of 12% (w/v, db). By integrating the grain pearling technology in rye and triticale with very high gravity fermentations (0.30 g solids mL^{-1} supernatant) the ethanol concentration was increased to around 16% (v/v) [31]. Partial removal of outer grain solids in an alcohol plant would also improve plant efficiency and decrease energy requirements for mash heating, mash cooling and ethanol distillation. In addition, the bran byproduct fractions containing pure grain layers or mixtures of them may be used as functional food ingredients or as raw materials to extract value-added products (e.g. enzymes, phytic acid, tocopherols, oil, proteins, wheat germ glycerides, agglutinin, arabinoxylans, β-glucan), contributing significant revenue for the development of cost-competitive biorefineries.

8.2.3.2 Air Classification

Air classifiers are rotary machines that are used in dry milling operations to separate a particulate feed into a fine and coarse fraction, using mainly air to entrain the fine product and a rotor to reject any airborne coarser particles [32]. The application of air classification in dry CFP can lead to the enrichment of milling fractions with specific components. The main advantage of air classification is that the procedure can easily be scaled up using a commercially available large air classifier without the clogging of screens by fine particles in a sieving method [33].

Letang et al. [34] reported that the combination of jet milling with air classification of soft wheat could produce a starch-enriched stream with only 2% protein content and reduced lipid and pentosan contents. Wu and Doehlert [33] enhanced the β-glucan content (200 g kg^{-1}) in oat bran fractions by applying a combination of pin milling, air classification and sieving. Similar results were obtained when air classification was applied to enrich the β-glucan content in milled fractions of barley [35] and oat groats [36].

8.2.4
Biorefinery Based on Novel Dry Fractionation Processes of Wheat

A potential wheat-based biorefinery (Fig. 8.4) could utilize a pearling system to produce a bran-rich fraction containing pericarp, seed coat, aleurone cells and germ layers from the wheat kernel. This fraction could be significantly enriched in bran by separating flour particles for further processing by the application of air classification. The bran-enriched fraction could be then used for the production of various coproducts, including natural polymers (e.g. arabinoxylans, β-glucans), monomers (e.g. glucose, xylose, arabinose, ferulic acid) or oil components (e.g. triglycerides, sterols). The selection of coproducts that will be eventually derived from the bran-rich fraction would be dependent on process economics, available technologies and existence of markets for their disposal.

Pearled wheat grains could be ground in a hammer mill and the resulting bran-free flour could be used for gluten extraction by the Martin, the Batter or a modified version of these processing schemes. The bran-free and gluten-free flour suspension resulting from the gluten extraction stage could be used for

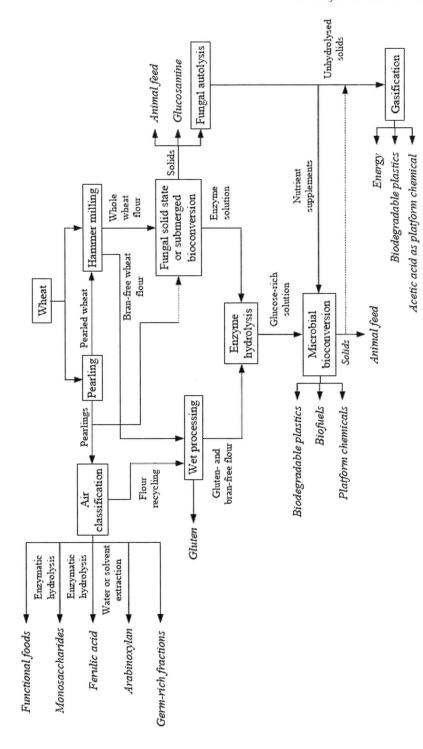

Fig. 8.4 Schematic diagram of a wheat-based biorefinery employing pearling and air classification.

the production of a glucose-rich solution to provide the carbon and energy source in subsequent microbial bioconversions. The enzymes required to hydrolyze this stream could be produced by submerged or solid state fungal bioconversions on whole wheat flour and pearlings, respectively. Remaining fermentation solids could be used as animal feed, glucosamine/N-acetyl-D-glucosamine extraction or for the production of nutrient supplements by exploiting fungal autolysis that occurs under oxygen-limiting conditions. Unhydrolyzed solids could be gasified for the production of energy or other value-added products. The generic feedstock formulated by mixing the glucose-rich solution with nutrient supplements produced by fungal autolysis can be used in microbial bioconversions for the production of biofuels, platform chemicals and biodegradable plastics.

8.2.4.1 Potential Value-added Byproducts from Wheat Bran-rich Fractions

Arabinoxylans Wheat bran and especially the aleurone layer contain high amounts of arabinoxylans and lower quantities of β-glucans. Arabinoxylan is a polysaccharide comprised of a backbone formed by xylose residues connected together with β-$(1 \rightarrow 4)$ bonds. The xylose residues are highly substituted with primarily single a-$(1 \rightarrow 3)$ and/or a-$(1 \rightarrow 2)$-linked L-arabinose residues as well as short arabinooligosaccharides, D-galactose, D-4-O-methylglucuronic acid and ferulic acid residues.

Phenolic acids, such as ferulic acid, play a significant role in the linkage of hemicelluloses with other cell wall components, especially lignin, through ester and ether bonds [37]. In addition, ferulic acid assists in the formation of covalently crosslinked arabinoxylans with well developed networks that exert an interesting water-holding capacity [38]. Different concentrations of ferulic acids would correspond to varying gelling potential of arabinoxylans. Arabinoxylan properties in solution are also dependent on the degree of polymerization of the xylan backbone.

The use of enzymatic oxidizing systems such as laccase, horseradish peroxidase or manganese peroxidase could dimerize the esterified ferulic acids causing gelation of the water-extractable arabinoxylans from wheat flour [39]. The high viscosity of aqueous solutions containing water-extractable arabinoxylans that have undergone oxidative gelation after they were treated with laccase and/or manganese peroxidase has a positive effect in breadmaking [40]. In particular, water-soluble arabinoxylans can absorb water, influence dough rheology and affect such bread characteristics as loaf volume, crumb firmness and staling events [41]. Arabinoxylans could also be potential ingredients for wound-care applications [42]. Sterigel is an arabinoxylan-based product that is used as wound management aid.

Ferulic Acid Ferulic acid could be released from bran-rich fractions by the synergistic action of various enzymes, such as esterase and xylanase [43]. Extraction of arabinoxylans located at the outer bran layers, seed coat and pericarp, may be more difficult than the ones located in the aleurone and nucellar layers [44]. The aleurone-free wheat bran is more resistant to enzymatic hydrolysis because it contains higher amounts of lignin, cellulose and glucuronoarabinoxylans than the aleurone layer. Increased crosslinking among cell wall components creates a rigid cell wall network and decreases the effectiveness of enzymatic hydrolysis.

Ferulic acid could be used as a natural food preservative due to its ability to inhibit peroxidation of fatty acids. The acid and its derivatives, steryl ferulates, have antioxidant properties. A commercial product, γ-oryzanol, with cholesterol lowering properties containing steryl ferulates has been extracted from rice bran [45]. Wheat bran fractions may contain up to 0.34 mg g^{-1} total steryl ferulates, which is significantly higher that the 0.063 mg g^{-1} content in the whole wheat grain [45]. Ferulic acid is currently used as an ingredient in many skin lotions, sunscreens and wound dressings [43]. The antioxidant potential of ferulic acid could be enhanced by converting it enzymatically into cafeic acid by using a microbial cell extract from the anaerobic bacterium *Clostridium methoxybenzovorans* SR3 [46]. Another commercial option is the bioconversion of ferulic acid into vanillin by *Streptomyces setonii*. Muheim and Lerch [47] reported that shake flask cultures of *S. setonii* resulted in the production of 6 g L^{-1} vanillin at a molar conversion yield from ferulic acid to vanillin of 68%.

Hwang et al. [48] patented a process separating ferulic acid and arabinoxylan from cereal brans by extrusion and subsequent treatment with plant cell wall hydrolyzing enzymes.

Wheat Germ   Most wheat germ currently produced by flour mills is used as animal feed contributing a very low revenue. Wheat germ could be upgraded into a useful byproduct if it is used for the extraction of various value-added materials, such as proteins, oils, vitamins and enzymes [24]. Oil extraction could be achieved simply by mechanical pressure or solvent extraction. The germ oil could be used as a specialty food or gourmet cooking oil. A commercial application of oil extracts has been introduced by the French company Bertin, which extracts these oils by cold pressing at 4,000 bars in sunflower oil as solvent [49]. The purified wheat germ oil (10^4 kg year^{-1}) is called heliogerme and is sold as an ingredient in cosmetics at a price ranging between £ 5–8 kg^{-1}. In the case that wheat germ is processed by solvent extraction, the functional properties of germ protein are retained enabling its commercialization as food grade protein. The extraction of micro components (e.g. enzymes, vitamins, flavonoids) from wheat germ may open additional market opportunities but additional research and market/process evaluation is required [24].

The bran-rich fraction produced by wheat pearling would contain a large amount, if not all, of the wheat germ. Thus, the utilization of the pearling technology in a wheat biorefinery may decrease the cost currently required by traditional flour mills to isolate the wheat germ fraction.

Monosaccharide Production Another potential market outlet would be the fractionation of pearlings into oil components and polysaccharides, which can be subsequently converted enzymatically into a spectrum of monomers, the most important of which would be glucose, xylose, arabinose and ferulic acid. The monosaccharides could be either utilized as a carbon source in microbial bioprocesses or converted catalytically into various chemicals currently derived from petrochemicals. For instance, glucose could be hydrogenated to sorbitol, which in turn could be catalytically converted to propylene glycol. Xylene and arabinose could also be catalytically converted to ethylene glycol, propylene glycol and xylitol.

Functional Foods Supplementation of human diets with wheat bran may enhance the prevention of a range of cancers due to the presence of various functional components, such as dietary fiber, phytic acid, lignans, oligosaccharides, antioxidants, phytoestrogens [50]. Reddy et al. [51] reported that the lipid fraction of wheat bran has strong colon tumor inhibitory properties and further studies are required to identify biologically active constituents of wheat bran lipid fractions and their relative role in colon tumor inhibition. The insoluble dietary fiber content of wheat bran may be responsible for their significant bile acid binding properties that cause decrease in the plasma cholesterol level in humans [52]. In turn, Cui et al. [19] reported that bran-rich fractions enriched in soluble fiber could be superior to AACC standard wheat bran, which contains 46.85% insoluble fiber and 2.8% soluble fiber [19]. Pearling may be employed to produce bran-rich fractions enriched in either soluble or insoluble dietary fiber depending on the requirements of end-product composition.

Pearling could be exploited for the sequential removal of individual wheat layers. Fenech et al. [53] reported that pearling could lead to the production of an aleurone-rich fraction that contains high amounts ($5~\mu g~g^{-1}$) of folate. Bran- and germ-rich fractions produced by pearling could potentially be used to enrich the mineral content of pan breads [54]. In addition, the quality of wheat bread, in terms of loaf volume, crumb structure, shelf life, starch structure and flavor, can be significantly improved when it is supplemented with wheat bran pre-fermented with yeast and/or lactic acid bacteria [55].

8.2.4.2 Exploitation of the Pearled Wheat Kernel

Vital Wheat Gluten Pearled wheat kernels could be used for the extraction of vital wheat gluten as a valuable co-product. Gluten can be separated from wheat flour by mixing endosperm particles with water that initiates the formation of protein microfibrils. The formation of dough from the mixture of flour and water is dependent on the water to flour ratio used and mixing. The main processes for the separation of vital wheat gluten from flour (e.g. Posner, Alfa-Laval/Raisio, Hydrocyclone, Pillsbury Hydromilling, Far-Mar-Co., High-Pressure Disintegration) could be categorized into those based on either the Martin or the Batter process [56, 57]. Such processes utilize a spectrum of raw materials (e.g. wheat, flour), solvents, equipments and wheat flour to water ratio. Weight for weight, gluten is more valuable than starch and could therefore improve the economics of biorefineries based on wheat. In general, 10 tonnes of wheat will give 6–7 tonnes of starch and 1–1.5 tonnes of gluten. The major impediments in gluten separation processes are the operational effectiveness of processing, the high cost required for drying vital gluten and waste treatment costs.

Gluten has many applications particularly in the food industry, such as in bread-making, specialty baked goods, pet foods, breakfast cereals, meat and cheese sub-stitutes and pizza [57]. Other industrial uses include production of hydrolysates, wheat protein isolate and deaminated gluten. The gradual decrease of gluten price in the last 10 years has shown that a potential large-scale utilization of wheat for non-food applications will saturate the current gluten market reducing its current price even lower. Identifying novel uses for gluten could provide more commercial outlets and higher revenue for this value-added co-product. Gluten could be used for the production of biodegradable or edible films and packaging materials [58]. It could also be used for the manufacture of biodegradable high-performance engi-neering plastics and composites when thiol-terminated, star-branched molecules are incorporated directly into the protein structure [59].

Microbial Feedstock Production and Bioconversion Processes After gluten extrac-tion, the remaining aqueous suspension is rich in starch. Starch has many ap-plications in numerous industries such as paper sizing/coating, thickening/gel-ling agent in food applications, industrial glues and pastes, dusting agent, slip-ping agent in oil drilling, water retention agent, biodegradable plastics, building panels, cosmetic applications, encapsulating polymers, packing material, edible packaging and feedstock for fermentation processes. This study will concentrate on the utilization of starch as a raw material for the production of fuels, chemi-cals and plastics by microbial bioconversion. To produce a nutrient-complete medium for microbial fermentations, three steps are required (Fig. 8.4):
1. on-site enzyme production via submerged or solid state fermentations;
2. enzymatic hydrolysis of gluten-free and bran-free flour suspensions; and
3. production of nutrient supplements (fungal extract) via fungal autolysis.

In many existing microbial fermentations, commercial (purified) starch is enzy-matically hydrolyzed into directly assimilable glucose by unnecessarily pure commercial enzyme formulations. Cost reduction could be achieved by utilizing a much less refined process involving on-site production of crude enzyme mix-tures via fungal fermentations conducted by single or combined fungal strains belonging to the genus *Aspergilli* (*A. awamori*, *A. oryzae*). The medium for the fungal fermentations could be whole cereal flour or pearlings depending on the bioprocess employed, which might be carried out in submerged or solid state, respectively. The solid residue from the enzyme producing fermentation, which contains mainly fungal cells and any undigested wheat particles, could be con-verted into nutrient supplements via fungal cell autolysis. A similar process that generates a generic microbial feedstock from whole wheat is described and cost evaluated in previous publications [60–62].

The generic microbial feedstock can be used for the bioproduction of several organic chemicals, including platform intermediates for chemical synthesis, ingredients for a spectrum of commercial products, biofuels, biodegradable plastics and solvents. This process could lead to the production of both commodities and specialties depending on market outlets and cost competitiveness. Potential bioconversion products, the large-scale bioproduction of which have or will incur low environmental and high societal and industrial impacts are [16]:

1. lactic acid, succinic acid and 3-hydroxypropionic acid as platform molecules and industrial ingredients;
2. 1,3-propanediol as a monomer for the production of novel plastics;
3. butanol as platform molecule, solvent, industrial ingredient and biobased transport fuel;
4. PHA as biodegradable plastics;
5. bioethanol as a platform intermediate and biofuel;
6. L-lysine as animal feed additive and industrial ingredient.

Remaining solids from fungal fermentation could also be used as animal feed or for the extraction of value-added coproducts, such as glucosamine and N-acetyl-D-glucosamine. The fungal cell walls contain chitin, which is an unbranched homopolymer of N-acetyl-D-glucosamine. Bohlmann et al. [63] used enzymatic and chemical methods for the recovery of N-acetyl-D-glucosamine from fungal biomass (A. niger) that was produced from a citric acid fermentation. The efficient degradation of chitin and glucan required the synergistic action of chitinases, β-N-acetylglucosaminidases and glucanases. Fan et al. [64] have also used various fungal species (Aspergillus, Penicillium, Mucor) for the production of glucosamine. Fungal autolysis might evolve into an effective and economic processing route for releasing glucosamine or/and N-acetyl-D-glucosamine from fungal cell walls.

It is strongly believed that glucosamine provides joint health benefits and pain relief. The US National Institute of Health is currently conducting research in order to assess the effectiveness of glucosamine on patients with osteoarthritis. The US retail market for nutritional supplements containing glucosamine is more that $ 10^9$/year [65]. Demand for bulk glucosamine has been growing in excess of 20% annually and global consumption exceeds 5×10^6 kg [65]. Apart from glucosamine, N-acetylglucosamine is used as health supplement as well as in cosmetic and pharmaceutical applications.

Unhydrolyzed solids from the fungal autolysis stage and solids from the microbial bioconversion could be gasified at various combinations of high temperatures, pressures and oxygen for the production of synthesis gas that is constituted of various compositions of CO, CO_2, H_2 and CH_4 depending on the conditions applied. Synthesis gas can be subsequently used either for energy generation or biological/chemical conversion into a spectrum of chemicals. Potential bioderived products from synthesis gas are bioethanol [66], biodegradable plastics [67], acetic acid and methanol [16].

8.3
A Biorefinery Based on Oats

8.3.1
Oat Structure and Composition

Like all cereal grains, oats have a complex structure and constitution (Table 8.2). The oat groat, consisting of endosperm, germ and bran, is encompassed in a fibrous hull structure that contains approximately 50% hemicellulose, 40% crude cellulose and 10% crude lignin. The main sections of oat groats are the trichomes (hairs), pericarp, nucellar tissues, aleurone, endosperm, embryo and scutellum. The composition of each layer varies significantly. In addition, the location and concentration of components in oats depend upon cultivar and environmental conditions. The chemical composition of oat groats and respective layers has been given by Webster [68] and Wood [69].

8.3.2
Layout of a Potential Oat-based Fractionation Process

The high value of oat bran necessitates its separation prior to further processing of the rest of the grain. Figure 8.5 presents a schematic diagram of a proposed biorefinery based on oat groats, employing pearling and air classification. Significant information in the formulation of this processing scheme was taken from Paton et al. [70] who used pearling to remove outer oat layers (1–15% of the oat kernel). Pearlings were used to produce the following products:
1. a highly concentrated anti-irritant and a light oat oil extracted successively by a volatile aqueous polar solvent and a nonpolar solvent;
2. a dark high quality oil and a highly stable lipase-active powder extracted by a nonpolar solvent;

Table 8.2 Oat nutrients and their location in the kernel.

Constituent		Function	Mass[a]	Composition
Hull		Encases oat groat	30[b]	Fiber, some protein, some antioxidants
Pericarp		Protect the grain	–	Fiber, protein, antioxidants, K, P, Mg, Ca
Seed coat and nucellus	Bran		–	
Aleurone layer		Encases endosperm	–	Protein, β-glucan, niacin, antioxidants, lipids, phytin, aromatic amines, minerals (especially P)
Endosperm		Stores food	55–70[c]	Starch, protein, β-glucan, lipids, minerals
Embryo		Root and shoot	2.8–3.7[c]	Similar to bran excluding niacin and aromatic amines
Scutellum		Stores food		

a) Mass fraction of the constituent within the kernel as % on a dry basis (db)
b) Content as related to dry weight of the complete oat kernel (hulls plus groat)
c) Content as related to the dry weight of the oat groat

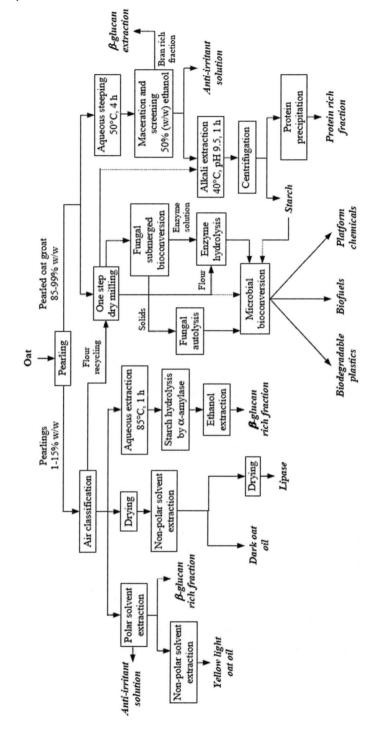

Fig. 8.5 Schematic diagram of a biorefinery based on oat groats employing pearling and air classification.

3. a β-glucan-rich fraction extracted by successive aqueous steeping of bran, starch removal by enzymatic hydrolysis, bran removal by screening/centrifugation and alcoholic extraction.

Pearled oat kernels could be either converted into a feedstock for subsequent microbial bioconversions or fractionated into various coproducts. Steeping the pearled oat groats in water would facilitate the maceration of bran and flour fractions accomplished by aqueous ethanol extraction. The bran fraction is used for the extraction of β-glucan, while the flour fraction is divided into starch and protein. From the remaining pearled oat groat extract, an oat anti-irritant can be recovered. Flour from pearled oat kernels or starch could be used in some fungal bioconversions for the production of chemicals without hydrolysis. For instance, *Rhizopus oryzae* can utilize starch for the production of lactic acid [71].

8.3.2.1 Potential Value-added Byproducts from Oat Bran-rich Fractions

Oat Gum: β-Glucan   β-Glucans are linear homopolysaccharides of glucose units linked via a mixture of $(1 \rightarrow 4)$- and $(1 \rightarrow 3)$-β-D-glycopyranosyl units. Water-soluble β-glucans have potential nutritional and health benefits. β-Glucan preparations exhibit blood serum cholesterol lowering capabilities when consumed daily [72]. A potential mechanism for β-glucan cholesterol lowering capability is their high molecular weight, which increases the luminal viscosity in the gastrointestinal tract [73]. Viscous water-soluble β-glucan preparations have hypoglycemic effects assisting in the metabolic control of diabetes [74]. It was recently reported that β-glucans could potentially be used in biomedical applications because of their abilities to:

1. activate host defense mechanisms against microbial and parasitic infections [75]; and
2. reduce the glycemic index, making them a useful food ingredient for decreasing postprandial glycemia while, at the same time, maintaining the food palatability [76].

Research has also focused on the investigation of the rheological properties of β-glucan extracts aiming at the creation of novel products for food purposes, such as stabilizers, thickeners, textural agents and fat replacers in food products, and medical as well as cosmetic applications [73]. In addition, oligosaccharides from β-glucan hydrolysis exhibit prebiotic properties and are considered as food ingredients in probiotic and synbiotic preparations.

Malkki and Virtanen [77] stressed that the health effects of β-glucans on cholesterol reduction, improved gastrointestinal function and glucose metabolism would require a daily consumption of 10 g oat β-glucan. This means that the daily digestion of adequate amounts of β-glucans requires consumption of substantial amounts of conventional oat products, which contain 35–50 g kg^{-1} β-glucan. Thus, the commercialization of concentrated oat bran products is necessary in order to provide consumers with the daily requirements for β-glucan. The presence of β-glucan in the pericarp, aleurone and sub-aleurone layers indicates that the application of a pearling technology would be ideal for the separation of β-glucan rich fractions [24]. However, distribution of β-glucan in the oat kernel is dependent on the oat cultivar used. Thus, oat cultivars should be screened so as to identify the ones that will provide β-glucan enriched fractions through pearling.

The market price, functional properties and concentration of β-glucan commercial preparations will be dependent on the final application and the fractionation process employed. For instance, purified β-glucan could reach a value of $ 55 kg^{-1}, while its use as thickening agent would compete with guar and xanthan gums, the market price of which is $ 0.78 kg^{-1} and $ 12 kg^{-1}, respectively [24].

Antioxidants Oats contain various compounds with antioxidant activities, such as tocols, phytic acid, phenolic acids, avenanthramides, flavonoids and sterols. A comprehensive review of these oat antioxidants has been published by [78]. Antioxidants are mainly located in the outer groat layers but each compound with antioxidant properties can be predominantly located in a specific outer layer, in the whole bran fraction or even in the hull. Some problems that are related to the extraction of antioxidants from cereal grains have to do with:

1. heat treatment to deactivate lipase prior to milling;
2. the localization of specific components with high antioxidant activities;
3. the production of cereal fractions containing botanical constituents enriched in antioxidants; and
4. the selection of analytical assays that can realistically measure the antioxidant activities of cereal fractions.

The selection of analytical assays is crucial in the detection of antioxidant activities because of the presence of both antioxidants and pro-oxidants in any cereal fraction and the fact that it measures the inhibition of oxidation of case-specific reactions depending on the combination of the various micro components with antioxidant properties [79].

Several researchers have shown that pearling could be an important tool in the production of bran-rich fractions enriched in compounds with antioxidant activities. Handelman et al. [25] fractionated oats by either pearling or conventional dry milling, with further enrichment by air classification to identify their antioxidant activities. Pearlings exhibited the highest antioxidant content in comparison to flour, trichome and bran fractions. Even the trichome fraction, that is the outer (hairy) surface of the groat, exhibited relatively high antioxidant activity. Peterson et al. [27] compared the antioxidant activity of bran-rich fractions produced through pearling for between 5 and 180 s, concluding that the antioxidant activity of 80% ethanol extract and the concentration of total phenolic compounds and specific phenolic acids (e.g. ferulic acid, *p*-coumaric acid) was higher in short-pearling-time fractions, and decreased at prolonged pearling times as more endosperm tissue was included. The results reported by Peterson et al. [27] about pearling fractions were reinforced by two other studies [79, 80].

The numerous functionalities of oat antioxidants including growth regulation, good emulsifying properties, defense against parasites, inhibition of oxidative degradation of unsaturated fatty acids, prevention of cardiovascular diseases, cholesterol lowering capabilities, prevention of specific cancers, and provision of color/aroma/stability/nutritional value in cereal food products, can impact many industries [27, 78]. Oil-rich fractions extracted from groats or oat bran could be used as emulsifiers or as ingredients in health foods, skin-care preparations, specialized food oils and pharmaceuticals [81].

8.4
Summary

This chapter presents some potential cereal-based biorefineries that can be employed for the production of fuels, chemicals and plastics, as well as many value-added byproducts derived from cereal bran. Cereals are complex biological entities and will represent a major category of the core photosynthetic raw materials that will replace petroleum in the production of commodities as well as specialties. The creation of viable biorefineries based on cereals will require the exploitation of all the botanical constituents of the grain as well as, if possible, the non-grain components such as straw, stalks and hulls. Novel processing routes for starch and protein in the production of a generic feedstock for microbial bioconversions have been presented and various products that could be derived from wheat and oats have been identified. The cost-competitiveness of such cereal-based biorefineries will depend on the range of high value end products and their integration with the much larger volume low to mid-value products, and could be further improved by exploiting straw, hulls and other non-grain components of the crop, either for the production of more value-added byproducts or simply for the generation of energy.

References

1 Morrison, R., Policy alternatives for the development of the cereal processing industry, A report issued from Winnipeg by Agriculture and Agri-Food Canada's Policy Branch under the Grains 2000 program, November, 1995.

2 Audsley, E. and Sells, J.E. Determining the profitability of a wholecrop biorefinery. In: Campbell GM, Webb C, McKee SL (eds) Cereals: Novel Uses and Processes, Plenum press, New York, pp 191–204.

3 Dobraszczyk, B.J. Wheat and flour. In D.A.V. Dendy and B.J. Dobraszczyk (Eds.), Cereals and cereal products: Chemistry and technology. Gaithersburg, MD: Aspen Publishers Inc. (1994) 100–139.

4 Pomeranz, Y. Chemical composition of kernel structures. In: Wheat: Chemistry and Technology. Vol. I. Pomeranz, Y. ed. AACC: St. Paul, Minnesota, USA (1988) pp. 97–158.

5 MacMasters, M. M., Hinton, J. J. C. and Bradbury, D. Microscopic structure and composition of the wheat kernel. In: Wheat: Chemistry and Technology, 2nd Ed. (1971) pp. 51–113.

6 Lintas, C. (1988). Durum wheat vitamins and minerals. In: Durum wheat: Chemistry and Technology. Fabriani, G. and Lintas, C. ed. AACC: St. Paul, Minnesota, USA (1988) pp. 149–160.

7 Stevens, D. J. Free sugars of wheat aleurone cells. Journal of Science in Food and Agriculture 21 (1970) pp. 31–34.

8 Hargin, K. D., Morrison, W. R. and Fulcher, R. G. Triglyceride deposits in the starchy endosperm of wheat. Cereal Chemistry 57 (1980) pp. 320–325.

9 Kent, N. L. Subaleurone endosperm cells of high protein content. Cereal Chemistry 43 (1966) pp. 585–601.

10 Mares, D. J., and Stone, B. A. Wheat endosperm. I. Chemical composition and ultrastructure of the cell walls. Australian Journal of Biological Sciences 26 (1973) pp. 793–812.

11 Kornegay, E. T. Digestion of phosphorus and other nutrients: The role of phytases and factors influencing their activity. In: Enzymes in farm animal nutrition. Bedford, M., Partridge, G. (eds). Finnfeeds International, UK (2001)

12 Abelson, P. H. A potential phosphate crisis. Science 283 (1999) 2015

13 Reade, A. E., Smith, R. H. and Palmer, R. M. Production of protein for nonruminant feeding by growing filamentous fungi on barley. Biochemical Journal 127 (1972) 32p

14 Reed, G. and Nagodawithana, T. Enzymes, Biomass, Food and Feed. Wiley-VCH, Weinheim, (2001) p. 174

15 Koutinas, A. A., Wang, R.-H. and Webb C. Development of a process for the production of nutrient supplements for fermentations based on fungal autolysis. Enzyme and Microbial Technology (in press)

16 Paster, M., Pellegrino, J. L. and Carole, T. M. Industrial bioproducts: Today and tomorrow. Energetics, Incorporated for the US Department of Energy, Office of Energy Efficiency and Renewable Energy, Office of the Biomass Program, Washington, DC (2003)

17 Zeikus, J. G., Jain, M. K., Elankovan, P. Biotechnology of succinic acid production and markets for derived industrial products. Applied Microbiology and Biotechnology 51 (1999) 545–552.

18 Dexter, J. E. and Wood, P. J. Recent applications of debranning of wheat before milling. Trends in Food Science and Technology 7 (1996) 35–41.

19 Cui, W., Wood, P. J., Weisz, J. and Beer, M. U. Nonstarch polysaccharides from preprocessed wheat bran: carbohydrate analysis and novel rheological properties. Cereal Chemistry 76 (1999) 129–133.

20 Tkac, J. J. Process for removing bran layers from wheat kernels. (1992) US Patent 5,082,680.

21 Wellman, W. Process for milling cereal grains. (1993) US Patent 5,186,968.

22 Satake, S., Ishii, T. and Tokui, Y. Vertical pearling machines and apparatus for preliminary treatment prior to flour milling using such pearling machines. (1995) US Patent 5,390,589.

23 Gills, J. M. and McGee, B. C. Advances in durum semolina milling. British Pasta Products Association, Technical Seminar, London (1999) http://www.satake-usa.com/brochures/Durum_ Milling_ Advances.pdf

24 Anonymous. Fractionation processes: Descriptions, merits and deficiencies. Agriculture and Agri-Food Canada, Threshold Technologies Company and POS Pilot Plant, CANUC Database (1995).

25 Handelman, G. J., Cao, G., Walter, M. F., Nightingale, Z. D., Paul, G. L., Prior, R. L. and Blumberg, J. B. Antioxidant capacity of oat (Avena sativa L.) extracts. 1. Inhibition of low-density lipoprotein oxidation and oxygen radical absorbance capacity. Journal of Agriculture and Food Chemistry 47 (1999) 4888–4893.

26 Marconi, E., Graziano, M. and Cubadda R. Composition and utilization of barley pearling byproducts for making functional pastas rich in dietary fiber and β-glucans. Cereal Chemistry 77 (2000) 133–139.

27 Peterson, D.M., Emmons, C.L. and Hibbs, A.H. Phenolic antioxidants and antioxidant activity in pearling fractions of oat groats. *Journal of Cereal Science* **33** (2001) 97–103.

28 Seog, H.-M., Seo, M.-S., Kim, Y.-S. and Lee, Y.-T. Physicochemical properties of barley bran, germ and broken kernel as pearling byproducts. *Food Science and Biotechnology* **11** (2002) 623–627.

29 Posner, E.S., Seib, P.A. and Qiang, Z. Process for dry milling of wheat to obtain gluten and starch. (1992) US Patent 5,164,013.

30 Wang, S., Sosulski, K., Sosulski, F. and Ingledew, M. Effect of sequential abrasion on starch composition of five cereals for ethanol fermentation. *Food Research International* **30** (1997) 603–609.

31 Wang, S. Thomas, K.C., Sosulski, K., Ingledew, W.M. and Sosulski, F.W. Grain pearling and very high gravity (VHG) fermentation technologies for fuel alcohol production from rye and triticale. *Process Biochemistry* **34** (1999) 421–428.

32 Klumpar, I.V. Measuring and optimizing air classifier performance. *Separations Technology* **2** (1992) 124–135.

33 Wu, Y.V. and Doehlert, D.C. Enrichment of β-glucan in oat bran by fine grinding and air classification. *Lebensmittel-Wissenschaft und Technologie* **35** (2002) 30–33.

34 Letang, C., Samson, M.-F., Lasserre, T.-M., Chaurand, M., Abecassis, J. Production of starch with very low protein content from soft and hard wheat flours by jet milling and air classification. *Cereal Chemistry* **79** (2002) 535–543.

35 Andersson, A.A.M., Andersson, R. and Aman, P. Air classification of barley flours. *Cereal Chemistry* **77** (2000) 463–467.

36 Wu, Y.V. and Stringfellow, A.C. Enriched protein and β-glucan fractions from high-protein oats by air classification. *Cereal Chemistry* **72** (1995) 132–134.

37 Saulnier, L., Vigouroux, J. and Thibault, J.-F. Isolation and partial characterization of feruloylated oligosaccharides from maize bran. *Carbohydrate Research* **272** (1995) 241–253.

38 Saulnier, L. and Thibault, J.-F. Ferulic acid and diferulic acids as components of sugar-beet pectins and maize bran heteroxylans. *Journal of the Science of Food and Agriculture* **79** (1999) 396–402.

39 Peyron, S., Abecassis, J., Autran, J.-C. and Rouau, X. Enzymatic oxidative treatments of wheat bran layers: Effects on ferulic acid composition and mechanical properties. *Journal of Agriculture and Food Chemistry* **49** (2001) 4694–4699.

40 Labat, E., Morel, M.H. and Rouau, X. Effect of laccase and manganese peroxidase on wheat gluten and pentosans during mixing. *Food Hydrocolloids* **15** (2001) 47–52.

41 Rattan, O., Izydorczyk, M.S. and Biliaderis, C.G. Structure and rheological behavior of arabinoxylans from Canadian bread wheat flours. *Food Science and Technology (London)* **27** (1994) 550–555.

42 Lloyd, L.L., Kennedy, J.F., Methacanona, P., Methacanon, P., Paterson, M. and Knill, C.J. Carbohydrate polymers as wound management aids. *Carbohydrate Polymers* **37** (1998) 315–322.

43 Sancho, A.I., Bartolome, B., Gomez-Cordoves, C., Williamson, G. and Faulds, C.B. Release of ferulic acid from cereal residues by barley enzymatic extracts. *Journal of Cereal Science* **34** (2001) 173–179.

44 Benamrouche, S., Cronier, D., Debeire, P. and Chabbert, B. A chemical and histological study on the effect of (1→4)-β-endo-xylanase treatment on wheat bran. *Journal of Cereal Science* **36** (2002) 253–260.

45 Hakala, P., Lampi, A.-M., Ollilainen, V., Werner, U., Murkovic, M., Wahala, K., Karkola, S. and Piironen, V. Steryl phenolic acid esters in cereals and their milling fractions. *Journal of Agriculture and Food Chemistry* **50** (2002) 5300–5307.

46 Micard, V., Landazuri, T., Surget, A., Moukha, S., Labat, M. and Rouau, X. Demethylation of ferulic acid and feruloyl-arabinoxylan by microbial cell extracts. *Lebensmittel-Wissenschaft und -Technologie* **35** (2002) 272–276.

47 Muheim, A. and Lerch, K. Towards a high-yield bioconversion of ferulic acid to vanillin. *Applied Microbiology Biotechnology* **51** (1999) 456–461.

48 Hwang, J., Park, B. and Yun, J. Biologically active materials such as ferulic acid and arabinoxylan obtained from cereal bran by extrusion and enzyme treatment. (2001) PCT International Applications WO 01/67891 A1.

49 Anonymous. Report from the state of France forming part of the IENICA project. Interactive European Network for Industrial Crops and their Applications (IENICA). Agency for Environment and Energy Management (ADEME) (1999).

50 Ferguson, L. R. and Harris, P. J. Protection against cancer by wheat bran: role of dietary fibre and phytochemicals. *European Journal of Cancer Prevention* **8** (1999) 17–25.

51 Reddy, B.S., Hirose, Y., Cohen, L.A., Simi, B., Cooma, I. and Rao, C.V. Preventive potential of wheat bran fractions against experimental colon carcinogenesis: implications for human colon cancer prevention. *Cancer Research* **60** (2000) 4792–4797.

52 Kahlon, T.S. and Woodruff, C.L. In vitro binding of bile acids by rice bran, oat bran, barley and β-glucan enriched barley. *Cereal Chemistry* **80** (2003) 260–263.

53 Fenech, M., Noakes, M., Clifton, P. and Topping, D. Aleurone flour is a rich source of bioavailable folate in humans. *Journal of Nutrition* **129** (1999) 1114–1119.

54 Sidbu, J.S., Al-Saqer, J.M. and Al-Hooti, S.N. Mineral composition of high-fiber pan bread formulations containing bran and germ fractions. *AFS, Advances in Food Sciences* **23** (2001) 108–112.

55 Salmenkallio-Marttila, M., Katina, K. and Autio, K. Effects of bran fermentation on quality and microstructure of high-fiber wheat bread. *Cereal Chemistry* **78** (2001) 429–435.

56 Czuchajowska, Z. and Pomeranz, Y. Process for fractionating wheat flours to obtain protein concentrates and prime starch. (1995) US Patent 5,439,526.

57 Sayaslan, A. Wet-milling of wheat flour: industrial processes and small-scale test methods. *Lebensmittel-Wissenschaft und -Technologie* **37** (2004) 499–515.

58 Bassi, S., Maningat, C.C., Chinnaswamy, R., Nie, L., Weibel, M.K. and Watson,

J.J. Modified wheat glutens for use in fabrication of films. (1999) US Patent 5,747,648.

59 Woerdeman, D.L., Veraverbeke, W.S., Parnas, R.S., Johnson, D., Delcour, J.A., Verpoest, I., Plummer, C.J.G. Designing new materials from wheat protein. *Biomacromolecules* **5** (2004) 1262–1269.

60 Webb C., and Wang R. (1997) Development of a generic fermentation feedstock from whole wheat flour. In: Campbell GM, Webb C, McKee SL (eds) Cereals: Novel Uses and Processes, Plenum press, New York, pp 205–218

61 Koutinas, A.A., Wang, R.–H. and Webb, C. Restructuring upstream bioprocessing: Technological and economical aspects for the production of a generic microbial feedstock from wheat. *Biotechnology and Bioengineering* **85** (2004) 524–538.

62 Webb, C., Koutinas, A.A. and Wang, R.-H. Developing a sustainable bioprocessing strategy based on a generic feedstock. In: Scheper T (Series ed), Zhong J-J (volume ed) Biomanufacturing. Advances in Biochemical Engineering/Biotechnology. Springer–Verlag Berlin **87** (2004) 196–268

63 Bohlmann, J.A., Schisler, D.O., Hwang, K.-O., Henning, J.P., Trinkle, J.R., Anderson, T.B., Steinke, J.D. and Vanderhoff, A. Enzymic process for producing N-acetyl-D-glucosamine from spent fungal biomass. (2003) PCT International Applications WO 03/13435 A2.

64 Ian, W., Bohlmann, J.A., Trinkle, J.R., Steinke, J.D., Hwang, K.-O. and Henning, J.P. Glucosamine from microbial biomass. (2002) US Patent 2002115639.

65 McCoy, M. Betting on glucosamine. *Chemical and Engineering News* **81** (No 7) (2003) 27–28.

66 Datar, R.P., Shenkman, R.M., Cateni, B.G., Huhnke, R.L., Lewis R.S. Fermentation of biomass-generated producer gas to ethanol. *Biotechnology and Bioengineering* **86** (2004) 587–594

67 Weaver, P.F. and Maness P.-C. Photoconversion of gasified organic materials into biologically-degradable plastics (1993) US Patent 5,250,427

68 Webster, F. H. Oats: Chemistry and technology. (1986) AACC, St Paul, Minnesota, USA

69 Wood, P. J. Oat bran. (1993) AACC, St Paul, Minnesota, USA.

70 Paton, D., Reaney, M. J. T. and Tyler, N. J. Methods for processing oat groats and products thereof. (2000) US patent 6,113,908.

71 Tay, A. and Yang, S.-T. Production of L(+)-lactic acid from glucose and starch by immobilized cells of Rhizopus oryzae in a rotating fibrous bed reactor. *Biotechnology and Bioengineering* **80** (2002) pp. 1–12.

72 Maki, K. C., Shinnick, F. S., Marlyn, A., Veith, P. E., Quinn, L. C., Hallissey, P. J., Temer, A. and Davidson, M. H. Food products containing free tall oil-based phytosterols and oat β-glucan lower serum total and LDL cholesterol in hypercholesterolemic adults. *Journal of Nutrition* **133** (2003) 808–813.

73 Colleoni-Sirghie, M., Kovalenko, I. V., Briggs, J. L., Fulton, B. and White, P. J. Rheological and molecular properties of water soluble (1,3) (1,4)-β-β-glucans from high-β-glucan and traditional oat lines. *Carbohydrate Polymers* **52** (2003) 439–447.

74 Wursch, P. and Pi-Sunyer, E. X. The role of viscous soluble fiber in the metabolic control of diabetes. *Diabetes Care* **20** (1997) 1774–1780.

75 Yun, C.-H., Estrada, A., Van Kessel, A., Park, B.-C. and Laarveld, B. β-Glucan, extracted from oat, enhances disease resistance against bacterial and parasitic infections. *FEMS Immunology and Medical Microbiology* **35** (2003) 67–75.

76 Jenkins, A. L., Jenkins, D. J. A., Zdravkovic, U., Wursch, P. and Vuksan, V. Depression of the glycemic index by high levels of β-glucan fiber in two functional foods tested in type 2 diabetes. *European Journal of Clinical Nutrition* **56** (2002) 622–628.

77 Malkki, Y. and Virtanen, E. Gastrointestinal effects of oat bran and oat gum: A review. *Lebensmittel-Wissenschaft und -Technologie* **34** (2001) 337–347.

78 Peterson, D. M. Oat Antioxidants. *Journal of Cereal Science* **33** (2001) 115–129.

79 Emmons, C. L., Peterson, D. M. and Paul, G. L. Antioxidant capacity of oat (Avena sativa L.) extracts. 2. In vitro antioxidant activity and contents of phenolic and tocol antioxidants. *Journal of Agricultural and Food Chemistry* **47** (1999) 4894–4898.

80 Gray, D. A., Auerbach, R. H., Hill, S., Wang, R., Campbell, G. M., Webb C. and South, J. B. Enrichment of oat antioxidant activity by dry milling and sieving. *Journal of Cereal Science* **32** (2000) 89–98.

81 Peterson, D. M. Composition, separation and applications. *Lipid Technology* **14** (2002) 56–59

Fuel-oriented Biorefineries

9

Iogen's Demonstration Process for Producing Ethanol from Cellulosic Biomass

Jeffrey S. Tolan

9.1
Introduction

The production of fuel alcohol from cellulosic biomass is of growing interest around the world. Cellulosic biomass can be used to produce transportation fuel, with the overall process having little net production of greenhouse gases. Biomass is available as agricultural residues or as a byproduct of many processes, or can be potentially produced from dedicated energy crops. The technology for biomass conversion has many significant technical and economic challenges that have delayed its commercialization. However, significant progress has allowed Iogen Corporation of Ottawa, Canada to produce up to 2000 gallons day^{-1} of ethanol from wheat straw since April 2004 to demonstrate the technology.

9.2
Process Overview

The basic process steps of Iogen's Ottawa plant are shown in Fig. 9.1. This is a demonstration plant that produces up to 2000 gallons day^{-1} of ethanol from wheat straw. A full scale plant would produce about 170 000 gallons of ethanol per day (60 million gallons year^{-1}).

A cellulosic feedstock material such as wheat straw or other straws, corn stover, or grass is subjected to *pretreatment*, that is, cooked in the presence of acid to break down its fibrous structure. After pretreatment, the material has a muddy texture. Cellulase enzymes are added to the pretreated material to hydro-

Biorefineries – Industrial Processes and Products. Status Quo and Future Directions. Vol. 1
Edited by Birgit Kamm, Patrick R. Gruber, Michael Kamm
Copyright © 2006 WILEY-VCH Verlag GmbH & Co. KGaA, Weinheim
ISBN: 3-527-31027-4

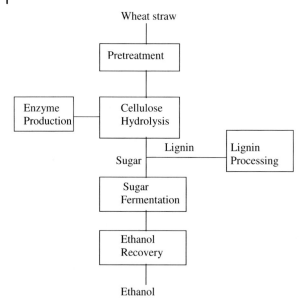

Fig. 9.1 Iogen's process for converting wheat straw to ethanol.

lyze the cellulose to the simple sugar glucose; this is known as *cellulose hydroly-sis*. The cellulase enzymes are made at the plant site by using a wood-rotting fungus in large fermentation vessels. This is known as *cellulase enzyme produc-tion*. After cellulose hydrolysis, the sugars are separated from the unhydrolyzed solids, which include lignin and residual cellulose. These solids are burned to provide energy for the entire process (*lignin processing*). The sugars are ferment-ed (*sugar fermentation*) to ethanol using recently developed recombinant *Sacchar-omyces* yeast from Purdue University to ferment the glucose and the more diffi-cult sugar to ferment, xylose. In *ethanol recovery*, the ethanol is recovered by con-ventional distillation, denatured, and blended into gasoline.

The remainder of this chapter describes the process steps and related technol-ogies in more detail.

9.3
Feedstock Selection

9.3.1
Feedstock Composition

The term "cellulosic biomass" refers to potential feedstocks that have *cellulose* as a primary constituent. Other major constituents of these materials include *hemi-cellulose* and *lignin*. Minor constituents include proteins, ash, starch, and various other organic compounds that are not carbohydrates.

Cellulose comprises 35% to 50% of most plant material. Cellulose is a polymer of glucose, of dp (degree of polymerization, or chain length) of 1000 to 10000. Cellulose is a linear, unbranched polymer, with glucose joined together by beta-1,4-linkages. Individual polymer chains run parallel to each other and form hydrogen bonds with each other, up to three per monomeric glucose unit. Several such chains form a *microfibril*. A microfibril region that has the full degree of hydrogen bonding forms a roughly cubic, 3-dimensional lattice. Such a region is *crystalline* cellulose and is very stable against attack by enzymes or acid. Other regions are not hydrogen-bonded to nearly this extent, and in the extreme are simply random configurations of glucose polymers. This is *amorphous* cellulose. Most natural cellulose is primarily crystalline cellulose.

The main source of ethanol is from the glucose, originating from the cellulose. However, a second source of ethanol is from the simple sugars that comprise the hemicellulose. Hemicellulose is a mixture of linear and branched polymers of the five-carbon sugars xylose and arabinose and (less importantly) the six-carbon sugars glucose, mannose, and galactose. Hemicellulose is readily dissolved and hydrolyzed to its simple sugars in dilute acid at moderate temperatures, for example, 120 °C. Hemicellulose comprises 15–25% of most plant material.

Lignin differs from cellulose and hemicellulose in that lignin is not comprised of carbohydrates, but rather consists of a complex three-dimensional matrix of phenolic propane units. Lignin confers water resistance and stiffness to the fiber and protection against microbial attack. Lignin does not participate in the pretreatment or hydrolysis processes except with a decrease in the degree of polymerization. The burning of lignin is the mode of energy generation for the process. Lignin comprises 15–30% of most plant materials.

In normal operation, the minor constituents exert only a minor impact on the process. The protein is degraded by pretreatment to the point where it cannot be recovered economically. The ash must not be at too high a level as to be abrasive to the process equipment. Such can be the case if large amounts of silica (sand) are present due to the harvest practices or the natural silica uptake by the plant. The starch is easily hydrolyzed to glucose and increases the overall

Table 9.1 Feedstock composition (mg g^{-1} total solids) (from Foody et al. 1999 [1]).

Feedstock	Cellulose	Starch	Xylan	Arabinan	Lignin	Ash	Protein
Barley straw	406	20	161	28	168	82	64
Wheat straw	455	9	165	25	204	83	64
Wheat chaff	391	14	200	36	160	121	33
Switch grass	399	3	184	38	183	48	54
Corn stover	408	3	128	35	127	60	81
Maple wood	500	4	150	5	276	6	6
Pine wood	648	1	33	14	320	0	2

ethanol yield. Table 9.1 shows the composition of several typical lignocellulosic materials.

9.3.2
Feedstock Selection

The scope of feedstocks considered by Iogen for ethanol production are listed in Table 9.2.

These potential feedstocks are evaluated based on the desired feedstock properties. The desired qualities of a feedstock are:

1. Low cost. Naturally, the cost of the feedstock is an important part of the overall cost. A desired feedstock can be obtained and transported to the plant at low cost. This rules out primary and secondary tree growth, sawdust, and waste paper, all of which have existing markets and high cost.
2. Availability. A feedstock must be in sufficient quantity to supply a commercial plant. This requires perhaps $800\,000$ tons year^{-1}, which is not available from bagasse in many locations.
3. Uniformity. For a high-speed production process, foreign matter present in municipal waste is unacceptable.
4. Cleanliness. High levels of silica can abrade equipment, as stated above. A high degree of microbial contamination is unacceptable. High levels of toxic or inhibitory materials are not acceptable.
5. High potential ethanol yield. The main constituents, cellulose and hemicellulose, must be present in high enough levels to produce ethanol. This is a disadvantage of forestry waste, which is high in bark that is mostly lignin and phenolic acids.
6. High efficiency of conversion. The efficiency of conversion to glucose (following Iogen's pretreatment process) is proportional to the arabino-xylan content

Table 9.2 Potential feedstocks.

Material	Subclass	Comments
Wood	Native forest	Difficult to process, especially softwood
	Tree farms	Too expensive due to demands of other markets
	Forest waste (bark)	Cellulose/hemicellulose content is too low
	Mill waste (sawdust)	Too expensive due to pulp and paper market
Agricultural residues	Straws (wheat, barley, oat, rice)	Leading candidate feedstocks
	Bagasse (cane)	Localized feedstock of interest
	Corn stover	Leading candidate feedstock
Energy crops	Grass	Possible second generation feedstock
Waste cellulose	Municipal waste	Not uniform enough to process
	Waste paper	Too expensive due to paper demand

of the feedstock [1]. The arabino-xylan content is roughly the sum of the arabinan and xylan content listed in Table 9.1. Feedstocks with a low arabino-xylan content, such as softwood, demand unacceptably high levels of enzyme for conversion to cellulose.

Matching the feedstock list with the desired properties results in the feedstocks used by Iogen, which are agricultural residues such as straws and stover and energy crops such as grasses. The energy crops, such as grass, are not currently harvested in a large scale, as this will require large scale demonstration of the technology before people commit to these as crops. The grasses are therefore second-generation feedstocks.

9.3.3
Ethanol from Starch or Sucrose

Starch-based or sucrose-based processes are already widely used to make ethanol. The leading starch-based material is corn, which is widely used to make ethanol in the US. Starch is converted to glucose by grinding corn kernels (in a dry milling process) or by steeping kernels in dilute sulfurous acid (in a wet milling process), then using starch-degrading enzymes known as amylases. The glucose is then fermented to ethanol. Sucrose-based feedstocks include sugar cane (Brazil) and sugar beets (Europe). These feedstocks are pressed and washed with water to extract the sucrose, which is then fermented to ethanol by yeast. Other feedstocks used to make small amounts of fuel ethanol in some regions include potatoes and Jerusalem artichokes.

Many cellulosic materials, including straw and grass, contain up to 10% starch. Wheat straw fed to Iogen's plant is 3–4% starch. This is converted to glucose during pretreatment and carried through to sugar fermentation, where it is converted to ethanol.

9.3.4
Advantages of Making Ethanol from Cellulosic Biomass

The conversion of cellulosic biomass to ethanol is more difficult than starch or sucrose, and this has limited commercialization of the technology. However, cellulosic biomass is available in much greater quantity and offers the potential for much greater ethanol production than the other feedstocks. In addition, ethanol production from starch and sucrose faces competition for the feedstock from the food and cattle feed industries, which exerts pressure on the price of the ethanol. Most cellulosic biomass is free of competition from other uses. Cellulosic biomass can be grown in a wider variety of climates and soils than starch and sucrose and therefore represent a potential new agricultural opportunity in many areas.

The most important advantage of making ethanol from cellulosic biomass is that the production and use of the ethanol does not add to the emission of greenhouse gases. Producing ethanol from corn, sugar cane, or sugar beets requires large amounts of energy-intensive fertilizers. The use of these feedstocks results in significantly less net energy generation from the lignin byproduct than that from using cellulosic biomass. These two areas (fertilizer and process energy) require significant input of fossil fuels in ethanol plants using corn, sugar cane, or sugar beets. By contrast, ethanol made from cellulosic biomass is not a net user of fossil fuels. The neutral fossil fuel usage is why ethanol from cellulose is expected to be neutral relative to the production of greenhouse gases [2].

An additional benefit of biomass conversion arises from the fact that corn, sugar cane, and sugar beets all contain 5–15% cellulose and hemicellulose. Cellulose conversion technology represents an opportunity to improve the ethanol yields and decrease the wastes from these processes.

9.4
Pretreatment

9.4.1
Process

Pretreatment is the process by which surface area of the feedstock is opened up for the subsequent enzymatic attack. In the absence of pretreatment, the requirement for cellulase enzymes is too high to be practical.

The basis for Iogen's pretreatment is steam explosion [3]. In the Iogen demonstration plant, wheat straw in bales is chopped and milled, then conveyed to the pretreatment reactor. High pressure steam and sulfuric acid are added to the feedstock to reach 180–260 °C with 0.5–2% sulfuric acid. The material is maintained at this condition for 0.5–5 min. The pressure is then released rapidly.

As a result of pretreatment, the fibrous structure of the feedstock is destroyed. The pretreated material has a muddy texture and a slightly sweet smell, with a dark brown color. Among different feedstocks, the cooking time varies while most of the other conditions are maintained relatively constant. The appearance of pretreated material is similar among different feedstocks.

9.4.2
Chemical Reactions

Of the major components, the first to react is the hemicellulose. The xylan portion is depolymerized and solubilized, and then hydrolyzed to xylose by the reaction:

$$(C_5H_8O_4)_n + H_2O \ \rightarrow \ (C_5H_8O_4)_{n-1} + C_5H_{10}O_5 \tag{1}$$

The presence of exogenous sulfuric acid is particularly important in the formation of monomeric xylose. In the absence of exogenous acid, xylose oligomers are formed. Further, the added acid improves the uniformity of the process, because natural acid levels vary considerably among feedstocks or batches of a given feedstock.

If the pretreatment reaction proceeds further, the xylose is dewatered to produce furfural (Eq. 2), which is undesirable.

$$C_5H_{10}O_5 \rightarrow C_5H_4O_2 + 3H_2O \tag{2}$$

Arabinose undergoes analogous reactions, but more slowly than xylose. Acetic acid is released from the hydrolysis of acetyl groups attached to the xylan.

Removing hemicellulose from the feedstock accomplishes two objectives. First, it makes the simple sugars that can potentially be fermented to ethanol. Second and more importantly, it opens up surface area on the feedstock, thereby allowing the cellulase enzyme to digest the cellulose more efficiently.

A small amount of cellulose reacts to form glucose, which is degraded to hydroxymethylfurfural, by Eqs (3) and (4):

$$(C_6H_{10}O_5)_n + H_2O \rightarrow (C_6H_{10}O_5)_{n-1} + C_6H_{12}O_6 \tag{3}$$

$$C_6H_{12}O_6 \rightarrow C_6H_6O_3 + 3H_2O \tag{4}$$

Only a small amount of cellulose hydrolysis (<20%) is desired in the pretreatment. More than this results in a decrease in glucose yield and accessibility of the enzyme to the cellulose. The older acid hydrolysis process carried out a much harsher acid hydrolysis and will be described below.

The lignin undergoes a depolymerization during pretreatment, but remains insoluble in water or acid. Protein is destroyed and starch is hydrolyzed to glucose in the pretreatment.

One can draw an analogy to cooking a turkey to describe the trade-off between time and temperature in the pretreatment: the longer the time, the lower the temperature. Acid also acts to decrease the temperature or time required for pretreatment.

The choice of reactor for this pretreatment is only important insofar as the desired chemistry must be delivered to the system. Numerous guns, vessels, and tubes have been proposed and built to carry this out.

9.4.3
Other Pretreatment Processes

Katzen et al. [4] published a detailed review of pretreatment that will only be summarized here. Pretreatment processes may be divided into (1) those that produce a stream directly for fermentation to ethanol and (2) those that are followed by enzymatic hydrolysis. The former are necessarily harsher and have a longer history.

Direct sugar production in pretreatment has been carried out using concentrated chemicals and dilute acid.

Concentrated chemical pretreatment represents the cellulose conversion technology with the longest history, dating back to 1890 or earlier in Germany. The concentrated chemicals include acids, bases, and salts. The principle behind the use of concentrated chemicals is to disrupt the crystalline cellulose structure, thereby dissolving and depolymerizing the cellulose. Among the chemicals used are 72% sulfuric acid, 40% hydrochloric acid, 40% sodium hydroxide, 65% zinc chloride, 40% calcium chloride. These methods have very high yields and low operating temperatures. Unfortunately, the economics of the process dictate that recovery and reuse of the pretreatment chemicals is critically important. The inability to obtain the necessary recoveries of order 99.9% has hindered the commercialization of these processes. A second problem is the exotic materials required to handle these streams.

Dilute acid hydrolysis represents the cellulose conversion technology with the most commercial experience. In dilute acid hydrolysis, the feedstock is treated at perhaps 180–200 °C for 1–4 h with 1 to 4% sulfuric acid. A glucose yield of 50% of the cellulose or higher is obtained. This process was used for ethanol production by Germany during World War II, Russia in the late 1940s, and pilot plants in the 1950s in Switzerland and Springfield, Oregon. All of these plants have been plagued by corrosion, low yields, high investments, and overall poor returns. Several plants of up to 10 t day^{-1} built in Russia in the 1950s still operate with this process.

Pretreatment followed by enzymatic hydrolysis is newer than direct pretreatment, as cellulase enzymes were only identified and worked with after World War II. The milder pretreatments carried out in preparation for enzymatic hydrolysis include mechanical action, solvent-based pretreatments, alkali treatments, and acid prehydrolysis.

Mechanical action was first tried at the U.S. Army laboratory in Natick, Massachusetts in the 1960s. The principle behind mechanical action is to increase the surface area of the feedstock particles. However, beyond producing small particles for uniform distribution of acid, there is no real advantage to further milling of the feedstock.

In solvent-based pretreatments, organic solvents such as ethanol and methanol are used to dissolve a portion of the lignin, thereby freeing up the cellulose for enzymatic attack. However, recovery of the solvent is difficult, and partial delignification is not of significant benefit in the hydrolysis.

In alkali pretreatments, such as with sodium hydroxide or ammonia, the crystalline cellulose is converted to a different form, cellulose II or III respectively. These forms of cellulose can be more easily hydrolyzed than native cellulose. However, destruction of the hemicellulose is reported in these systems, and they are not yet used commercially.

Acid prehydrolysis is preferred by Iogen because it has fewer of these problems than the other methods. The levels of acid are low enough that recovery is not needed and corrosion is not a problem. The process provides a selective hydrolysis of hemicellulose and produces a cellulosic substrate with a high surface area suitable for enzymatic hydrolysis.

9.5
Cellulase Enzyme Production

9.5.1
Production of Cellulase Enzymes

Cellulase enzymes convert cellulose to glucose, which can then be fermented to ethanol. Cellulase enzymes are made by a wide variety of microbes, but those best suited to cellulose hydrolysis are made by the wood-rotting fungus *Trichoderma*. This fungus was isolated during World War II in rotted U.S. Army cotton tents in the South Pacific. Researchers led by Elwyn Reese and Mary Mandels at the U.S. Army laboratory in Natick, Massachusetts determined that the microbe responsible for the destruction of the cotton was secreting a mixture of enzymes that hydrolyzed the cotton. Reese and Mandels determined cultivation conditions for production of cellulase in liquid culture. Selection of *Trichoderma* strains with higher productivities of cellulase was successfully carried out by Montenecourt at Lehigh University in the 1970s. Despite research and development of cellulase production from other microbes, *Trichoderma* remains the organism of choice to produce cellulase for ethanol production.

Cellulase is made at Iogen's commercial enzyme plant in Ottawa in a submerged liquid culture, as is used by Genencor International, Novozym Biotech, Rohm AB, and other commercial cellulase manufacturers. The fermentation vessels are similar to those used for producing antibiotics. The fermenters are 50 000 gallons and are maintained free of contaminating microbes. The liquid broth contains carbon source, salts, complex nutrients such as corn steep liquor, and other nutrients in water. The most important nutrient is the carbon source. Glucose promotes growth of the organism but not cellulase production. The carbon source must include an inducing sugar to promote cellulase production. Well known inducers of cellulase include the sugars cellobiose, lactose, sophorose, and other low molecular weight oligomers of glucose.

The nutrient broth is sterilized before the start of the fermentation by heating with steam. The fermenter is inoculated with the enzyme production strain once the liquid broth has cooled down. The operating conditions are 30 °C, pH 4 to 5, and these are maintained by the addition of cooling water in external coils and by alkali, respectively. Trichoderma is highly aerobic and a constant stream of air or oxygen is used to maintain aerobic conditions. A cellulase enzyme production run lasts about one week. At the end of the run, the broth is filtered across a cloth to remove cells. The spent cell mass is destroyed and disposed of by landfilling.

The resulting enzyme broth is a clear, light brown liquid, similar in appearance to weak tea.

9.5.2
Enzyme Production on the Ethanol Plant Site

Iogen has the unique advantage of operating an ethanol plant on a cellulase production site. In this case, the crude fermentation broth containing cellulase is simply added to the cellulose hydrolysis tanks. If the cellulase is to be stored for long periods before use, it must be stabilized against (1) microbial contamination, which uses preservatives such as sodium benzoate, and (2) protein denaturation, which uses compounds such as glycerol.

The production and use of cellulase on the ethanol plant site therefore has the advantage that the cost of preservatives and stabilizers, as well as transportation of the enzyme, is avoided. This is a big cost advantage for on-site enzyme production.

9.5.3
Commercial Status of Cellulase

There is an ongoing business in cellulase enzymes besides that used for cellulose hydrolysis. Cellulase sales are roughly $ 100 million annually to the textiles, detergent, animal feed, beverage, and pulp and paper industries [5].

These commercial cellulase enzymes are made by several microbes, including *Humicola*, *Aspergillus*, and *Penicillium* fungi, and *Bacillus* bacteria in addition to *Trichoderma*. Ethanol production requires aggressive action of cellulase to destroy cellulose, for which *Trichoderma* cellulase is superior. The other industries often require milder action and/or specific conditions better suited to other cellulases. For example, the textile industry uses cellulase to soften denim blue jeans. *Humicola* cellulases can be less aggressive in this application than *Trichoderma* cellulases, though *Trichoderma* cellulases can be modified to improve their performance. Detergents require alkaline conditions that are not easily accessible to *Trichoderma* enzymes.

9.6
Cellulose Hydrolysis

9.6.1
Process Description

In cellulose hydrolysis, cellulase enzymes convert the cellulose to glucose. The pretreated feedstock is conveyed to the hydrolysis tanks in a slurry that is 5–15% total solids (as high as can be handled). The slurry is adjusted to pH 5 with alkali and maintained at 50 °C. A single hydrolysis tank has a volume of 200,000 gallons. Crude cellulase broth is added as a liquid at a dosage of 100 liters per tonne of cellulose. The contents of the tank are agitated to move the material and keep it dispersed, but not nearly as agitated as a fermentation vessel.

The hydrolysis proceeds for 5–7 days. As it proceeds, the viscosity of the slurry drops, and the remaining insoluble particles, which are lignin in increasing proportion, diminish in size. At the end of the hydrolysis, 90% to 98% of the cellulose is converted to glucose. The remainder is insoluble and contained within the unhydrolyzed particles, which are mostly lignin.

9.6.2
Kinetics of Cellulose Hydrolysis

Trichoderma cellulase is a mixture of three types of enzymes: *cellobiohydrolase(CBH), endoglucanase (EG),* and *beta-glucosidase (BG).* CBH enzymes act sequentially along the cellulose. *Trichoderma* cellulase includes two CBH enzymes, CBHI and CBHII, which together account for 80% of the total cellulase protein. EG enzymes act to cut random locations on the fiber. *Trichoderma* makes at least 4 different EG enzymes: EGI, EGII, EGIII, and EGV. The EG enzymes account for about 20% of the cellulase protein. The third type of enzyme, beta-glucosidase, hydrolyzes the glucose dimer cellobiose to glucose.

The enzymatic hydrolysis of cellulose proceeds as two consecutive reactions:

$$(C_5H_{10}O_5)_n + H_2O \;\rightarrow\; (C_5H_{10}O_5)_{n-2} + C_{12}H_{22}O_{11} \tag{5}$$

$$C_{12}H_{22}O_{11} + H_2O \;\rightarrow\; 2C_6H_{12}O_6 \tag{6}$$

Eq. (5) depicts the hydrolysis of cellulose to its soluble dimer, cellobiose. This reaction is catalyzed by the CBH and EG enzymes. The CBH and EG enzymes work synergistically to hydrolyze cellulose. Reaction (6) is the hydrolysis of cellobiose to glucose. This reaction is catalyzed by the soluble enzyme beta-glucosidase and proceeds according to standard Michaelis-Menten kinetics. BG accounts for less than 1% of the total cellulase protein. Hydrolysis of the cellobiose is important because glucose can be readily fermented to ethanol while cellobiose is not. In addition, cellobiose is a potent inhibitor of CBH and EG, so the accumulation of even 5 g L^{-1} cellobiose slows down the hydrolysis significantly.

The properties of the *Trichoderma* cellulase enzymes are summarized in Table 9.3.

There are several inherent difficulties in cellulose hydrolysis that have been the focus of much research. The first is the inherent shortage of BG, both because of its low concentration and because it is inhibited by its product glucose. With a shortage of BG, cellobiose accumulates, thereby inhibiting the action of CBH and EG in hydrolyzing cellulose.

Three approaches have been proposed to overcoming the shortage of BG. The first is to produce BG in a separate fermentation by *Aspergillus* spp. The disadvantage of this is the added process cost of a second fermentation.

The second and most widely discussed approach is to carry out a simultaneous saccharification and fermentation (SSF) process. In SSF, the enzymatic

Table 9.3 Trichoderma cellulase enzymes.

Enzyme	Mol. wt.	Isoelectric point	Family	Concn. (%)	Ref.
CBHI	63 000	4.3	7	50–60	6
CBHII	58 000	6.0	6	15–18	7
EGI	53 000	4.6	7	12–15	8
EGII	50 000	5.3	5	9–11	9
EGIII	25 000	7.4	12	0–3	10
EGV	23 000	3.7	45	0–3	11

hydrolysis and glucose fermentation are run simultaneously, with the notion that the yeast consumes the glucose to prevent inhibition of BG, which can then hydrolyze cellobiose and lift the inhibition of CBH/EG. In Iogen's research, SSF systems have achieved poor results, because the enzyme's optimum temperature is 50 °C and the yeast runs best at 28 °C, so a compromise temperature of 37 °C is used. In addition to the loss of rate, microbial contamination is observed at 37 °C. We have put this approach aside.

The third option is to develop *Trichoderma* strains with high beta-glucosidase production included in the CBH/EG. This has been carried out at Iogen [12] and has largely overcome the shortage of BG.

Other important difficulties in the hydrolysis are the decrease in rate as hydrolysis proceeds and the diminishing returns with enzyme dosage, i.e. doubling the amount of enzyme does not double the extent of conversion achieved. These issues, which are probably linked, are not well understood and differ substantially from Michaelis-Menten kinetics. These effects can, however, be characterized empirically.

The enzyme components initially must adsorb to the surface of the insoluble substrate cellulose. An equilibrium corresponding roughly to a Langmuir adsorption isotherm is reached within a few minutes. The adsorbed enzyme then acts on the cellulose at a rapid initial rate. The rate declines significantly after the first few minutes of hydrolysis, and after 24 h is less than 2% of the initial rate. The hydrolysis continues over several days at ever decreasing rates. Depending on the enzyme dosage used and the duration of the hydrolysis, the final cellulose conversion is 90% to 98%.

The reason the rate slows down is not fully known. Speculation in the literature has centered on: end-product inhibition; an increasingly difficulty in hydrolyzing the substrate (substrate recalcitrance); and denaturation of the cellulase protein over time. However, straightforward experiments demonstrate that none of these factors account for more than a small fraction of the drop in rate. Further research continues in this area.

9.6.3
Improvements in Enzymatic Hydrolysis

Despite many years of research, cellulose hydrolysis remains the least efficient part of the process. To illustrate the problem, hydrolysis of pretreated cellulose requires 100-fold more enzyme than hydrolysis of starch. The enzyme manufacturing cost is still sufficiently high that the trade-off between enzyme dosage and hydrolysis time favors longer times and lower dosages.

One approach to potentially decrease the cost of enzymatic hydrolysis is to recycle enzyme and/or substrate. These ideas have not been fully explored. The cellulase enzyme adsorbs to the substrate, so recycle of unconsumed cellulose would be one way to reuse the enzyme. Reuse of the enzyme in solution is also a possibility. The current configuration of Iogen's plant does not carry out these recycles, but upgrades are under way to allow the demonstration plant to evaluate these options.

Another approach to reducing the cost of hydrolysis is to use fed-batch of substrate or of enzyme. Again, these are ideas with a sound basis that have not been explored. Fed batch systems are especially interesting because they might allow high cellulose concentrations to be maintained at all times.

The development of superior cellulase enzymes has been explored extensively at several research labs, with as yet no cellulases found that are superior to *Trichoderma* cellulase. However, the new tools of molecular biology, such as protein engineering, can be brought to bear on this problem and might lead to success. Large development efforts are under way at Iogen and at Genencor International, Novozym Biotech, and Diversa to address this area.

Another area that has been widely explored is novel hydrolysis reactors, such as trickling bed, high shear, etc. Some improvements in efficiency have been reported, but not easily generalized across feedstocks and enzymes. A better understanding of the nature of the enzyme's action will be helpful in evaluating these reactors.

Taking a wider point of view, better hydrolysis would be a direct benefit of better pretreatment. Pretreatment has been widely studied, but there are always new ideas on the horizon.

9.7
Lignin Processing

9.7.1
Process Description

The hydrolysis slurry contains glucose, xylose, arabinose, and other compounds dissolved in the aqueous phase, and insoluble lignin and unconsumed cellulose. The insoluble particles are separated by a plate and frame filter, with the cake washed with water to obtain a high sugar recovery. The sugar stream is pumped to the fermentation tanks. The lignin cake is disposed of. In a full-scale ethanol plant, the lignin would be burned on site to generate power and steam to run the plant, with excess electricity sold to the power grid.

9.7.2
Alternative Uses for Lignin

Lignin is a lattice of phenolic propane units. Lignin has been the object of much study, and a good review of applications of lignin is provided by Chum et al. [13]. The potential applications of lignin fall into the broad categories of insoluble and chemically modified. Insoluble lignin is limited to high-volume, low value applications such as an ingredient in roads or cement. In these applications, lignin is a filler and competes with corn cobs, gravel, and ground bark.

Chemically modified lignin has a much wider variety of potential markets. The major types of chemical modifications are to solubilize the lignin, by reaction with i.e. sulfurous acid, or to crosslink the lignin, by reaction with i.e. phenol. Crosslinked lignin is suitable for resins, glues, and other such materials, where it competes with phenol–formaldehyde resins. Solubilized lignin, i.e. sodium lignosulfonate, is used in surfactants, detergents, and biocides.

9.8
Sugar Fermentation and Ethanol Recovery

The hydrolysis sugars, which consist of glucose, xylose, arabinose, and various organic impurities in aqueous solution, are pumped to the sugar fermenters for ethanol production. The fermenters are large tanks with gentle agitation, sufficient to keep the contents moving. The fermenters are inoculated with *Saccharomyces* yeast, which readily ferment the glucose to ethanol, and have been genetically modified for metabolism and fermentation of xylose. These yeast strains have been developed at Purdue University [14]. The advantage of these strains over others is that the plant operations (contamination control, cell recycle, and markets for spent cells) involving *Saccharomyces* yeast are well developed, and the ethanol tolerance of the strains are good. The areas for further improvement include developing the inability to ferment arabinose to ethanol and increasing the yields and rates of xylose fermentation.

In addition to *Saccharomyces* yeast, other microbes are under development to ferment xylose to ethanol, which is not carried out naturally in high efficiency. *Pichia* yeast have a natural ability for xylose uptake, but require genetic modification to ferment the xylose to ethanol. This strategy is carried out at the University of Wisconsin [15]. In addition, *Zymomonas* bacteria have been genetically modified for xylose uptake and metabolism. This strategy is carried out by the National Renewable Energy Laboratory in Boulder, Colorado [16]. Two other strategies for pentose fermentation include genetically modified enteric bacteria such as *E. coli* and *Klebsiella*, carried out at the University of Florida [17–19], and thermostable *Bacillus* strains developed at Imperial College.

After fermentation, the broth containing ethanol and unfermented sugar is pumped to a distillation column. The ethanol is distilled off the top and dehydrated. The ethanol yield is about 75 gallons per tonne wheat straw. The ethanol is denatured with 1% gasoline. The denatured ethanol is then blended into gasoline in 10% or 85% ethanol mixtures. The still bottoms are disposed of. Tests are under way to determine whether the still bottoms can be recovered for byproducts.

References

1 Foody, B., Tolan, J. S., Bernstein, J., *Pretreatment process for conversion of cellulose to fuel ethanol*, US Patent 5,916,780 issued June 29, **1999**.

2 Singh, L., *Scenarios of U.S. Carbon Reductions: Potential Impacts of Energy Technologies by 2010 and Beyond*, Interlaboratory Working Group on Energy Efficient and Low-Carbon Technologies (ORNL, LBNL, PNNL, NREL, ANL), **1997**.

3 Foody, P., *Method for Increasing the accessibility of cellulose in lignocellulosic materials, particularly hardwoods, agricultural residues, and the like*, US patent 4,461,648 issued July 24, **1984**.

4 Katzen, R., Madsen, P. W., Monceaux, D. A., Bevernitz, K., *Use of Cellulosic Feedstocks for Alcohol Production*, Chapter 5 of The Alcohol Textbook, edited by T. P. Lyons, D. R. Kelsall, and J. E. Murtagh, **1990**.

5 Godfrey, T., Industrial Enzymology, Chapter 1, **1996**.

6 Shoemaker et al., *Molecular cloning of exo-cellobiohydrolase I derived from Trichoderma reesei strain L27*, Bio/technology, **1983**, 1, 691–696.

7 Chen et al., *Nucleotide sequence and deduced primary structure of cellobiohydrolase II from Trichoderma reesei*, Bio/technology, **1987**, 5, 274–278.

8 Penttila et al., *Homology between cellulase genes of Trichoderma reesei: complete nucleotide sequence of the endoglucanase I gene*, Gene, **1986**, 45, 253–263.

9 Saloheimo et al., *EGIII, a new endoglucanase from Trichoderma reesei: the characterization of both gene and enzyme*, Gene, **1988**, 63, 11–21.

10 Ward, M., Clarkson, K. A., Larenas, E. A., Lorch, J. D., Weiss, G. L., *DNA Sequence Encoding Endoglucanase III Cellulase*, US patent 5,475,101 issued Dec. 12, **1995**.

11 Saloheimo et al., *A novel, small endoglucanase gene, egl5, from Trichoderma reesei isolated by expression in yeast*, Molecular Microbiology, **1993**, 61, 1090–1097.

12 White, T. C., Hindle, C., *Genetic constructs and genetically modified microbes for enhanced production of beta-glucosidase.* US patent 6,015,703 issued January 18, **2000**.

13 Chum, H. L., Parker, S. K., Feinberg, D. A., Wright, J. D., Rice, P. A., Sinclair, S. A., Glasser, W. G., *The Economic Contribution of Lignins to Ethanol Production from Biomass*, National Renewable Energy Lab, Golden, Colo., **1985**.

14 Ho, N. W. Y., Chen, Z.-D., *Stable Recombinant Yeasts for Fermenting Xylose to Ethanol*, PCT patent application WO 97/42307, **1997**.

15 Cho, J., Jeffries, T. J., *Pichia stipitis Genes for Alcohol Dehydrogenase with Fermentative and Respirative Functions*, Appl. Environ. Microbiol., **1998**, 64(4), 1350–1358.

16 Mohagheghi, A., Evans, K., Finkelstein, M., Zhang, M., *Cofermentation of Glucose, Xylose, and Arabinose by Mixed Cultures of Two Genetically Engineered Zymomonas mobilis Strains*, Applied Biochem. Biotechnol., **1998**, 70–72, 285.

17 Ingram, L. O., Conway, T., Clark, D. P., Sewall, G. W., Preston, J. F., *Genetic Engineering of Ethanol Production in Escherichia coli*, Appl. Environ. Microbiol., **1987**, 53(10), 2420–2425.

18 Ohta, K., Alterthum, F., Ingram, L. O., *Effects of Environmental Conditions on Xy-*

lose Fermentation by Recombinant Escherichia coli, Appl. Environ. Micro., **1990**, 56(2), 463–465.

19 Ohta, K., Beall, D. S., Mejia, J. P., Shanmugam, K. T., Ingram, L. O., *Genetic Improvement of Escherichia coli for Ethanol Production: chromosomal integration of Zymomonas mobilis genes encoding pyruvate decarboxylase and alcohol dehydrogenase II*, Appl. Environ. Micro., **1991**, 57(4), 893–900.

10

Sugar-based Biorefinery –
Technology for Integrated Production
of Poly(3-hydroxybutyrate), Sugar, and Ethanol

Carlos Eduardo Vaz Rossell, Paulo E. Mantelatto, José A. M. Agnelli, and Jefter Nascimento

10.1
Introduction

Poly(3-hydroxybutyric acid) polymer (PHB) and related copolymers such as poly(3-hydroxybutyric-*co*-3-hydroxyvaleric) are natural polyesters synthesized by a wide range of organisms, particularly some bacterial strains. They have very interesting properties, for example they are totally and rapidly biodegraded to carbon dioxide and water by many different microorganisms and are biocompatible. These polyesters can be compounded to thermoplastic resins whose physicochemical and mechanical properties are quite similar to petrochemical-based polymers such as polyethylene and polypropylene. PHB can be produced in an environmentally safe way integrated to a sugar mill. This context, with its large quantities of readily available and comparatively low-cost sugar, and accessible thermal, mechanical, and electrical energy obtained from renewable agricultural sources, could be the optimum place to introduce a large-scale facility for its production.

10.2
Sugar Cane Agro Industry in Brazil – Historical Outline

10.2.1
Sugar and Ethanol Production

During the last quarter of the 20th century, Brazil's sugar cane agroindustry underwent major changes. This initially traditional sector, previously devoted specifically to the production of sugar and occasionally to by-products, recovering or producing very few new products from available sugar or molasses, shifted its scope to diversify its production lines. In 1975, after the international oil crisis and the rise of oil prices, the Brazilian government launched the National

Biorefineries – Industrial Processes and Products. Status Quo and Future Directions. Vol. 1
Edited by Birgit Kamm, Patrick R. Gruber, Michael Kamm
Copyright © 2006 WILEY-VCH Verlag GmbH & Co. KGaA, Weinheim
ISBN: 3-527-31027-4

Fuel Ethanol Program, with the objective of replacing oil imports with sugar cane-based ethanol as an alternative fuel. Many mills began to produce aqueous ethanol, for direct use in converted car engines, or anhydrous ethanol to add to gasoline as a fuel enhancer. The scale of production increased substantially, agricultural and industrial productivity grew, and production costs dropped.

This new situation, which led to a favorable change in the country's energy balance, caused the production of an excess of bagasse, which has been used as primary fuel by the mills or has been sold to third parties. Today, Brazil is the largest worldwide producer of sugar and sugar cane-based ethanol and, on the basis of cultivated area and income, sugar cane is one of the most important agricultural activities. This statement is confirmed by figures from the 2003/ 2004 season – sugar cane production was 338 316 619. metric tons. Ethanol production was 14 107 873 m^3, 8 577 410 m^3 of which was anhydrous fuel grade and the remaining 5 530 468 m^3 aqueous fuel grade. Sugar production rose to 23 404 703 tons, of which 12 914 468 tons were exported, accounting for revenues of US $ 2 140 002 217 [1].

10.2.2
The Sugar Cane Agroindustry and the Green Cycle

The modern sugar agroindustry, which tends to operate as a "green cycle", can achieve a unique condition as a source of renewable raw materials if a continuous effort is made to keep its production practices environmentally friendly. The basis of this sector is sugar cane (*Saccharum officinarum*), a subtropical gramineous plant cultivated on a large scale in Brazil's south central region with productivity averaging 85 tonnes per hectare per year and for which production costs are low. Sugar cane captures solar energy and converts atmospheric carbon dioxide into biomass. Macedo [2] produced an inventory of carbon dioxide released during sugar cane processing into final products and, after fuel ethanol combustion, concluded that the net balance was positive and that atmospheric carbon dioxide is effectively removed by cane crops. Macedo also demonstrated that the balance between energy available from final products such as fuel ethanol, bagasse and electrical power generated versus energy consumption during cane culture and industrial processing is positive [3, 4].

The sugar mills operating in Brazil today are very large units functioning as autonomous industrial complexes. Their main products are sugar and fuel ethanol, and bagasse – the fibrous fraction of sugar cane – is the primary fuel. Bagasse burned in high-pressure boilers provides mechanical power for driving mill tandems, electrical power to meet the requirements of sugar and ethanol production, and the heat demand involved in processing cane into final products. Mills whose energy production is well planned and optimized exceed their energy requirements, generating excess electrical power and bagasse. Modern mills have large facilities for processing and cooling water, and systems for recycling liquid and effluent to irrigate and/or fertilize crops. Vinasse from ethanol distillation, condensed water from sugar processing, filter sludge resulting from

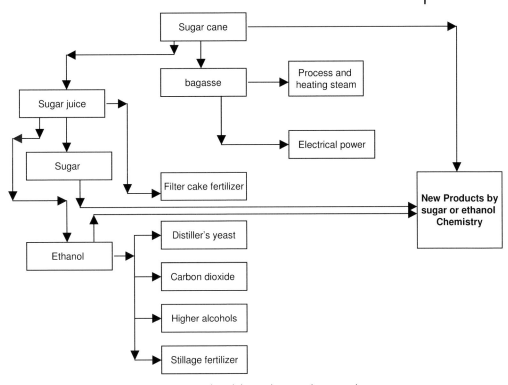

Fig. 10.1 Sugar cane processing to sucrose, ethanol, by-products, and new products.

juice treatment, and ashes and carbon residue captured in the treatment of boiler exhaust gases are disposed of in this way.

The idea of integrating the production of new products with that of sugar is not new. Sugar cane is a renewable agricultural resource and its processing yields sugar, cane juice, syrup, and molasses, a very rich substrate that is convertible by fermentation into higher value chemicals such as organic acids, amino acids, and biopolymers, etc. Sugar, a highly reactive molecule, can be chemically converted into valuable products, as indicated by Kahn [5]. Ethanol, the other main product of Brazilian sugar mills, is the starting molecule of ethanol chemistry, whereby important basic chemicals such as aldehyde, acetic acid, and acetates are produced. Paturau [6] describes some successful examples of integration at sugar mills whose processing involves products such as citric acid, fodder yeast and yeast products, acetic acid, vinegar and cellulose, paper, and bagasse-based fiberboard.

The block diagram in Fig. 10.1 illustrates the context of green cycle production from renewable agricultural raw materials.

10.3
Biodegradable Plastics from Sugar Cane

10.3.1
Poly(3-Hydroxybutyric Acid)

10.3.1.1 Biodegradable Plastics and the Environment

A wide variety of synthetic plastics have been applied in many products, replacing metal, wood, natural rubber, and other materials, and developing into a base industry in industrialized countries since the early 20th century. Today, the production of plastics amounts to 150 million tonnes $year^{-1}$ and the trend is still upward [7, 8]. The main polymeric materials are oil-derived, and the world's growing population has led to increasing oil consumption, which may lead to its depletion as a natural resource [7]. Another problem is the environmental pollution resulting from the disposal of polymeric materials, which may take hundreds of years to decompose. This, with the world's growing environmental awareness, renders the characteristic of nondeterioration desired for a material's use an inconvenience during its disposal.

Although attempts have been made to solve this environmental problem by recycling techniques, despite its wide acceptability, recycling alone has proved insufficient to solve environmental problems, because it is impossible to recover all discarded plastic by this process. The recycling of loaded materials and multicomponents is usually a more complex process. One relevant aspect is that such processes usually consume substantial amounts of energy [7, 8]. Another means of treating solid residues (discarded plastics) is by incineration; this also generates environmental problems, for example air and water pollution, because it releases aggressive chemical agents and causes global warming by release of carbon dioxide. These effects are not restricted to the places where such techniques are employed but are spread around the globe [7, 8].

In this context, the search for a material that is durable while in use and degradable after disposal has led to the emergence of biodegradable plastics – materials that decompose into low molar mass compounds as a result of the action of microorganisms (bacteria, fungi). Biodegradable materials were initially used in medical applications such as sutures, prostheses, controlled drug-release systems, vascular grafts, etc., owing to their biocompatibility, their ability to dissolve and be absorbed by the body, and because their mechanical properties were appropriate for such applications. More recently, biodegradable plastics have been applied elsewhere, including packaging and agriculture (plant containers, controlled release of chemical substances, etc.) [10, 11]. According to U. J. Hänggi [12], because of their higher costs, biodegradable plastics should not be used as a substitute for traditional materials but in applications where traditional plastics are inappropriate. It is worth noting that biodegradable plastics cannot yet compete with traditional plastics because of their higher cost, and that some types are limited to products which are stored for less than one year [12].

10.3.1.2 **General Aspects of Biodegradability**

It is important to clearly define the concepts of degradation and biodegradation. According to the ASTM D-833 there are [13]:

- degradable plastic which, under specific environmental conditions, undergoes significant changes in chemical structure, resulting in loss of some of its properties, and
- biodegradable plastic, degradation of which also results from the action of naturally occurring microorganisms such as bacteria, fungi, and algae.

Biodegradable plastic must initially be broken down into fragments of low-molecular-mass by chemical reactions, after which they can be absorbed by microorganisms, because they are inert to microorganism attack in their original form [8]. These reactions can be induced by oxidative enzymes, which cause superficial erosion, or by abiotic mechanisms (without the presence of living organisms), through hydrolytic or oxidative reactions. In the former process a bacterial or fungal colony on the surface of the material releases an extracellular degrading enzyme which breaks down the polymer into smaller units (monomers or oligomers) which are then absorbed by the microorganisms' cell walls and metabolized as a source of nutrients (carbon). It has been proposed that this mechanism first hydrolyzes the chains of the amorphous phase of PHB and then proceeds to attack the chains in the crystalline state. The enzymatic degradation rate decreases as the crystallinity increases [14, 15]. In the latter situation, hydrolytic and oxidative mechanisms occur in the absence of living microorganisms and are restricted to the amorphous phase and the borders of the crystals, because the crystalline regions are almost impermeable to water and oxygen. The action of the microorganisms begins after the polymeric chains have been broken down.

Although the phenomenon of biodegradation seems simple, it is actually quite complex, for it is affected by several factors which are often interrelated. The rate of biodegradation of these materials may vary over time and depends on the material and on environmental factors, for example the type of repeating unit (nature of the functional group and its complexity), morphology (crystallinity, size of the spherulites), hydrophilicity, surface area, presence of additives, and environment (humidity, temperature, pH, etc.) [9, 15]. A complete understanding of the degradation process will enable us to optimize the entire life cycle of the materials obtained [16]. The products resulting from the biodegradation process are carbon dioxide and water in aerobic environments and carbon dioxide and methane in anaerobic environments [17].

10.3.2
Poly(3-Hydroxybutyric Acid) Polymer

10.3.2.1 General Characteristics of Poly(3-hydroxybutyric acid)
and its Copolymer Poly(3-hydroxybutyric Acid-co-3-hydroxyvaleric Acid)

PHB is an environmentally degradable material belonging to the polyhydroxyal-kanoates (PHA) family, alkanoic acid polyesters which were first described in 1926 by Lemoigne [18]. Figure 10.2 shows the general chemical structure of the PHA and the biodegradable PHB plastic.

This is a material with a unique characteristic among thermoplastics because it presents a complete cycle starting from sugar cane and bacterial fermentative synthesis. PHB is produced, molded, and, after a period of use, discarded and transformed into compost, thus completing the natural cycle. In the absence of microorganisms biodegradability the hydrolysis of PHB in aqueous environments is slow, because of its hydrophobicity. Thus, in principle, the lifetime of a stored PHB product is unlimited; after its disposal, however, PHB becomes clearly biodegradable in domestic effluent-treatment systems [19].

PHB is a biocompatible, biodegradable, thermoplastic, hydrophobic, and stereospecific material. It has a high molecular mass, high crystallinity (55 to 75%), good chemical resistance, and its barrier properties enable practical packaging applications [20, 21]. Table 10.1 lists the physical and thermal characteristics of this polymer.

This material has unit cells with an orthorhombic structure, with the lattice parameters $a = 5.76$ Å, $b = 13.20$ Å, $c = 5.96$ Å [22]. Many of the physical and mechanical characteristics of PHB are similar to those of polypropylene (PP), among them [14]:

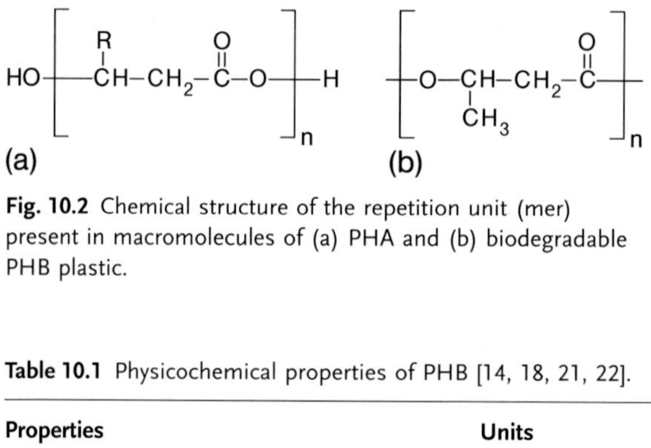

Fig. 10.2 Chemical structure of the repetition unit (mer) present in macromolecules of (a) PHA and (b) biodegradable PHB plastic.

Table 10.1 Physicochemical properties of PHB [14, 18, 21, 22].

Properties	Units	Reference values
Mean weighted molar mass	Dalton (Da)	200 000 to 600 000
Crystalline melting temperature (T_m)	°C	165 to 175
Vitreous transition temperature (T_g)	°C	0 to 5
Theoretical density of 100% crystalline PHB	kg m^{-3}	1260
Density of amorphous PHB	kg m^{-3}	1180

- Young's modulus 2.5–3.5 GPa (comparable with PP or PET)
- tensile strength 20–40 MPa
- Elongation at rupture 3–5%.

The processibility, high crystallinity, and high T_m value of PHB can be altered by bacterial fermentation or use of polymer blends. The various copolyesters (PHBV) include random copolyester (R)-3-hydroxybutyrate with (R)-3-hydroxyvalerate, P(3HB-co-3HV), and random copolyester (R)-3-hydroxybutyrate with (R)-4-hydroxybutyrate, P(3HB-co-4HB). The copolyesters are characterized by their lower crystalline melting point, hardness, tensile strength, and crystallinity (hence, greater ductility and elasticity) than pure PHB. Their physical and thermal properties can be adjusted by varying the HV content of P(3HB-co-3HV) and the 4-HB content of P(3HB-co-4HB). Simply varying the copolymer content [15, 21] enables production of a material with elastomeric characteristics from one which is rigid and highly crystalline. For P(3HB-co-3HV) the crystallinity usually decreases with increasing HV content. The T_m of PHB of approximately 175 °C drops to 71 °C for P(3HB-co-3HV) with a 3HV molar mass of 40%. The T_g of P(3HV) varies from −10 to −12 °C and the T_m varies from 107 to 112 °C [14].

Although copolymers such as PHBV can be used to prevent thermal degradation (lower melting point), the comonomer must be inserted homogeneously into the polymeric chains. For example, for a comonomer content of 16 mol% HV inserted homogeneously into the polymeric chains the corresponding T_m is approximately 140 °C and a single melting peak is obtained for the copolymer in differential scanning calorimetry (DSC) thermal curves. If the comonomer is not inserted uniformly into the PHB chains, however, multiple melting peaks will appear, and the highest-melting peak among these multiple peaks will be located at a temperature exceeding that at which the material is thermally stable (below 160 °C). The HV content is therefore important for the reduction of the system's T_m; equally important is reduction of the heterogeneity of the HV content in the copolymer [23].

The physical properties of copolymers can be altered by varying the comonomer content, but the use of polymeric blends and incorporation of plasticizers are preferable alternatives, because they enable greater versatility in the modification of properties. The synthesis of copolymers is also a more complex process.

10.3.2.2 Processing of Poly(Hydroxybutyrates)

Poly(hydroxybutyrate) can be processed as a conventional thermoplastic in most industrial transformation processes, including extrusion, injection, and thermopressing. By extrusion, PHB can be transformed into rigid shapes (for example pipes) and films for packaging. PHB can also be modified by extrusion by incorporation of additives (stabilizers, plasticizers, and pigments), immiscible additives (e.g. wood and starch powder), or by mixing with other plastics. Because poly(hydroxybutyrate) undergoes thermal degradation at temperatures above 190 °C, the extruder's temperature profile must be as low as possible (approx.

150 °C), and the screw speed must be appropriate. Because of the need for strict control, the processing window of PHB is narrow in comparison with that of conventional plastics. It should be pointed out that virgin PHB is supplied in the powder form, requiring an appropriate screw profile to enable it to be processed efficaciously.

Poly(hydroxybutyrate) is highly versatile when used in the injection process and is easily molded into pieces of varying shapes and sizes, which may range from a few grams to several kilograms. The main uses of this material include injectable packaging for cosmetics and food, agrotoxic packaging and tubettes, and medical and veterinary implants. As in extrusion, injection of poly(hydroxybutyrate) should be conducted with a nonaggressive temperature profile and a low injection pressure to prevent the appearance of burrs.

PHB can also be thermopressed into sheets or other flat shapes. Because characteristics that affect the speed of biodegradation (for example crystallinity, physical shape, molar mass distribution, and compaction of the material) can be altered during processing, PHB samples that have undergone different types of processing may not biodegrade at the same rate. When using most types of conventional equipment, without inclusion of special modifications such as screws or matrixes with specific designs, several operating procedures must be observed if products with satisfactory end quality are to be obtained. Extrusion or injection processes can use typical polyolefin processing screws (L/D 20:1) designed to minimize the exposure time of the melted biopolymer. After use the equipment can be purged using low-density polyethylene resin as vehicle. To prevent marked thermal degradation poly(3-hydroxybutyric acid) should not be exposed to temperatures exceeding 160 to 170 °C for more than 5 min. The polymer's "window of processibility" is relatively narrow compared with that of olefinic polymers, so precise control of the processing temperature is required to prevent temperature peaks in the heating resistances, which would lead to rapid degradation of the material. The "window of processibility" can be monitored by observation of the surface characteristics of the molded component, for example rugosity and shine, which are highly indicative for this polymer.

When using multistage injection equipment, it is advisable to fill the mold cavity rapidly, using high injection velocities combined with high pressures, and ensuring that the injection pressure applied does not lead to the appearance of defects such as burrs and rugosity, because the fluidity index of poly(3-hydroxybutyric acid) drops rapidly when the mass is subjected to high shearing rates. Poly(3-hydroxybutyric acid) does not usually require long cooling times in the mold in comparison with polyolefins. To minimize PHB-molding "cycle times" it is advisable to use injection molds heated to approximately 50 °C rather than injection molds with cold water systems at approximately 10 °C; this enables faster crystallization, with direct consequences on the thermomechanical properties of the molded component. This mold temperature is appropriate, because it is approximately 50 °C higher than the polymer's vitreous transition temperature. The use of this procedure improves the characteristics of ejectability of the molded component, resulting in a gain in "cycle times".

10.4
Poly(3-Hydroxybutyric Acid) Production Process

Poly(3-hydroxybutyric acid) is produced in an aerobic fermentation process in which the sugar carbon source is converted into biopolymer by means of the microorganism *Ralstonia eutropha*. Biopolymer stored in cells as a carbon reserve is recovered by an extraction and purification process described by Derenzo et al. [24]. A description of the fermentation process, microorganism strains, culture media, and the fermentation procedure has been given by Braunegg [25].

10.4.1
Sugar Fermentation to Poly(3-Hydroxybutyric acid) by *Ralstonia eutropha*

The fermentation process follows the procedure described by Bueno et al. [26]. A strain of *Ralstonia eutropha* is grown under aerobic conditions to furnish a high-cell-density culture. After this step the culture conditions are altered and the metabolic pathway is shifted to biosynthesis and intracellular storage of poly(3-hydroxybutyric acid). The block diagram in Fig. 10.3 illustrates the fermentation process; its main characteristics are listed in Table 10.2.

Industrial strains of the *Ralstonia* genus, for example those described by Braunegg [25], are employed in fermentation. Some varieties are highly productive and can store up to 80% of their dry weight as biopolymer. When cultured in a medium containing sugar, ammonium, phosphorus, and salts with a low carbon-to-nitrogen ratio they produce mainly biomass; when cultured with a high carbon to nitrogen ratio, however, their growth phase stops and they begin synthesizing biopolymer.

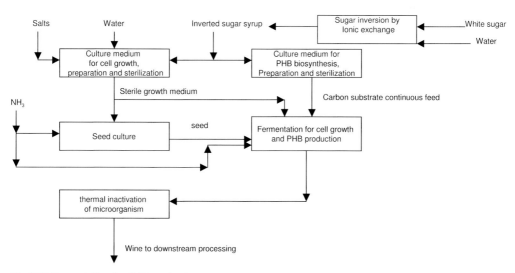

Fig. 10.3 Fermentation for PHB production.

Table 10.2 Fermentation process data.

Biomass concentration in final culture (dry basis)	150 kg m^{-3}
Poly(3-hydroxybutyric acid) content of biomass	75%
Fermentation yield	98%
Fermentation productivity	1.89 kg m^{-3} h^{-1}
Remaining reducing sugars in culture	10 kg m^{-3}
Fermentation temperature	32–34 °C
Fermentation pH	6.8
Molecular weight of poly(3-hydroxybutyric acid) obtained	1200 kDa

Fermentation is by a fed-batch procedure at temperatures of 32–34 °C and pH 6.8. Vigorous aeration and stirring must be provided to accommodate the high oxygen uptake of the biomass. The cell growth stage is highly exothermic and requires the assistance of an efficient cooling system. The growth phase lasts from 24 to 28 h and is followed by the polymer biosynthesis stage, which lasts 30–35 h. At the end of fermentation, when the poly(3-hydroxybutyric acid) content has reached 75% of the dry biomass weight, the microorganisms are inactivated by heating to 105 °C for 5 min to prevent polymer loss, because starved *Ralstonia* use it as a carbon source in the absence of reducing sugars. The final culture is then ready for the polymer recovery stage.

10.4.2
Downstream Processing for Recovery and Purification of Intracellular Poly(3-Hydroxybutyric Acid)

10.4.2.1 Processes for Extraction and Purification of Poly(hydroxyalkanoates)
Recovery of poly(hydroxyalkanoates) in biomass from fermentation involves several complex steps, for example microorganism cell breakdown, removal of impurities, and purification of the final product. These steps are critical from the standpoint of production cost and polymer quality [28]. Use of organic solvents, some of them chlorinated, therefore is unavoidable, at least during the final steps of purification. These solvents are usually hazardous to human health and the environment. The large-scale production of a biodegradable and biocompatible product using environmentally aggressive procedures is contrary to common sense. Poly(hydroxyalkanoate) production should be conducted according to a green cycle, using renewable materials and energy, to avoid impact on the environment [27]. The product recovery process can follow two main routes – biomass digestion and solvent extraction [29].

10.4.2.2 Chemical Digestion
Chemical digestion of microorganism cells using strong oxidants such as sodium hypochlorite was one of the initial procedures for recovering intracellular poly(hydroxyalkanoates) [31]. The granules obtained were washed with solvents such as

diethyl ether or methanol to increase their purity. A drawback of this procedure is the possibility of partial breakage of the polymer, reducing its molecular weight and the purity of the final product. Improvements introduced in this procedure, mainly an organic solvent wash of the polymer granules [32–34], yielded a 95% pure product with a molecular weight of 600 kDa. The main disadvantage of chemical digestion is the resulting harmful and heavily polluting effluents.

10.4.2.3 Enzymatic Digestion

This procedure, which was introduced by Imperial Chemical Industries [35–37] for commercial production of poly(3-hydroxybutyrate-co-valerate), consists of enzymatic digestion of biomass to recover polymer granules. Biomass cells are subjected to thermal treatment at 100–150 °C and pH 6.8 to dissolve the nucleic acid and denature proteins. After this pretreatment, the material is digested with a mixture containing enzymes such as phospholipidase, proteinase, and alkalase. The granules thus obtained are 90% pure, containing 6–7% of proteinaceous material and 3–4% of peptidoglycan as impurities. To obtain a polymer with the required purity, the procedure must include a solvent-treatment step. The solvent step increases production costs and requires the use of environmentally harmful solvents.

10.4.2.4 Solvent Extraction

Many extraction and purification procedures using solvents have been reported [30]. The dry biomass is treated with a chlorinated solvent such as chloroform [38–43], dichloroethane [45, 46], 1,1,2-trichloroethane [46], dichloromethane [47, 48], and/or propylene carbonate [48]. The polymer is dissolved by the solvent, suspended insoluble material is then removed by filtration, and the poly(hydroxyalkanoates) are recovered from the solution by precipitation with methanol, diethyl ether, or hexane. This procedure yields a highly pure final product, but requires the use of undesirable toxic compounds.

Extraction Process in Brazilian Patent PI 9302312-0 Extraction using a renewable, biodegradable solvent is described in the Brazilian patent PI 9302312-0. Figure 10.4 illustrates the solvent extraction and purification of poly(3-hydroxybutyric acid) with isoamyl alcohol, a byproduct of ethanol fermentation [50].

Thermally inactivated fermentation liquor is diluted with water and then coagulated by adding phosphoric acid and lime. A polyelectrolyte is added to flocculate particles, which are recovered by settling and centrifugation. A sludge containing 25 to 35% solids is recovered and sent to the extraction stage. Extraction is performed in a set of multistage continuous stirred-tank reactors coupled with hydrocyclones. Vaporized solvent and liquid are fed continuously countercurrent to the biomass flow. Extraction is performed at the boiling point of the binary mixture. This condition makes it possible to remove excess water, break the cell wall, and remove the polymer with the aid of the solvent.

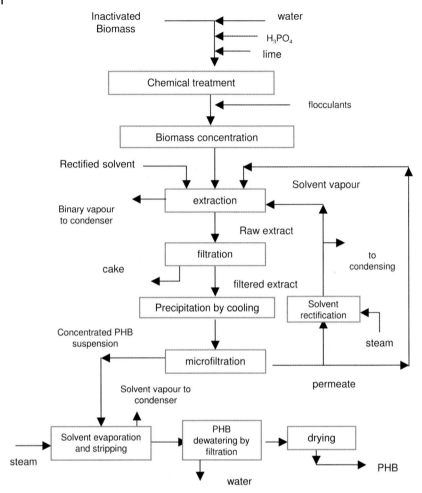

Fig. 10.4 Downstream processing of PHB.

Raw extract of Poly(3-hydroxybutyric acid) leaving the extraction stage contains suspended material such as cell debris and calcium salts, which are removed by deep filtration in a bed of diatomaceous material. The clarified extract is cooled to precipitate the polymer and the debris cake is sent to the solvent-recovery section. The solvent-free cake, consisting of biomass debris and filter aid, is composted and applied to cane crops.

The poly(3-hydroxybutyric acid) suspended in isoamyl alcohol is preconcentrated by membrane microfiltration, raising the concentration from 1.5 to 4%. The solvent permeate is recovered by distillation and the main stream of the polymer suspension is concentrated in a multistage evaporation system to which steam and water are added to distil the solvent as a binary mixture. A final stripping step completes the removal of the solvent. The poly(3-hydroxybutyric acid) is washed, dewatered, and carefully dried to avoid thermal breakage of the polymer. The moisture content after drying and cooling is less than 0.3%. A white powder of 100 to 200 mesh size and 500 to 800 kDa molecular weight is obtained. The fraction of degraded polymer of molecular weight < 300 kDa is less than 3%.

This procedure yields a highly pure polymer by solvent extraction, avoiding the negative environmental impacts of other processes.

10.4.3
Integration of Poly(3-Hydroxybutyric Acid) Production in a Sugar Mill

Production of poly(3-hydroxybutyric acid) is integrated with that of sugar and ethanol and with the generation and consumption of energy at the sugar mill. The production of poly(hydroxybutyrates) from sugar cane is conceived by us as a process to be integrated into sugar mill operations, using not only sugar substrate but also all the facilities the mill can advantageously offer, for example heating and cooling, electric power, water, and effluent treatment and disposal. Figure 10.5 shows a flow diagram for simultaneous processing of sugar cane to sugar, ethanol, and PHB in a typical Brazilian sugar mill in which a milling capacity of 12 000 tons of sugar cane per day is used for production of sugar (55% of total milling) and the rest for fuel ethanol, and where PHB production is to be installed. The milling season last 180 days whereas PHB facilities work all year round, a total of 330 working days.

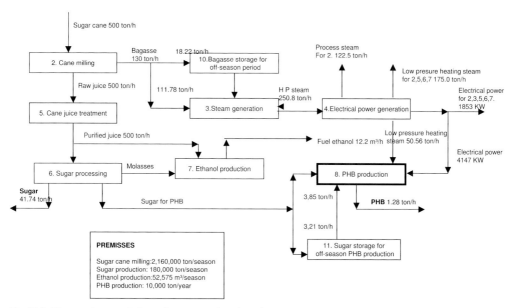

Fig. 10.5 Mass and energy balance for sugar, ethanol, and PHB.

Sugar cane processing begins with extraction of cane juice by mill tandems, leaving behind bagasse, the fibrous material that is sent to the boiler house and to storage. The cane juice is treated physically and chemically to purify it. Most of this juice is used for production of sugar and the rest goes to the fermentation plant to produce ethanol. In the sugar-processing sector, this juice is concentrated in multiple effect evaporators, yielding thick syrup consisting of nearly 65% soluble solids. The syrup is then boiled in vacuum pans until sugar crystals are produced by evaporation–crystallization, which is usually performed in two stages. White sugar of various standards is recovered in this step; the molasses by-product, left over noncrystallizable thick impure sugar syrup, is normally fermented and converted into ethanol.

Part of the sugar production will be used to produce PHB, and sent to the PHB plant for direct use or stored for use during the off-season. At the cane juice fermentation plant, the molasses and sugar syrup are blended to formulate the fermenting must. The must then undergoes ethanol fermentation, yielding the final liquor, which is distilled into aqueous and anhydrous fuel ethanol. By-products such as fusel oil and yeast are recovered in the ethanol production sector. Meanwhile, at the PHB production facility, medium quality standard sugar is processed into PHB by the aforementioned procedure.

Sugar cane milling and ethanol and PHB processing are energy-intensive processes that require mechanical and electrical power and thermal energy in the form of low-pressure steam. Recovered bagasse is burned in a high-pressure boiler, producing superheated steam at 60 bar and 450 °C. This primary steam is expanded in high efficiency multistage turbines equipped with electricity generators, providing the electricity consumed by the manufacturing complex. Medium pressure steam at 20 bar is extracted from multistage turbines and used as the primary mover for mechanical power generation in the milling step involving cane cutters, defibrators, and extraction tandems. Low-pressure steam extracted from the turbines is used as the source of thermal energy for sugar, ethanol, and PHB processing.

The solid effluents from the PHB process will be composted and spread over sugar cane fields as filtering mud from the juice treatment. Liquid effluents, for example the final fermentation liquor and the washing water left behind after removal of microorganism cells containing PHB, will be sprayed on the cane crops like vinasse from ethanol distillation.

10.4.4
Investment and Production Cost of Poly(3-Hydroxybutyric Acid) in a Sugar Mill

A preliminary analysis has been made of the investments required for, and the production costs involved in, sugar-derived PHB. The purpose of the work was to determine the economical feasibility of biodegradable production integrated with an existing sugar mill. The analysis was based on two scenarios – an autonomous unit producing 10 000 tons of PHB per year, located outside the mill site, and an integrated unit having the same production capacity. Construc-

Table 10.3 Investment and production cost of the PHB process.

	Investment in US $	%
Buildings and civil works	3 000 000.00	7.9
Fermentation unit	15 000 000.00	39.5
Downstream processing unit	15 000 000.00	39.5
Utilities	5 000.00	13.2
Total	38 000 000.00	
Production cost breakdown		
Depreciation over buildings and equipment		11
Sugar substrate		29
Other raw materials and chemicals		15.5
Bagasse for energy needs		4.9
Salaries		12.3
Maintenance		5.1
Others		8.6

tion of a manufacturing unit for a production capacity of 10 000 tons per year requires a large investment. Table 10.3 gives a breakdown of investments and costs, with installed equipment totaling US $ 38 000 000. The production cost of PHB is highly dependent on the price of sugar, which is the major factor, accounting for almost 29% of the final cost.

The production cost for a basic 99% pure poly(3-hydroxybutyrate) chemical is estimated at US $ 2.25 to 2.75 kg^{-1}, depending on the price of sugar, other chemicals, and bagasse. It is worth noting that a similar calculation for an autonomous PHB unit shows the production cost rises to US $ 2.50 to 3.00 kg^{-1}, indicating the advantages of integrating PHB production with an existing mill. Comparing our cost data with Lee's [51] estimate of $US 2.65 kg^{-1} and Bertrand's [52] of US $ 5.85 kg^{-1}, we conclude that our proposed scenario is feasible.

10.5
Outlook and Perspectives

Expectations of the development of industrial poly(3-hydroxybutyric acid) production by the sugar cane agroindustry are high. There is a large margin for improvement of the current production process, which will result in lower capital and production costs, less generation of solid and liquid effluents, and lower consumption of energy. Poly(hydroxyalkanoate) production technology will undergo significant improvements when novel microorganisms are obtained by selection or by genetic engineering. One target is microorganisms that can directly assimilate more complex carbon sources, for example sucrose, or even metabolize pentose sugar. Other targets are simultaneous growth and polymer production steps and larger percentages of intracellular stored PHB. Efficient synthesis of heteropolymers other than poly(3-hydroxybutyrate) and fermentation at higher temperatures and lower medium pH will also affect the fermentation technology favorably.

Steinbuchel [53] reviewed bacterial strains and possible genetically modified organisms to improve PHB production. Vicente [54, 55] gave examples of the construction of genetically modified bacteria for poly(3-hydroxybutyric acid) biosynthesis. Poly(3-hydroxybutyric acid) production costs could be significantly reduced by optimizing production processes. Moreover, fermentation could be improved to increase the PHB content of the cells to 80%. There is also a margin for increasing the concentration of biomass in the final liquor to 200 kg m^{-3}, assuming the oxygen transfer rate in fomenters is improved. The technology available today limits fermenter capacity to less than 500 m^{-3}; overcoming this obstacle will lead to increasing gains resulting from scale. The fermentation cycle can be optimized by reducing the content of reducing sugars in the final liquor from the current 1 to 0.2%.

There is a broad range of possibilities for optimizing and reducing the cost of technology available for the extraction and purification of poly(3-hydroxybutyrate). The consumption of thermal energy and the power requirements in downstream processing could be reduced. Polymer extraction and purification should be reviewed to improve the processing stages and to obtain a purer product of higher molecular weight and a lower poly dispersion index. A survey of new extraction solvents is required to identify nontoxic and environmentally friendly solvents that can dissolve more polymer and less undesirable impurities.

A milestone in poly(hydroxyalkanoate) production will be reached when it becomes possible to replace sucrose with carbohydrates contained in the lignin–cellulose biomass component of sugar cane. The bagasse or trash left behind after cane harvesting are lower-cost substrates than sugar and, according to Macedo [3], will be available in large quantities. Depending on the extent of optimization of energy production and available consumption cycles, the amount of bagasse will range from 39 to 67 kg ton^{-1} sugar cane. Biomass availability in trash is estimated to be 56 to 98 kg ton^{-1} cane, depending on the harvesting method employed. In the near future, when the hydrolytic process is commercially ready, this lignin cellulose-based material will be transformed into hexose and pentose sugars, replacing sucrose in PHB fermentation. Da Silva [56] reports on the biosynthesis of poly(3-hydroxybutyric acid) by strains of *Bhukolderia Spp*, using hydrolysis liquor from an organosolve process that yields 65 to 75% total reducing sugars from bagasse. The *Bhukolderia* strain can ferment the pentose and hexose sugar contained in bagasse.

Other poly(hydroxyalkanoates) unlike poly(3-hydroxybutyric acid) and with superior functional properties will lead to improvement of biodegradable plastics. Long chain hydroxyacids and heteropolymer alkanoates can be produced by dosing specific carbon substrates in the polymer-biosynthesis step. Thus, the biological process could be engineered to produce new polymers with desirable properties.

References

1 ÚNICA, www.unica.com.br, **2004**.

2 I. Macedo, São Paulo State Government Report. March, **2004**.

3 I. Macedo, Copersucar Technical Bulletin. **1985**, 31:22–27.

4 I. Macedo, Biomass and Bioenergy. **1996**, 14:77–81.

5 R. Kahn, H. F. Jones, Chemistry and processing of sugar beet and sugar cane. M. A. Clarke, M. A. Godshall editors, **1988**, Elsevier Science Publishers B. V., Netherlands.

6 J. M. Paturau, By-products of the cane sugar industry. **1989**, Elsevier Science Publishers B. V., Netherlands.

7 M. Okada, Progress in Polymer Science. **2002**, 27, 88–103.

8 W. M. Pachekoski, Ms Sc. Thesis. UFS-CAR, SP, Brazil, **2001**

9 S. Karlsson, A. C. Alberton, Polymer Engineering and Science. **1998**, 38, 1251–1254.

10 R. Chandra, R. Rutsgi, Progress in Polymer Science. **1998**, 23, 1273–1335.

11 K. Van de Velde, P. Kiekens, Polymer Testing, **2002**, 21, 433–442.

12 U. J. Hänggi, International Symposium on Natural Polymer and Composites, 2. Proceedings, Embrapa, SP, Brazil. **1998**, 309–310.

13 ASTM. *D883*: Terminology relating to plastics. Filadélfia, **2002**, vol. 08.01.

14 C. Ha, W. J. Cho, Progress in Polymer Science. **2002**, 27, 759–809.

15 M. K. Cox, International Scientific Workshop on Biodegradable Polymers and Plastics, 2. Proceedings, Royal Society of Chemistry, Montpellier. **1992**, 95–100.

16 P. Gatenholm, A. Mathiason, Journal of Applied Polymer Science **1994**, 51, 1231–1237.

17 G. Swift, International Scientific Workshop on Biodegradable Plastics and Polymers. Proceedings, Tokio, Japan. **1994**, 228–236.

18 Y. Doi, International Scientific Workshop on Biodegradable Polymers and Plastics, 2. Proceedings, Royal Society of Chemistry, Montpellier. **1992**, 139–148.

19 G. J. M. Koning, Prospects of Bacterial Poly(R)-3-Hydroxyalkanoates, **1993**, 5–26.

20 M. K. Cox, International Scientific Workshop on Biodegradable Polymers and Plastics, 2. Proceedings, Royal Society of Chemistry, Osaka, Japan, **1994**, 120–135.

21 H. Sudesh, Progress in Polymer Science **2000**, 25, 1503–1555.

22 A. El-Hadi. Polymer Testing, **2002**, 21, 665–674.

23 M. Yamaguchi, Yokkaichi Research Laboratory Report. **2004**.

24 S. Derenzo, Brazilian Patent PI 9302312-0, **1993**.

25 Braunegg, J. Biotechnol. **1998**, 65, 127–161.

26 C. L. Bueno, Brazilian Patent PI 9103116-8, **1993**.

27 R. V. Nonato, Appl. Microbiol. Biotechnol. **2002**, 57, 1–5G.

28 A. J. Asenjo, Separation Processes in Biotechnology, Marcel Dekker, Inc., New York, USA, **1990**.

29 G. J. L. Griffin, Chemistry and Technology of Biodegradable Polymers, Blackie Academic and Professional, Glasgow, Scotland, **1994**.

30 E. Berger, Dr. Sc. Thesis, Ecole Polytechnique, Universite de Montreal, Canada, **1990**.

31 D. H. Williamson, J. F. Wilkinson, J. Gen. Microbiol., **1958**, 19, 198.

32 M. P. Nuti, Can. J. Microbiol., **1972**, 18, 1257.

33 E. Berger, Biotechnol. Tech., **1989**, 3 (4), 227.

34 B. A. Ramsay, Biotechnol. Technol. **1989**, 4 (4), 221.

35 J. M. Merrick, M. Dourdoroff, J. Bacteriol. 88(1), 60–71, **1964**.

36 P. A. Holmes, European Patent Application EP 46 335, **1985**.

37 P. A. Holmes, G. B. Lim, European Patent Application EP 145 233, **1985**.

38 Y. Inoue, N. Yoshie, Prog. Polym. Sci, **1992** 17, 517–610.

39 M. Lemoigne, C. R. Acad. Sci. **1925**, 180,1539.

40 M. Lemoigne, *Ann. Inst. Pasteur. Sci.* **1925**, 39, 144.

41 M. Lemoigne, Bull. Soc. Chim. Biol, **1925**, 8, 770.

42 M. Lemoigne, Ann. Inst. Pasteur Sci. **1925**, 41 ,148.

43 J. Walker, European Patent Application EP 0046017, **1982**.

44 Solvay and Co, European Patent Application EP 14490, **1979**.

45 P.J. Barham, A. Selwood, US Patent Application 4391766, **1982**.

46 P.J. Barham, A. Selwood, European Patent Application EP 0058480, **1982**.

47 J.N. Baptist, US Patent Application 3036959, **1962**.

48 J.N. Baptist, US Patent Application 3044942, **1962**.

49 J.N. Baptist, US Patent Application 3044942, **1962**.

50 S.Y. Lee, J. Choi, Polym Deg Stab, **1998**, 59, 387–393.

51 J.L. Bertrand, Dr. Sc. Thesis, Université de Montreal, Montreal, Canada, **1992**.

52 A. Steinbuchel, B. Fuchttenbusch, Tibtech. **1998**, 16, 419–427.

53 E.J. Vicente, Brazilian Patent PI 9806581-5, **1998**.

54 E.J. Vicente, Brazilian Patent PI 9805116-4, **1998**.

55 L.F. Da Silva, J. Ind. Microb. Biotechnol., **2004**, 31, 245–254.

Biorefineries Based on Thermochemical Processing

11
Biomass Refineries Based on Hybrid Thermochemical-Biological Processing – An Overview

Robert C. Brown

11.1
Introduction

The Biomass Research and Development Technical Advisory Committee (2002) of the US Departments of Energy and Agriculture defines a biorefinery as: "A processing and conversion facility that (1) efficiently separates its biomass raw material into individual components and (2) converts these components into marketplace products, including biofuels, biopower, and conventional and new bioproducts." Implicit in this definition is the assumption that grain will be fractionated into starch, oils, proteins, and fiber and lignocellulosic crops will be fractionated into cellulose, hemicellulose, lignin, and terpenes before these components are converted into market products. Certainly, this is the approach of modern wet corn milling plants and wood pulp and paper mills.

Another possibility for high fiber plant materials is, however, thermochemical processing into a uniform intermediate product that can be biologically converted into a biobased product. This alternative route to biobased products is known as hybrid thermochemical-biological processing or simply hybrid processing of biomass. There are two distinct approaches to hybrid processing:
- gasification followed by fermentation of the resulting gaseous mixture of carbon monoxide (CO), hydrogen (H_2) and carbon dioxide (CO_2), and
- rapid pyrolysis followed by hydrolysis and/or fermentation of the anhydrosugars found in the resulting bio-oil.

Biorefineries – Industrial Processes and Products. Status Quo and Future Directions. Vol. 1
Edited by Birgit Kamm, Patrick R. Gruber, Michael Kamm
Copyright © 2006 WILEY-VCH Verlag GmbH & Co. KGaA, Weinheim
ISBN: 3-527-31027-4

11.2
Historical Outline

The history of hybrid thermochemical-biological processing is brief. The concept only emerged in the 1980s and no such processes have been commercially introduced. Although hybrid refining has potential for overcoming some of the shortfalls of conventional fractionation of biomass, it has not drawn wide attraction, possibly because it crosses the disparate fields of high-temperature thermochemistry and biology. The following paragraphs give brief histories of the gasification and fast pyrolysis approaches to hybrid refining.

11.2.1
Origins of Biorefineries Based on Syngas Fermentation

Traditionally, the feedstocks for the manufacture of biotechnology products have been carbohydrates. Several anaerobic bacteria use C_1 compounds such CO, CO_2, and methanol (CH_3OH) and hydrogen as sources of carbon and energy for growth and metabolite production, however. Syngas, a mixture rich in CO, CO_2, and H_2, is produced by heating carbon-rich solids under high-temperature (600–1000 °C), oxygen-starved conditions. Its name derives from the fact that this gas mixture is used to synthesize a variety of industrially important organic compounds, for example acetic acid and methanol, by the application of metal catalysts and elevated temperatures and pressures. Zeikus and his colleagues (1985) at the Michigan Biotechnology Institute were among the first to propose substituting biocatalysts for the metal-based catalysts currently used to convert syngas into industrial chemicals. A few years later Gaddy and coworkers at the University of Arkansas published a series of papers detailing how a variety of products, including methane, acetic acid, and ethanol, might be fermented from syngas (Ko et al. 1989; Vega et al. 1989 a, b, c, d). Because of the US Department of Energy's interest in developing alternative transportation fuels from biomass, much of the early work in syngas fermentation focused on alcohol production. By 1991, the Michigan Biotechnology Institute had identified the Gram-positive, nonmotile, rod-shaped anaerobe *Butyribacterium methylotrophicum* as a possible candidate for production of alcohol from syngas (Worden et al. 1991) whereas the University of Arkansas focused on the Gram-positive, motile, rod-shaped anaerobe *Clostridium ljungdahlii* (Vega et al. 1989 d). These two groups published several papers in the 1990s although by 1993 Gaddy had started a company to commercialize syngas fermentation technology (Tobler 1994) and his group ceased publishing the results of their investigations.

Only a few other groups have explored syngas fermentation. Elmore and coworkers at Louisiana Tech University (Madhukar et al. 1996) isolated three unidentified rod-shaped, Gram-positive cultures that used mixtures of CO, CO_2, and H_2 (that is, simulated syngas) as their primary carbon source to produce acetate, ethanol, methanol, and smaller quantities of other alcohols and organic acids. Maness and Weaver at the National Renewable Energy Laboratory (1994) opened up new opportunities for syngas fermentation by exploring the conversion of CO and H_2 into poly(3-hydroxybutyrate) by photosynthetic bacteria. More recently, a team at the University of Oklahoma (Datar et al. 2004) has demonstrated the production of ethanol from clean syngas derived from a biomass gasifier and Iowa State University (Brown et al. 2003) is exploring the production of both hydrogen and polyesters from the purple non-sulfur bacteria *Rhodospirillus rubrum* under dark reaction conditions.

11.2.2
Origins of Biorefineries Based on Fermentation of Bio-oils

Bio-oil is a liquid mixture of oxygenated organic compounds produced by heating finely divided biomass in the absence of oxygen. The process, known as fast pyrolysis, involves lower temperatures and shorter reaction times than gasification with the result that it produces mostly liquid product (as much as 70% *w/w*) whereas gasification yields essentially all gas. The technology was developed in the 1980s with the goal of using bio-oil as a substitute for (petroleum-derived) fuel oil (Bridgwater and Peacocke 2000).

Scott and his coworkers at the University of Waterloo, Ontario (1989) discovered that the amount of anhydrosugars, particularly levoglucosan, in bio-oil could be dramatically increased by demineralizing the biomass before pyrolyzing it. Because levoglucosan is readily hydrolyzed to glucose, they suggested that fast pyrolysis be used as an alternative to acid or enzymatic hydrolysis for recovery of sugars from lignocellulosic biomass.

Recognizing that elimination of the hydrolysis step would improve the prospects for using bio-oil as substrate, Zhuang and coworkers (2001a) at the Chinese Academy of Sciences adapted a mutant of *A. niger* CBX-209 to directly ferment levoglucosan to citric acid. They demonstrated that levoglucosan was the sole source of carbon and energy for this fermentation.

So and Brown at Iowa State University (1999) performed an economic assessment that found the cost of ethanol from this fast pyrolysis route to be, within the uncertainty of the analysis, comparable to the cost of ethanol from acid hydrolysis or enzymatic hydrolysis of woody biomass. The prospects of producing both power and chemical products by fast pyrolysis of fibrous biomass, which would constitute a biorefinery, was recently evaluated by Sandvig and his collaborators (2004). One manifestation of this biorefinery included recovery, hydrolysis, and fermentation of levoglucosan. Although fast pyrolysis is a commercial technology, it has yet to be employed as part of a hybrid thermochemical-biological biorefinery.

11.3
Gasification-Based Systems

11.3.1
Fundamentals of Gasification

Gasification is the high-temperature (750–850 °C) conversion of solid, carbonaceous fuels into flammable gas mixtures, sometimes known as synthesis gas or syngas, consisting of CO, H_2, CO_2, methane (CH_4), nitrogen (N_2), and smaller quantities of higher hydrocarbons (Reed 1981). Not only can syngas be used for generation of heat and power, it can serve as feedstock for production of liquid fuels and chemicals. Because of this flexibility of application, gasification has been proposed as the basis for refineries that would provide a variety of energy and chemical products, including electricity and transportation fuels.

Gasification consists of several distinct processes: heating and drying of the fuel; pyrolysis of solid fuel to gases, condensable vapors, and char; solid-gas reactions that consume char; and gas-phase reactions that adjust the final chemical composition of the syngas. Pyrolysis, which begins between 300 °C and 400 °C, may convert up to 80% w/w of solid biomass into gases and vapors. The pyrolytic gases include CO, CO_2, H_2, H_2O, and CH_4 and the condensable vapors include a variety of hydrocarbons and oxygenated organic compounds. The solid-gas reactions produce CO, H_2, and CH_4 by the following reactions (Reed 1981):

Carbon-oxygen reaction:

$$C + \frac{1}{2}O_2 \leftrightarrow CO \qquad \Delta H_R = -110.5 \; MJ \; kmol^{-1}$$

Boudouard reaction:

$$C + CO_2 \leftrightarrow 2CO \qquad \Delta H_R = 172.4 \; MJ \; kmol^{-1}$$

Carbon-water reaction:

$$C + H_2O \leftrightarrow H_2 + CO \qquad \Delta H_R = 131.3 \; MJ \; kmol^{-1}$$

Hydrogenation reaction:

$$C + 2H_2 \leftrightarrow CH_4 \qquad \Delta H_R = -74.8 \; MJ \; kmol^{-1}$$

Two important gas-phase reactions also influence the overall gasification process:

Water-gas shift reaction:

$$CO + H_2O \leftrightarrow H_2 + CO_2 \qquad \Delta H_R = -41.1 \; MJ \; kmol^{-1}$$

Methanation:

$$CO + 3H_2 \leftrightarrow CH_4 + H_2O \qquad \Delta H_R = -206.1 \text{ MJ kmol}^{-1}$$

The final gas composition is highly dependent on the amount of oxygen and steam admitted to the reactor and the time and temperature of reaction. For sufficiently long reaction times chemical equilibrium is achieved and the products are essentially limited to the light gases CO, CO_2, H_2, and CH_4 (and nitrogen if air was used as a source of oxygen).

Gasifiers are usually classified according to the method of contacting fuel and gas. The three main types suitable for biomass gasification are illustrated in Fig. 11.1 (Brown 2003). Updraft gasifiers are the simplest, consisting of little more than a grate with chipped fuel admitted from above and insufficient air for complete combustion entering from below. This countercurrent flow of fuel and air results in producer gas with large quantities of undesirable tars. In downdraft gasifiers, fuel and gas move in the same direction with contemporary designs usually adding an arrangement of tuyeres that admit air or oxygen directly into a region known as the throat where combustion forms a bed of hot char. This design assures that condensable gases released during pyrolysis are forced to flow through the hot char bed, where tars are cracked. A disadvantage is the need for tightly controlled fuel properties (particles sizes between 1 and 30 cm, low ash content, and moisture less than 30%) and an upper bound on gasifier size of approximately 2 MW thermal. In fluidized bed gasifiers a gas

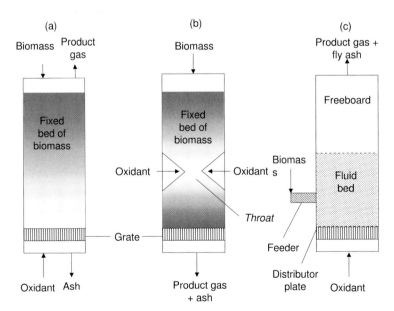

Fig. 11.1 Common types of biomass gasifier:
(a) updraft, (b) downdraft, (c) fluidized bed (Brown 2003).

stream passes vertically upward through a bed of inert particulate material to form a turbulent mixture of gas and solid. They are able to process a wide variety of fuels and are easily scaled to large sizes. Disadvantages include moderate tar loadings, high particulate loadings, and relatively high power consumption to run the air blower.

Overall, gasification is endothermic and requires either simultaneous burning of part of the fuel or an external source of heat to drive the process. Addition of air is called air-blown gasification and has the disadvantage of admitting nitrogen to the syngas, which dilutes the concentration of reactive compounds in the syngas and reduces its chemical enthalpy. Substitution of oxygen for air, known as oxygen-blown gasification, eliminates nitrogen as a diluent but is an extremely expensive solution to the problem.

Several researchers have developed methods for bringing sufficient heat to the gasifier without admitting air or oxygen, a process known as indirectly heated gasification (Bridgwater 1995). Chemical enthalpy from such gasifiers is typically 200% higher than from air-blown gasifiers.

Often gasifier temperatures and reaction times are not sufficient to achieve chemical equilibrium and the raw syngas contains various amounts of light hydrocarbons such as C_2H_2 and C_2H_4 and up to 10% w/w heavy hydrocarbons that condense to a black, viscous liquid known as "tar." Furthermore, two kinds of particulate matter often contaminate syngas. The first, known as ash, is mineral matter in the raw biomass that remains on completion of gasification. The second is char formed during pyrolysis but not consumed by solid-gas reactions. Taken together, ash and char are sometimes referred to as ash or gasification residue.

Typical gas concentrations and chemical enthalpies for syngas are compared in Table 11.1 for air-blown and indirectly heated gasifiers. Clearly, the higher concentrations of CO and H_2 from an indirectly heated gasifier reduce the size of bioreactors needed to convert these gases into organic compounds.

Table 11.1 Syngas composition from various kinds of gasifiers (Brown 2003).

Gasifier type	Gaseous constituents (% v/v, dry)					HHV (MJ m^{-3})	Gas quality	
	H_2	CO	CO_2	CH_4	N_2		Tars	Dust
Air-blown updraft	11	24	9	3	53	5.5	High (~ 10 g m^{-3})	Low
Air-blown downdraft	17	21	13	1	48	5.7	Low (~ 1 g m^{-3})	Medium
Air-blown fluidized bed	9	14	20	7	50	5.4	Medium (~ 10 g m^{-3})	High
Oxygen-blown downdraft	32	48	15	2	3	10.4	Low (~ 1 g m^{-3})	Low
Indirectly-heated fluid bed	31	48	0	21	0	17.4	Medium (~ 10 g m^{-3})	High

11.3.2
Fermentation of Syngas

Traditional fermentations rely on carbohydrates as the source of carbon and energy in the growth of microbial biomass and the production of commercially valuable metabolites. Several microorganisms, however, can use less expensive substrates for growth and production. These include autotrophs, which use C_1 compounds as their sole source of carbon and hydrogen as their energy source, and unicarbonotrophs, which use C_1 compounds as their sole source of both carbon and energy. Among suitable C_1 compounds are CO, CO_2, and methanol (CH_3OH), all of which can be produced by thermochemical processing of biomass.

Although both aerobic and anaerobic microorganisms can use C_1 substrates, anaerobes offer the most promising route to chemicals and fuels from syngas, because they employ very energy-efficient metabolic pathways – most of the chemical energy of the substrate appears in the products of fermentation.

Organisms that form the metabolic intermediary acetyl-CoA from carbonyl or carboxyl precursors are known as acetogens. Although many acetogens consume alcohols or fatty acids to produce acetate, CO_2, and H_2, some are able to utilize CO_2 and hydrogen (autotrophic acetogens) or CO (unicarbonotrophic acetogens) as substrates for growth and production of organic acids and, occasionally, alcohols (Grethlein and Jain 1993).

As illustrated in Fig. 11.2, metabolism of CO begins with the reaction of CO and H_2O via CO dehydrogenase to yield CO_2 and H_2; this is the biologically-mediated water-gas shift reaction. Subsequent steps include production of formate from CO_2 via formate dehydrogenase, several tetrahydrofolate-mediated dehydrogenase transformations resulting in a methyl-corrinoid complex, reaction of CO with CO dehydrogenase to form an enzyme-bound carbonyl moiety, and synthesis of acetyl-CoA from methyl and carbonyl groups bound to the CO dehydrogenase complex (Zeikus et al. 1985).

Metabolism of H_2 and CO_2 occurs by the same mechanism. As shown in Fig. 11.2, H_2 reduces CO_2 to a bound form of CO in a ferredoxin-dependent reaction. The resulting carbonyl group reacts with the methyl-corrinoid complex described previously via CO dehydrogenase to form acetyl-CoA (Zeikus et al. 1985). Acetyl-CoA is the chemical intermediate in the subsequent formation of biomass (growth) and metabolites (production), as subsequently described.

The autotrophs and unicarbonotrophs that convert single-carbon compounds into higher-molecular-weight products are dependent on enzymes and co-enzymes that contain nickel, cobalt, iron, tungsten, molybdenum, selenium, zinc, or combinations of these metals (Zeikus et al. 1985). Similarly, the petrochemical industry is dependent on metal-based catalysts to convert syngas into products. This includes nickel catalysts for steam reforming of hydrocarbons, iron-chromium and copper-zinc catalysts to produce hydrogen via the water-gas shift reaction, copper catalysts to produce methanol, and iron or chromium catalysts to produce hydrocarbons via the Fischer-Tropsch reaction (Spath and Dayton 2003).

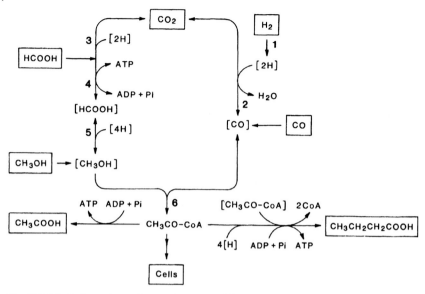

Fig. 11.2 Metabolic pathways for acetogenic bacteria that synthesize acetate or butyrate during growth on C_1 substrates or H_2 and CO_2. The symbols [CH_3OH] and [HCOOH] represent two oxidation states of C_1 units bound to tetrahydrofolate (THF) carriers whereas the chemical nature of [CO] remains undetermined. Numbers indicate the following enzymic activities: 1, hydrogenase; 2, CO dehydrogenase; 3, formate dehydrogenase; 4, formyl-THF synthetase; 5, other THF enzymes; and 6, one or more enzymes required for the synthesis of acetyl-CoA from [CO] and a methyl-corrinoid (Zeikus et al. 1985).

Biological routes to syngas fermentation have several potential advantages over conventional catalytic routes (Grethlein and Jain 1993). Most catalysts used in the petrochemical industry are readily poisoned by sulfur-bearing gases whereas syngas-consuming anaerobes are sulfur-tolerant; thus, expensive sulfur-gas clean-up can be eliminated by using biological catalysts. In conventional catalytic processing the CO/H_2 ratio of the syngas is critical to commercial operations. Because CO/H_2 ratios depend on the quality of the gasified feedstocks, water-gas shift reactors are required to make this adjustment. Biological catalysts are not sensitive to this ratio; indeed, the water-gas shift reaction is implicit in the metabolism of autotrophic and unicarbonotrophic anaerobes. Gas-phase catalysts typically employ temperatures of several hundreds of degrees Centigrade and at least ten atmospheres of pressure whereas syngas fermentation proceeds at near ambient conditions. Finally, biological catalysts tend to be more product specific than inorganic catalysts.

11.3.2.1 Production of Organic Acids

As illustrated in Fig. 11.2, the primary metabolites from the conversion of C_1 compounds by autotrophic and unicarbonotrophic anaerobes are organic acids. The chemical intermediate acetyl-CoA can produce either acetate via acetyl phosphate or butyryl-CoA and subsequently butyrate. The relative yields of these two organic acids depend on the type of organism and the substrate. For example, in studies with *Butyribacterium methylotrophicum* Worden et al. (1989) showed that the fraction of electrons going from CO into butyrate production could be increased from 6 to 70% at the expense of acetate production by reducing the pH from 6.9 to 6.0.

Representative species of acidogenic (acid-forming) anaerobes include *Clostridium thermoaceticum*, *Clostridium ljungdahlii*, *Peptostreptococcus productus*, *Acetobacterium woodii*, *Eubacterium limosum* and *Butyribacterium methylotrophicum* (Grethlein and Jain 1993), with some of these also forming alcohols, as subsequently described.

The metabolism of *B. methylotrophicum* is given as an example of the molar stoichiometric yields that can be expected (Bredwell et al. 1999). For CO substrate and acetate production, the molar stoichiometry, balanced for carbon and available electrons, is:

$$4CO \rightarrow 2.17CO_2 + 0.74CH_3COOH + 0.45Cell \tag{1}$$

where Cell indicates C-moles (carbon equivalents) in the cell mass produced. At least half of the CO must be oxidized to CO_2 to provide enough electrons to reduce the remaining CO to acetate and cell mass. For CO_2 and H_2 substrate and acetate production, the molar stoichiometry is:

$$2H_2 + 1.03CO \rightarrow 0.43CH_3COOH + 0.13Cell \tag{2}$$

11.3.2.2 Production of Alcohols

Although production of organic acids seems to dominate the metabolites from wild strains of autotrophic and unicarbonotrophic anaerobes, alcohols have also been produced from some organisms. For example, the wild strain of *Clostridium ljungdahlii*, a Gram-positive, motile, rod-shaped anaerobe, originally furnished ethanol/acetate ratios of only 0.05 with a maximum ethanol concentration of 0.1 g L^{-1} (Vega et al. 1989d). Adjustment of the fermentation conditions, notably reducing the pH, was reported by Gaddy and coworkers to essentially eliminate acetate production and produce ethanol concentrations as high as 48 g L^{-1} (Phillips et al. 1993).

Similarly, in continuous-culture experiments with *B. methylotrophicum*, Worden and coworkers (Grethlein et al. 1990) found increasing quantities of ethanol and butanol in the fermentation products as pH decreased. More generally, they found a trend toward more reduced products (acids with longer chain lengths and alcohols) as fermentation pH decreased. For example, at pH 6.8 the molar stoichiometry of the continuous fermentation of *B. methylotrophicum* was:

$$4CO \rightarrow 2.09CO_2 + 0.63CH_3COOH + 0.043C_3H_7COOH + 0.027C_2H_5OH$$
$$+ 0.43Cell \qquad (3)$$

whereas reducing the pH to 6.0 changed the molar stoichiometry to:

$$4CO \rightarrow 2.27CO_2 + 0.30CH_3COOH + 0.161C_3H_7COOH + 0.032C_2H_5OH$$
$$+ 0.029C_3H_7OH + 0.31Cell \qquad (4)$$

Worden et al. (1991) noted that acetone, butanol, and ethanol were once produced commercially from glucose by use of a biphasic process consisting of an acidogenic phase, which produced organic acids and H_2, followed by a solventogenic phase, in which the organic acids were reduced to alcohols. In this process acid production generates ATP but consumes no electrons while alcohol production consumes electrons but produces no ATP. They propose a similar scheme for syngas fermentation, with the first phase producing acetate and butyrate from CO (acidogenic phase) followed by alcohol production in a second phase, with reducing equivalents to convert the acids to alcohols coming from hydrogen in the syngas.

11.3.2.3 **Production of Polyesters**

Acetyl-CoA is the chemical intermediate not only for production of organic acids and alcohols by anaerobes but for growth of cell mass, including polyesters that serve as energy stores for the organism. Under conditions of stress, such as an imbalance in the supply of nutrients, many microorganisms synthesize polyhydroxyalkanoates (PHA), which are stored in the cells as discrete granules, as illustrated in Fig. 11.3, that can accumulate to levels as high as 30 to 80% of their cellular dry weight (Kim and Lenz 2001).

Most known polyhydroxyalkanoates are polymers of 3-hydroxyalkanoic acids, the monomeric unit of which is illustrated in Fig. 11.4. Although a wide range of alkanes of different carbon chain length between 4 and 14 carbon atoms can

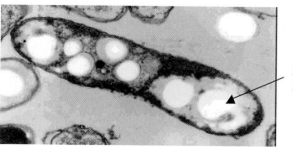

PHA
granules

Fig. 11.3 Photomicrograph showing the accumulation of PHA in *Rubrivivax gelatinosus* (Maness and Weaver 1994).

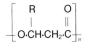

Fig. 11.4 Monomeric unit of poly(3-hydroxybutyrate).

be incorporated into PHA, the most commonly occurring in nature is poly(3-hy-droxybutyrate) (PHB). PHB can be synthesized by a variety of prokaryotes, including Gram-positives and Gram-negatives, aerobic and anaerobic chemo-orga-no-heterotrophs, chemo-litho-autotrophs, and aerobic and anaerobic phototrophs (Babel et al. 2001).

Although glucose is commonly used as the substrate for PHA production, a variety of carbon and energy sources, including CO and CO_2 and H_2, have been exploited by bacteria in production of PHA. The key enzyme in CO utilization, CO dehydrogenase, functions to oxidize CO to CO_2, synthesize acetyl-CoA, and cleave acetyl-CoA in a variety of energy-yielding pathways, depending on the microorganism (Ferry 1995). *Ralstonia eutropha* is an autotrophic bacterium that produces PHB from CO_2, H_2, and O_2 (Schlegel et al. 1961). *Synechococcus* sp. MA19 is a cyanobacteria capable of producing up to 20% PHB when cultivated in a nitrogen-free inorganic medium aerated with CO_2 (Miyake et al. 1996). The photosynthetic bacterium *Rubrivivax gelatinosus* has produced similar yields of PHA copolymers from syngas (Maness and Weaver 1994). *Rhodopseudomonas gelatinosa* can utilize CO as a sole carbon and energy source in the dark to produce PHA (Uffen 1983) and *Rhodospirillum rubrum* can accomplish this in either the presence or absence of light (Kerby et al. 1995).

Irrespective of the carbon source, synthesis of PHA is initiated from acetyl-CoA. The process is illustrated in Fig. 11.5 for synthesis of PHB (labeled poly(3HB)). The route from acetyl-CoA to PHB is thought to involve three steps (Babel et al. 2001). The first step, catalyzed by 3-ketothiolase, links two acetyl-CoA moieties to acetoacetyl-CoA. The second step produces D-(–)-3-hydroxybu-tyryl-CoA either through a single reaction catalyzed by reductase or a sequence of three reactions involving reductase and two hydratases. The final step, mediated by a polymerase, adds hydroxybutyryl monomer to the growing polymer chain to form PHB. Other steps shown in Fig. 11.5 are associated with the decomposition of PHB.

PHB was thought to be the only polyester produced by microorganisms. In 1974, however, other 3-hydroxyalkanoates, including 3-hydroxyvalerate (PHV) and 3-hydroxyhexanoate, were isolated from microorganisms in sewage sludge (Wallen and Rohwedder 1974). Since then a variety of polyesters containing 3-, 4-, and 5-hydroxyalkanoate units have been found to be synthesized by bacteria (Steinbuchel 2001). Most of these are obtained only if precursor substrates structurally related to the resulting PHA are provided to the bacteria as carbon sources, however. Although this might seem to preclude the synthesis of all but a few PHA from syngas, the volatile organic acids that can be generated from syngas by some anaerobes might prove suitable substrates for production of longer-chained hydroxyalkanoates.

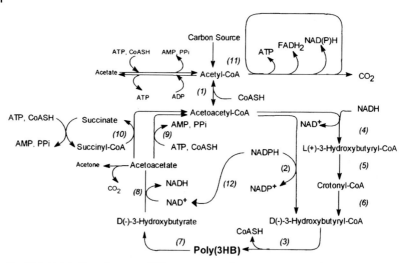

Fig. 11.5 Metabolic pathways to PHB synthesis and degradation (1) ketothiolase; (2) NADPH-dependent acetoacetyl-CoA reductase; (3) poly(3HB) synthase; (4) NADH-dependent acetoacetyl-CoA reductase; (5), (6) enolases; (7) depolymerize; (8) D-(−)-3-hydroxybutyrate dehydrogenase; (9) acetoacetyl-CoA synthetase; (10) succinyl-CoA transferase; (11) citrate synthase (Babel et al. 2001).

Yields of PHB and cell biomass from a given substrate can be determined by experiment or by calculation based on the known metabolic pathways involved. Recovery of this water-insoluble polymer can proceed by one of several methods. Solvent extraction gives high recovery but requires high capital investment and large quantities of solvent. Non-solvent alternatives disintegrate cells by heat shock followed by enzymatic and detergent digestive processes to solubilize the non-PHA components (Anderson and Dawes 1990).

PHB is structurally similar to polypropylene and has similar crystallinity and glass transition temperature. Their chemical properties are completely different, however, and PHB is stiffer and more brittle than polypropylene. These physical properties can be changed by forming copolymers from monomeric units of PHB and PHV. Thus, a range of properties can be engineered from copolymers, ranging from hard and brittle to soft and tough (Anderson and Dawes 1990).

Polyhydroxyalkanoates are attractive as biobased and biodegradable polymers. Specialty applications of PHA include hydrophobic coatings, specialty elastomers, medical implants, functionalized polymers for chromatography, microgranules for use as binders in paints or in blends that incorporate latexes, and as sources of chiral monomers (Kessler et al. 2001).

11.3.3
Biorefinery Based on Syngas Fermentation

One possible manifestation of a biorefinery based on syngas fermentation is illustrated in Fig. 11.6. Fibrous feedstock, for example switchgrass, woodchips, or
cornstover, is fed into an oxygen-blown or indirectly heated gasifier followed by
gas clean-up to remove particulates and char from the gas stream. Removal of
trace contaminants, for example sulfur, chlorine, ammonia, and alkali, is probably unnecessary because they are not thought to poison the anaerobes used in
the fermentation process. The cleaned gas is cooled and passed through a bioreactor where CO is dissolved in the fermentation media and taken up by a
suitable unicarbonotroph, for example *Rhodospirillum rubrum*. In the analysis
that follows, it is assumed that 20% w/w CO is used for growth (formation of
cellular biomass) and 80% w/w of CO goes to metabolite production (H_2 generation via the biologically-mediated water-gas shift reaction). It is further assumed that 40% w/w of the cellular biomass is in the form of storage polymer
(PHA). The actual values for these yields are not well known but these assumed
values are within the expected ranges (Dispirito 2004). Although the diagram
shows gas recycle, it is not clear whether this will be necessary, because the process may not be thermodynamically limited as it is for Fischer-Tropsch and
other types of syngas-to-chemicals catalytic reactors. PHA is recovered and the
hydrogen-rich gas-stream leaving the reactor is used for either on-site or distributed power production via fuel cells.

Brown et al. (2003) have performed a preliminary economic assessment of a
biorefinery producing 20 tpd of PHA and 50 tpd of hydrogen. The capital costs
for this biorefinery, detailed in Table 11.2, are estimated to be $103 million, with
60% of the cost associated with the fermentation equipment. The operating
costs for this plant are detailed in Table 11.3. In this analysis, PHA is taken to
be the primary product with hydrogen a co-product, providing a credit of

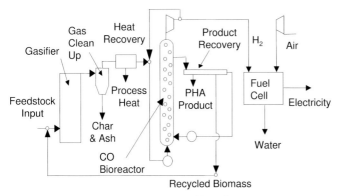

Fig. 11.6 Conceptual schematic diagram of biorefinery to
produce hydrogen and PHA coproducts from fibrous biomass
(Brown et al. 2003).

Table 11.2 Estimated capital costs for a biorefinery to produce hydrogen and PHA coproducts from fibrous biomass (Brown et al. 2003).

Gasifier	$ 18.6 million	Estimated from: Larson and Svenningsson (1990)
Fermenter	$ 59.1 million	Estimated as 25% of total cost of an ethanol plant
Separation equipment	$ 25.3 million	Estimated as 30% of total costs of a fermentation plant
Basic Capital	**$ 103 million**	

Table 11.3 Estimated operating costs for biorefinery to produce hydrogen and PHA coproducts from fibrous biomass (Brown et al. 2003).

Annual H_2 output	16.4×10^6 kg	Assumes 20% CO to cell mass; 40% cell mass to PHA
Annual PHA output	6.6×10^6 kg	
Annual input (switchgrass)	192×10^6 kg	90% capacity factor
Total Capital	$ 119 million	
Raw materials (switchgrass)	$ 9.6 million	Purchased at $ 0.05 kg^{-1}
Credit for H_2	($ 42.8 million)	Assumed to sell for $ 2.60 kg^{-1} (DOE target price)
Labor, utilities, maintenance	$ 16.0 million	
Indirect costs	$ 11.5 million	
Annual capital charges	$ 13.9 million	10% interest, 20 years
Annual operating costs	$ 8.2 million	
PHA Production costs	**$ 1.24 kg^{-1}**	

$ 2.60 kg^{-1}, which is based on a US Department of Energy target price for this fuel. The cost of producing PHA through syngas fermentation is estimated to be $ 1.24 kg^{-1}, which is in the range of many petroleum-derived polymers and considerably cheaper than the production cost of PHA from glucose, which may be as much as $ 5–7 kg^{-1}. Until more complete information is available on yields of H_2 and PHA from syngas, however, this cost of production should be considered an approximate estimate.

11.3.4
Enabling Technology

In a comprehensive review on the prospects of obtaining ethanol from cellulosic biomass, Lynd (1996) noted that syngas fermentation represents an "end run" with regard to acid or enzymatic hydrolysis of biomass, because it avoids the costly and complicated steps of extracting monosaccharide from lignocellulose. Syngas fermentation, by virtue of reducing all feedstocks to a common set of low-molecular-weight building blocks, is able to accept a wide variety of biomass feedstocks, irrespective of their chemical composition. It also has the potential for being more energy-efficient, because it effectively utilizes all the constituents of the feedstock, whether cellulose, hemicellulose, lignin, starch, oil, or protein.

Nevertheless, as described by Grethlein and Jain, syngas fermentation has several barriers to overcome before it can be commercialized (1993). Among these are relatively low rates of growth and production by anaerobes, difficulties in maintaining anaerobic fermentations, product inhibition by acids and alcohols, and difficulties in transferring relatively insoluble CO and H_2 from the gas phase to the liquid phase, where the anaerobes can utilize the gas. Of these, mass-transfer limitations are probably the main bottleneck to commercializing this technology. Studies by Worden and coworkers (1997), however, give encouragement that the use of non-toxic surfactants and novel dispersion devices can enhance mass transfer through the generation of microbubbles to carry syngas into bioreactors.

11.4
Fast Pyrolysis-based Systems

11.4.1
Fundamentals of Fast Pyrolysis

Fast pyrolysis is the rapid thermal decomposition of organic compounds in the absence of oxygen to produce liquids, gases, and char (Bridgwater and Peacocke 2000). The distribution of products depends on the biomass composition and the rate and duration of heating. The yield of pyrolytic liquid, also known as bio-oil, depends on pyrolysis conditions, including relatively short residence times (0.5–2 s), moderate temperatures (400–600 °C), and rapid quenching at the end of the process. Rapid quenching is essential if high-molecular-weight liquids are to be condensed rather than further decomposed to low molecular weight gases. Typical product yields for two kinds of wood are given in Table 11.4.

Bio-oil from fast pyrolysis is a low viscosity, dark-brown fluid containing up to 15 to 20% water, which contrasts with the black, tarry liquid resulting from slow pyrolysis or gasification (Piskorz et al. 1988). As indicated by Table 11.4, the bio-oil is a mixture of many compounds although most can be classified as acids, aldehydes, sugars, and furans, derived from the carbohydrate fraction, and phenolic compounds, aromatic acids, and aldehydes, derived from the lignin fraction. The liquid is highly oxygenated, approximating the elemental composition of the feedstock, which makes it highly unstable.

Despite the high water content of bio-oil, no appreciable phase separation is apparent (Scott et al. 1999). If an equal volume of water is added to the liquid, however, the high-molecular-weight, largely aromatic compounds, are precipitated. Because most of the aromatic compounds can be traced to the lignin content of the biomass, this precipitate is widely known as "pyrolytic lignin".

Table 11.4 Analysis of products from fast pyrolysis (Piskorz et al. 1988).

	White Spruce	Poplar	Type of compound
Moisture content, % w/w	7.0	3.3	
Particle size, μm (max)	1000	590	
Temperature	500	497	
Apparent residence time	0.65	0.48	
Product yields, % w/w, m.f.			
Water	11.6	12.2	
Char	12.2	7.7	
Gas	7.8	10.8	
Pyrolytic liquid (bio-oil)	66.5	65.7	
Gas composition, % w/w, m.f.			
H_2	0.02	–	
CO	3.82	5.34	
CO_2	3.37	4.78	
CH_4	0.38	0.41	
C2 hydrocarbons	0.20	0.19	
C3+ hydrocarbons	0.04	0.09	
Pyrolytic liquid composition, % w/w, m.f.			
Organic liquid	66.5	65.7	
Oligosaccharides	–	0.70	Saccharides
Glucose	0.99	0.41	
Other monosaccharides	2.27	1.32	
Levoglucosan	3.96	3.04	Anhydrosugars
1,6-anhydroglucofuranose	–	2.43	
Cellobiosan	2.49	1.30	
Glyoxal	2.47	2.18	Aldehydes
Methylglyoxal	–	0.65	
Formaldehyde	–	1.16	
Acetaldehyde	–	0.02	
Hydroxyacetaldehyde	7.67	10.03	
Furfural	0.30	–	Furans
Methylfurfural	0.05	–	
Acetol	1.24	1.40	Ketones
Methanol	1.11	0.12	Alcohols
Ethylene glycol	0.89	1.05	
Acetic acid	3.86	5.43	Carboxylic acids
Formic acid	7.15	3.09	
Water-soluble – Total above	34.5	34.3	
Pyrolytic lignin	20.6	16.2	
Amount not accounted for (losses, water soluble phenols, furans, etc.)	11.4	15.2	

Bio-oil has several undesirable characteristics (Oasmaa and Czernik 1999). The low pH of bio-oil, which arises from organic acids derived primarily from the hemi-cellulosic content of the feedstock, makes the liquid highly corrosive. The oil contains large quantities of non-volatile carbohydrates and oligomeric phenolic compounds, which prevents complete distillation of the bio-oil. The highly oxygenated product is chemically unstable, with polymerization of double-bonded compounds and etherification and esterification reactions proceeding over time. The liquid contains fine-particulate char, which is thought to promote polymerization.

The higher heating values of pyrolysis liquids range between 17 MJ kg^{-1} and 20 MJ kg^{-1} with liquid densities of about 1280 kg m^{-3}. Assuming conversion of 72% of the biomass feedstock to liquid on a weight basis, yield of pyrolysis oil is approximately 560 L ton^{-1}.

The mechanism by which cellulose, hemicellulose, and lignin in biomass are converted into liquids is not fully understood. Rapid pyrolysis of pure cellulose yields levoglucosan, an anhydrosugar with the same empirical formula as the monomeric building block of cellulose: $C_6H_{10}O_5$ (Evans and Milne 1987). Addition of a small amount of alkali inhibits the formation of levoglucosan and promotes the formation of hydroxyacetaldehyde (glycolaldehyde). Pyrolysis of pure cellulose at slower heating rates and lower temperatures favors the formation of char rather than liquids. These observations suggest the multiple reaction pathways for pyrolysis of cellulose illustrated in Fig. 11.7 (Bridgwater and Peacocke 2000). Low temperatures and slow heating rates favor dehydration reactions that ultimately convert the cellulose to char and water. At higher temperatures, depolymerization dominates, yielding levoglucosan as the primary product. The presence of alkali, however, catalyzes the dehydration route but yields hydroxyacetaldehyde instead of char and water if reaction products are removed fast enough. Similarly, hemicelluloses form furanoses and furans as primary reaction products whereas lignin forms monocyclic aromatics and non-condensed bicyclic aromatic materials with high phenolic content.

The mechanism by which reaction products are transported from the reaction zone and recovered as liquids is also uncertain (Daugaard and Brown 2004). Many of the reaction products, including levoglucosan, have very low vapor pressures, making vapor transport problematic, but this possibility has not been definitively disproved. Alternatives include transport of low-molecular-weight compounds that condense to higher molecular weight compounds outside the reactor and the elutriation of fine liquid droplets (aerosols) from the reactor.

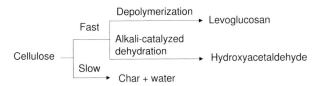

Fig. 11.7 Reaction pathways in fast pyrolysis.

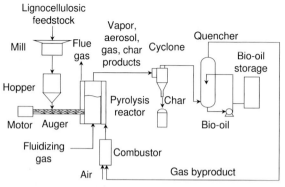

Fig. 11.8 Schematic diagram of fast-pyrolysis plant (Brown 2003).

Production of pyrolysis oils and its co-products is illustrated in Fig. 11.8 (Brown 2003). Lignocellulosic feedstocks, such as wood or agricultural residues, are milled to fine particles of less than 1 mm diameter to promote rapid reaction. The particles are entrained in an inert gas stream, which transports the material to the pyrolysis reactor, shown here as a fluidized bed, which provides the prerequisite high heat transfer rates. Within the reactor, the particles are rapidly heated and converted into condensable vapor, non-condensable gas, and solid charcoal. These products are transported out of the reactor into a cyclone operating above the condensation point of pyrolysis vapor where the charcoal is removed. Vapor and gas is transported to a direct-contact quench vessel where a spray of pyrolysis liquid cools and condenses the vapor. The non-condensable gas, which include the flammable gases CO, H_2, and methane (CH_4), are burned in air to provide heat for the pyrolysis reactor. A number of schemes have been developed for indirectly heating the reactor, including transport of solids into fluidized beds or cyclonic configurations to bring the particles into contact with hot surfaces.

There are several problems with bio-oil. Phase-separation and polymerization of the liquids and corrosion of containers make storage of these liquids difficult. The high oxygen and water content of bio-oil makes it incompatible with conventional hydrocarbon fuels. Furthermore, bio-oil is of much lower quality than even Bunker C heavy fuel oil, so upgrading is highly desirable.

11.4.2
Fermentation of Bio-oils

One possibility for upgrading bio-oil is to change the processing conditions to yield a product that is compatible with biochemical processing. Scott and co-workers (1989) at the University of Waterloo in Ontario, Canada recognized that alkali and alkaline earth metals in the biomass serve as catalysts that degrade lignocellulose to char. If these cations are removed by soaking the feedstock in dilute acid before pyrolysis, the lignocellulose is depolymerized to anhydrosu-

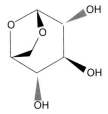

Fig. 11.9 Chemical structure for 1,6-anhydro-beta-D-glucose.

gars at very high yields. Anhydrosugar is a sugar from which one or more molecules of water have been removed, resulting in the formation of an internal acetal structure. The prevalent anhydrosugar from the fast pyrolysis of biomass is 1,6-Anhydro-beta-D-glucose. The chemical structure of this compound, commonly known as levoglucosan, is illustrated in Fig. 11.9. A dimer of levoglucosan, cellobiose, is also produced during fast pyrolysis, but in much lower concentrations. Anhydrosugar has prospects as a platform for chemical synthesis or as a substrate for fermentation.

In studies on woody biomass with and without cation removal Piskorz et al. (1997) found that levoglucosan increased from 3.04% in pyrolysis liquid from untreated poplar wood to 30.42% in bio-oil from pretreated poplar wood. Increases were more modest for cellobiose.

Brown and his collaborators (2001) evaluated the effect of alkali removal on the pyrolytic products of cornstover, an important herbaceous biomass. Three pretreatments were evaluated: acid hydrolysis, washing in dilute nitric acid, and washing in dilute nitric acid with addition of $(NH_4)_2SO_4$ as a pyrolytic catalyst. Although alkali compounds in plant materials are generally water-soluble, attempts to remove alkali by water washing did not prove effective in this study. On the other hand, all three acid treatments were able to substantially increase the yield of anhydrosugars, as shown in Table 11.5. Acid hydrolysis of this anhydrosugar yielded 5% solutions of glucose and other simple sugars.

The resulting glucose solutions can be fermented, as demonstrated by Prosen et al. (1993). However, the substrate derived from the bio-oil contains fermentation inhibitors that must be removed or neutralized by chemical or biological methods. Chemical methods that have been evaluated on bio-oil-derived substrate include solvent extraction, hydrophilic extraction, and adsorption extraction (Brown et al. 2000). The most effective of the chemical methods employed activated carbon. As a less expensive alternative, Khiyami (2003) explored biological treatments. He found that biofilms of *Pseudomonas putida* and *Streptomyces setonii* were able to remove toxins from substrates derived from bio-oil.

As an alternative to hydrolyzing levoglucosan to glucose, several microorganisms have been identified that directly ferment levoglucosan (Kitamura et al. 1991; Nakahara et al. 1994; Zhuang et al. 2001 a, b). This would eliminate the hydrolysis step and probably improve the economics of producing fermentation products from bio-oil.

Table 11.5 Products of pyrolysis for several different pretreatments of cornstover (Brown et al. 2001).

	No pretreatment	Acid hydrolysis	Demineralization	Demineralization with catalyst
Pyrolysis products (% *w/w* maf)				
Char	15.8	13.2	13.2	15.9
Water	2.57	10.6	10.4	7.96
Organics	59.1	67.2	68.5	67.7
Gases	22.6	9.02	7.88	8.44
Organics (% *w/w*)				
Cellobiosan	Trace	4.55	3.34	4.97
Levoglucosan	2.75	17.69	20.12	23.10
Hydroxyacetaldehyde	11.57	5.97	3.73	3.93
Formic acid	2.61	Trace	Trace	0.73
Acetic acid	3.40	1.51	1.26	0.40
Acetol	4.53	Trace	Trace	Trace
Formaldehyde	2.75	1.63	trace	0.70
Pyrolytic lignin	33.40	16.89	17.74	20.08

11.4.3
Biorefineries Based on Fast Pyrolysis

One manifestation of a biorefinery based on fermentation of bio-oil is illustrated in Fig. 11.10. Fibrous biomass is pretreated with dilute acid to simultaneously remove alkali and hydrolyzes the hemicellulose fraction to pentose. The remaining fraction, containing cellulose and lignin, is pyrolyzed at 500 °C to yield char, gas, and bio-oil. The bio-oil is separated into pyrolytic lignin and levoglucosan-rich aqueous phase. The char, gas, and lignin are burned to generate steam for distillation and other process heat requirements of the plant and the levoglucosan is hydrolyzed to hexose. The pentose and hexose are fermented to ethanol.

So and Brown (1999) compared the cost of producing ethanol from cellulosic biomass using fast pyrolysis combined with a fermentation step to acid hydrolysis and enzymatic hydrolysis technologies. The azeotropic ethanol production capacity used in this case study was 95 million L year^{-1} and the assumed cost for biomass was \$ 46 ton^{-1} (1997 US dollars). As summarized in Table 11.6, total capital investment for a plant based on fermentation of bio-oil was estimated to be \$ 69 million, while the annual operating cost was about \$ 39.2 million, resulting in an ethanol selling price of \$ 0.42 L^{-1}. This is about 23% higher than ethanol from plants based on acid hydrolysis and enzymatic hydrolysis of biomass, but well within the uncertainty of the analysis (30%).

A more advanced concept for a biorefinery based on fast pyrolysis is illustrated in Fig. 11.11 (Sandvig et al. 2004). This biorefinery integrates pyrolysis with combined cycle (IPCC) power. Biomass is first washed to remove alkali before it is pyrolyzed.

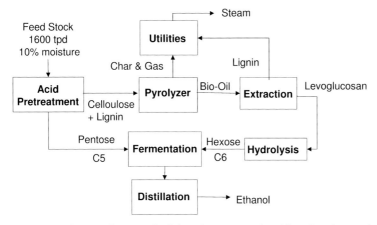

Fig. 11.10 Schematic diagram of cellulosic biomass-to-ethanol based on fast pyrolysis.

Table 11.6 Comparing production cost of ethanol from cellulosic biomass for three conversion technologies (1997 US $).

	Fast pyrolysis	SSF[a]	Acid hydrolysis
Annual ethanol output	95 million L	95 million L	95 million L
Annual biomass input	240×10^6 kg	244×10^6 kg	238×10^6 kg
Total capital	$ 69 million	$ 64 million	$ 67 million
Raw materials	$ 11.1 million	$ 11.3 million	$ 11.0 million
Labor, utilities[b], maintenance	$ 6.18 million	$ 0.9 million	$ 2.13 million
Indirect costs	$ 8.07 million	$ 7.13 million	$ 7.21 million
Annual capital charges	$ 13.8 million	$ 12.8 million	$ 13.3 million
Annual operating costs	$ 39.2 million	$ 32.1 million	$ 33.7 million
Production cost of ethanol	**$ 0.42 L^{-1}**	**$ 0.34 L^{-1}**	**$ 0.35 L^{-1}**

a) Simultaneous saccharification and fermentation (enzymatic hydrolysis)
b) Includes credit for steam generation for SSF and acid hydrolysis processes

Pyrolytic char is recovered for additional processing to activated carbon or marketed as a soil amendment. Pyrolytic gas is used to heat the pyrolysis reactor. Bio-oil is recovered in a specially designed quencher intended to fractionate the bio-oil into different chemicals, including levoglucosan. The levoglucosan-rich fraction is either purified or used as substrate for fermentation to additional chemical products (not illustrated). The other fractions of bio-oil are used to fire the gas turbine cycle to produce electricity. The waste heat from the gas turbine is directed to a waste heat recovery generator, which provides power to a Rankine steam turbine bottoming cycle.

Advantages of the biomass-fueled IPCC system include: cycle efficiency exceeding that of biomass-fired Rankine cycles; avoids need for high-pressure thermal

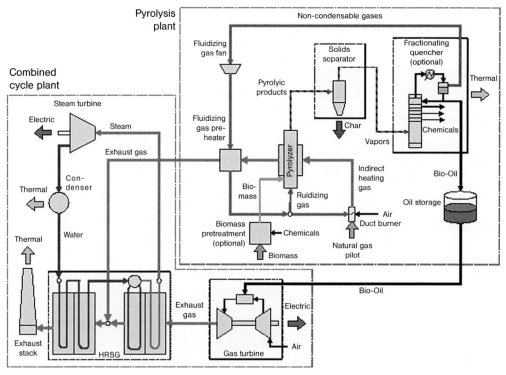

Fig. 11.11 Biorefinery based on fast pyrolysis incorporating combined cycle power and chemical recovery (Sandvig et al. 2004).

reactors; reduces the strong coupling between fuel processing and power generation typical of integrated power systems; and provides opportunities for recovering value-added products. The proposed IPCC system is estimated to have a total project cost of between $ 2300 and $ 2500 kW^{-1} based on a net combined cycle output of 7655 kW. This cost does not include the additional equipment required for production of value-added chemicals. This capital cost compares favorably with that of conventional biomass power systems in this range, which cost around $ 2000 for basic systems to over $ 3000 kW^{-1} for systems designed for higher efficiency and reliability. The cost of electricity for the IPCC plant is projected to be similar to the costs for conventional biomass power systems, approximately $ 0.02 kWh^{-1}.

11.4.4
Enabling Technologies

When Scott and coworkers (1989) first proposed a pyrolytic route to cellulosic ethanol, it was offered as a way of leapfrogging the barriers to fractionating biomass. In a simple, rapid process, fast pyrolysis was able to separate lignocellulose into a pyrolytic lignin and a carbohydrate-rich aqueous phase. The process introduces its own set of technical barriers that have yet to be fully solved, however.

Fast pyrolysis of pure cellulose produces, in principle, levoglucosan as its sole reaction product. In practice, the presence of lignin and a variety of inorganic compounds in fibrous biomass results in more than a hundred chemical products, many of which are not only unsuitable as a carbon and energy source for fermentation but are actually toxic to the microorganisms to be cultivated. Improved selectivity of pyrolytic reactions will be important to achieving high yields of fermentable carbohydrate. Understanding reaction pathways will be the key to success in this endeavor.

Like many of the pre-treatment processes used to facilitate fractionation by acid or enzymatic hydrolysis, fast pyrolysis generates biological inhibitors that must be removed before the bio-oil is used as a fermentation substrate. Methods that are more cost-effective than adsorption with activated carbon must be developed.

Like any process for the production of ethanol from biomass, efficient use of the hemicellulosic and lignin fractions of the lignocellulose will be essential to economic viability. In principle, the pentoses released during demineralization of the biomass can be fermented and the pyrolytic lignin can be used in the production of process steam. Effective use of these coproducts will require more attention to integrating the individual processes making up a system for pyrolytic production of cellulosic ethanol.

11.5
Outlook and Perspectives

Thermochemical processing of biomass to produce substrates suitable for fermentation is a relatively new and unexplored approach to biobased products. Two distinct routes for hybrid thermochemical-biological processing have been offered in this paper: (1) gasification then fermentation of the syngas, and (2) fast pyrolysis then hydrolysis and/or fermentation of the anhydrosugars in the resulting bio-oil. The syngas route, by transforming all the plant constituents into CO and H_2, is attractive for its efficient use of biomass. The fast pyrolysis route, by yielding a storable carbohydrate-rich liquid, enables processing of the solid biomass to be decoupled from fermentation and offers prospects for distributed processing of widely dispersed biomass resources. Both have an advantage over hydrolytic methods in that they are able to process a wider variety of feedstocks, although this is especially true for the gasification route.

Compared with acid and enzymatic hydrolysis, relatively few resources have been devoted to developing hybrid thermochemical-biological routes to biobased products. The reason for this circumstance is easy to understand – the original feedstocks of the fermentation industry were naturally occurring sugars and starches that were easily hydrolyzed to sugar. The fact that starch and cellulose are both polymers of glucose encouraged similar approaches to depolymerizing these two carbohydrates. In fact, cellulose is not only more recalcitrant than starch but it is imbedded in a matrix of lignin, which makes the process of releasing sugar from lignocellulose much more difficult than for starch. Considering these difficulties, hybrid thermochemical-biological approaches to biobased products deserves increased attention.

References

Anderson, A. J. and E. A. Dawes (1990). "Occurrence, Metabolism, Metabolic Role, and Industrial Uses of Bacterial Polyhydroxyalkanoates." *Microbiological Reviews* 54: 450–472.

Babel, W., J. Ackermann and U. Breuer (2001). "Regulation, and Limits of the Synthesis of Poly(3HB) Physiology." *Advances in Biochemical Engineering/Biotechnology* 71.

Biomass Research and Development Technical Advisory Committee of the US Departments of Energy and Agriculture (2002). Roadmap for Biomass Technologies in the United States, Biomass Research and Development Technical Advisory Committee.

Bredwell, M. D., P. Srivastava and R. M. Worden (1999). "Reactor design issues for synthesis-gas fermentations." *Biotechnology Progress* 15(5): 834–844.

Bridgwater, A. V. (1995). "The technical and economic feasibility of biomass gasification for power generation." *Fuel* 74: 631–653.

Bridgwater, A. V. and G. V. C. Peacocke (2000). "Fast pyrolysis processes for biomass." *Renewable and Sustainable Energy Reviews* 4: 1–73.

Brown, R. C. (2003). *Biorenewable Resources: Engineering New Products from Agriculture.* Ames, IA, Blackwell Publishing.

Brown, R. C., T. Heindel, A. Dispirito and B. Nikolau (2003). *Production of biopolymers and hydrogen via syngas fermentation.* National ACS Meeting, Anaheim, California.

Brown, R. C., A. L. Pometto, T. L. Peeples, M. Khiyami, B. Voss, J. W. Kim and S. Fischer (2000). "Strategies for pyrolytic conversion of herbaceous biomass to fermentation products." *Proceedings of the Ninth Biennial Bioenergy Conference, Buffalo, New York.*

Brown, R. C., D. Radlein and J. Piskorz (2001). Pretreatment Processes to Increase Pyrolytic Yield of Levoglucosan from Herbaceous Feedstocks. *Chemicals and Materials from Renewable Resources: ACS Symposium Series No. 784.* Washington, D.C., American Chemical Society: 123–132.

Datar, R. P., R. M. Shenkman, B. G. Cateni, R. L. Huhnke and R. S. Lewis (2004). "Fermentation of biomass-generated producer gas to ethanol." *Biotechnology and Bioengineering* 86(5): 587–594.

Daugaard, D. E. and R. C. Brown (2004). *The transport phase of pyrolytic oil exiting a fluidized bed reactor.* Science in Thermal and Chemical Biomass Conversion Conference, Victoria, British Columbia, Canada.

Dispirito, A. (2004). Personal communication.

Evans, R. J. and T. A. Milne (1987). "Molecular characterization of the pyrolysis of biomass." *Energy and Fuels* 1: 123–137.

Ferry, J. G. (1995). "CO dehydrogenase." *Annual Review of Microbiology* 49: 305–333.

Grethlein, A. J. and M. K. Jain (1993). "Bioprocessing of coal-derived synthesis gases by anaerobic bacteria." *Trends in Biotechnology* 10: 418–423.

Grethlein, A. J., R. M. Worden, M. K. Jain and R. Datta (1990). *Applied Biochemistry and Biotechnology* 24/25: 875.

Kerby, R. L., P. W. Ludden and G. P. Roberts (1995). "Carbon monoxide-dependent growth of Rhodospirillum rubrum." *J. Bacteriology* 177: 2241–2244.

Kessler, B., R. Weusthuis, B. Witholt and G. Eggink (2001). "Production of Microbial Polyesters: Fermentation and Downstream Processes." *Advances in Biochemical Engineering/Biotechnology and Bioengineering* 71: 159–182.

Khiyami, M.A. (2003). Biological methods for detoxification of corn stover and corn starch pyrolysis liquors, Ph.D. Thesis, Iowa State University.

Kim, Y.B. and R.W. Lenz (2001). "Polyesters from Microorganisms." *Advances in Biochemical Engineering/Biotechnology* 71: 51–79.

Kitamura, Y., Y. Abe and T. Yasui (1991). "Metabolism of levoglucosan (1,6-Anhydro-β-D-glucopyranose) in microorganisms." *Agric. Biol. Chem.* 55: 515–521.

Ko, C.W., J.L. Vega, E.C. Clausen and J.L. Gaddy (1989). "Effect of high-pressure on a co-culture for the production of methane from coal synthesis gas." *Chemical Engineering Communications* 77: 155–169.

Larson, E.D. and P. Svenningsson (1990). *Development of biomass gasification systems for gas turbine power generation.* Energy from Biomass and Wastes XIV, Lake Buena Vista, FL, USA. Published by Inst Gas Technology, Chicago, FL, USA, pp. 1–19.

Lynd, L.R. (1996). "Overview and evaluation of fuel ethanol from cellulosic biomass: technology, economics, the environment, and policy." *Annu. Rev. Energy Environ.* 21: 403–465.

Madhukar, G.R., B.B. Elmore and H.K. Huckabay (1996). "Microbial conversion of synthesis gas components to useful fuels and chemicals." *Applied Biochemistry and Biotechnology* 57/58: 243–251.

Maness, P.C. and P.F. Weaver (1994). "Production of Poly-3-Hydroxyalkanoates from CO and H$_2$ by a Novel Photosynthetic Bacterium." *Applied Biochemistry and Biotechnology* 45/46: 395–406.

Miyake, M., M. Erata and Y. Asada (1996). *J. Fermentation Bioengineering* 82: 512.

Nakahara, K., Y. Kitamura, Y. Yamagishi and H. Shoun (1994). "Levoglucosan dehydrogenase involved in the assimilation of levoglucosan in *Arthrobacter* sp. I-552." *Biosci. Biotech. Biochem.* 58: 2193–2196.

Oasmaa, A. and S. Czernik (1999). "Fuel oil quality of biomass pyrolysis oils – State of the art for the end users." *Energy and Fuels* 13: 914–921.

Phillips, J.R., K.T. Klasson, E.C. Clausen and J.L. Gaddy (1993). "Biological production of ethanol from coal synthesis gas." *Applied Biochemistry and Biotechnology* 39/40: 559–571.

Piskorz, J., P. Majerski, D. Radlein, D.S. Scott, Y.P. Landriault, R.P. Notarfonzo and D.K. Vijh (1997). *Economics of the Production of Fermentable Sugars from Biomass by Fast Pyrolysis.* Third Biomass Conference of the Americas, Montreal, Ontario, Canada.

Piskorz, J., D.S. Scott and D. Radlein (1988). Pyrolysis Oils from Biomass. *ACS Symposium Series 376.* E.J. Soltes and T.A. Milne. Washington, DC, American Chemical Society: 167–178.

Prosen, E.M., D. Radlein, J. Piskorz, D.S. Scott and R.L. Legge (1993). "Microbial utilization of levoglucosan in wood pyrolysate as a carbon and energy source." *Biotechnol. and Bioengineering* 42: 538–541.

Reed, T. (1981). *Biomass Gasification: Principles and Technology.* Park Ridge, N.J., Noyes Data Corp.

Sandvig, E., G. Walling, D.E. Daugaard, R.J. Pletka, D. Radlein, W. Johnson and R.C. Brown (2004). "The prospects for integrating fast pyrolysis into biomass power systems." *International Journal of Power and Energy Systems* 24(3): 228–238.

Schlegel, H.G., G. Gottschalk and R. von Bartha (1961). *Nature* 191: 463.

Scott, D.S., S. Czernik, J. Piskorz and D. Radlein (1989). *Sugars from biomass cellulose by a thermal conversion process.* Energy from Biomass and Wastes XIII, New Orleans, LA, USA, Published by Inst of Gas Technology, Chicago, IL, USA, pp. 1349–1362.

Scott, D.S., P. Majerski, J. Piskorz and D. Radlein (1999). "A second look at fast pyrolysis of biomass – the RTI process." *J. Analytical and Applied Pyrolysis* 51: 23–37.

So, K. and R.C. Brown (1999). "Economic analysis of selected lignocellulose-to-ethanol conversion technologies." *Applied Biochemistry and Biotechnology* 77–79: 633–640.

Spath, P.L. and D.C. Dayton (2003). Preliminary Screening – Technical and Economic Assessment of Synthesis Gas to Fuels and Chemicals with Emphasis on the Potential for Biomass-Derived Syngas. National Renewable Energy Laboratory, Technical Report NREL/TP-510-34929, Golden, CO, USA.

Steinbuchel, A. (2001). "Perspectives for biotechnological production and utilization of biopolymers: metabolic engineering of polyhydroxyalkanoate biosynthesis pathways as a successful example." *Macromolecular Bioscience* 1: 1–14.

Tobler, C. (1994). Genesis gives Birth to another company. *Arkansas Business*, February 28.

Uffen, R. L. (1983). "Metabolism of carbon monoxide by *Rhodopseudomonas gelatinosa*: cell growth and properties of the oxidation system." *J. Bacteriology* 155: 956–965.

Vega, J. L., G. M. Antorrena and E. C. Clausen (1989a). "Study of gaseous substrate fermentations: Carbon monoxide conversion to acetate. 2. Continuous culture." *Biotechnology and Bioengineering* 34: 785–793.

Vega, J. L., E. C. Clausen and J. L. Gaddy (1989b). "Study of gaseous substrate fermentations: Carbon monoxide conversion to acetate. 1. Batch culture." *Biotechnology and Bioengineering* 34(6): 774–784.

Vega, J. L., V. L. Holmberg, E. C. Clausen and J. L. Gaddy (1989c). "Fermentation parameters of peptostreptococcus-productus on gaseous substrates (CO, H$_2$/CO$_2$)." *Archives of Microbiology* 151(1): 65–70.

Vega, J. L., S. Prieto, B. B. Elmore, E. C. Clausen and J. L. Gaddy (1989d). "The biological production of ethanol from synthe-

sis gas." *Applied Biochemistry and Biotechnology* 20/21: 781–797.

Wallen, L. L. and W. K. Rohwedder (1974). "Poly-beta-hydroxyalkanoate from activated sludge." *Environ Sci Technol* 8: 576–579.

Worden, R. M., M. D. Bredwell and A. J. Grethlein (1997). Engineering Issues in Synthesis-Gas Fermentations. *Fuels and Chemicals from Biomass*. Washington, D.C., American Chemical Society. ACS Symposium Series No. 666: 320–336.

Worden, R. M., A. J. Grethlein, M. K. Jain and R. Datta (1991). "Production of butanol and ethanol from synthesis gas via fermentation." *Fuel* 70(5): 615–619.

Worden, R. M., A. J. Grethlein, J. G. Zeikus and R. Datta (1989). *Applied Biochemistry and Biotechnology* 20/21: 687.

Zeikus, J. G., R. Kerby and J. A. Krzycki (1985). "Single-carbon chemistry of acetogenic and methanogenic bacteria." *Science* 227: 1167–1173.

Zhuang, X. L., H. X. Zhang and J. J. Tang (2001a). "Levoglucosan kinase involved in citric acid fermentation by Aspergillus niger CBX-209 using levoglucosan as sole carbon and energy source." *Biomass and Bioenergy* 21: 53–60.

Zhuang, X. L., H. X. Zhang, J. Z. Yang and H. Y. Qi (2001b). "Preparation of levoglucosan by pyrolysis of cellulose and its citric acid fermentation." *Bioresource Technology* 79(1): 63–66.

Green Biorefineries

12
The Green Biorefinery Concept – Fundamentals and Potential

Stefan Kromus, Birgit Kamm, Michael Kamm, Paul Fowler,
and Michael Narodoslawsky

12.1
Introduction

Green biorefineries are integrated technologies and technology systems for production of materials and energy processing of green plants and parts of green
plants. Above all, green biorefinery technologies are based on traditional technologies of green forage preservation, leaf-protein extraction, chlorophyll production, and modern biotechnological and chemical conversion methods.

The main raw material of green biorefineries are green plants, for example
grass, alfalfa, and immature (green) grain or green plant parts, for example
leaves. Green plant parts are a virtually inexhaustible raw material reservoir,
which is fast-growing, available world-wide, and may have ecological advantages.
Considering alfalfa alone, 32 million hectares are currently cultivated and converted into green pellets or forage flour worldwide.

By means of primary photosynthesis green C3 plants can yield up to 20 tons
dry matter with up to four tons of proteins in temperate climates each year. C4
plants in tropical zones can, however, produce up to 80 tons dry matter with six
tons of proteins per hectare per year. Green plants are, moreover, rich in carbohydrates, proteins, lipids, lignin, and a group of secondary plant substances and
phytochemicals. Green plants and green plant parts may therefore be seen as a
chemical plant with a huge potential. In comparison with other vegetable biomass green plants are characterized by a high content of aqueous cell juice with
carbohydrates of low molecular weight, a large amount of enzymes (proteins)
for photosynthesis and a relatively low content of lignin in the cell walls.

For these reasons all technological concepts of green biorefineries include the
separation of the cell juice from the plant framework. Both fractions, the cell

Biorefineries – Industrial Processes and Products. Status Quo and Future Directions. Vol. 1
Edited by Birgit Kamm, Patrick R. Gruber, Michael Kamm
Copyright © 2006 WILEY-VCH Verlag GmbH & Co. KGaA, Weinheim
ISBN: 3-527-31027-4

juice and the cellulose-containing leaf cells are subjected to different biotechnological and physicochemical conversion methods.

12.2
Historical Outline

12.2.1
The Inceptions

The green parts of plants have been used by the human being for ages. Primarily ruminants use green plants as fodder. The relevance of green crop cultivation was already apparent from the occupation of the sons of Adam and Eve, Cain and Abel – Abel became a shepherd, Cain a farmer [1]. The direct use of green plants in the diet of humans is ancient. We are able to distinguish between use as nutrition or for salvation or as a natural stimulant. In Europe the consumption of spinach (*Spinacia oleracea*), stinging-nettle (*Urtica*), sorrels (*Rumex acetosa*), curly kale (*Brassica oleraceae var. Sabellica*), and leek (*Allium ampelobrasum*) is very common.

The chemical and biochemical scientific exploration of green plant leaves can be traced back to the 18th century. The French chemists G. F. and H. M. Roulle reported obtaining protein extracts from alfalfa leaves in 1773. Hillaire Marin Roulle in particular, a demonstrator at the royal garden in Paris since 1770, proved that the juices obtained by pressing the vegetable alfalfa contain a substance which coagulated when heated into a "cheesy" substance similar to animal material. The new coagulate, found by Roulle in the heated juice obtained by pressing different plants, was therefore called "vegato-animale" substance (today it is called leaf protein) [2].

Mild warming yielded a green colored fraction, further heating delivered an almost colorless precipitate. Chemical analysis of the colorless substance revealed it contained a larger amount of that new substance than the green coagulate. Also, by extraction of the green pigments with alcohol the green precipitate could be removed [2]. It is impressive that key procedures of modern protein separation of green biomass in green biorefineries were researched as early as 1773 [3–7]. The functional characteristic of thermal coagulation of proteins was, moreover, the first criterion for later definition of proteins as a class of substance [3].

12.2.2
First Production of Leaf Protein Concentrate

In the 20th century research on leaf protein concentrate (LPC) focused on use of the proteins for human nutrition [4–6], because of the widespread availability, high nutritional value, and high protein productivity in green plants, with its valuable spectrum of essential amino acids and the intensive growth of green plants under climatically favorable conditions. Technical manipulations are necessary to separate the leaf protein in a form digestible by humans, because the human being is not equipped with the opportunity to digest leaf cells and, particularly, their cellulose membrane as ruminants do.

Of special economic interest is a fraction expressed in the chloroplasts of green plants. The so called fraction-I-protein is the photosynthesis enzyme ribulose-1,5-biphosphatecarboxylase/oxygenase or rubisco, which can be regarded as the most widespread protein in the world. In spinach leaves, rubisco accounts for 75% of soluble proteins; in wheat and barley it is 53–75% and in corn and sweet sorghum (sugar millet) (*Sorghum dochna*) 15% [8, 9]. It must, however, be stressed that by means of electrophoresis approximately 250 to 300 different proteins and polypeptides can be detected in green-plant extracts [10, 11]. In alfalfa (*Medicago sativa L.*) rubisco amounts for 30–70% of the soluble proteins, depending on genotype and vegetation cycle [9, 12]. On the basis of the protein harvest from one hectare of arable land, alfalfa provides a 3 to 10-fold higher yield than oilseeds, grain legumes, or grain [9].

In times of crises, especially, the topic of leaf protein for nutrition has repeatedly been put on the nutrition agenda. For example, in 1917 the use of alfalfa flour for bread manufacture was reported in the "Literary digest". In 1920 and 1921 Osborne and Chibnell published their results of examinations of proteins in green leaves. Ereky proposed the utilization of leaf proteins for public nutrition in 1925 and Slade renewed this suggestion in 1937. Slade and Birkinshaw were the first to patent the utilization of grass and other green plants in 1939 [13].

These developments were favored by results from examinations which proved that green forage supplies ruminants with more proteins and essential amino acids than they can actually utilize. Ruminants like cows, oxen, and sheep need, on a dry matter basis, only 16% of crude protein in their feed. Alfalfa and grasses, however, contain 22–28% crude protein on dry matter basis [14]. The opportunity to simultaneously provide benefits for both animals and humans from green plants would result from removal of the "surplus" protein before feeding the green fodder to ruminants. This idea evolved for the first time during World War II. Because of the manure-nitrogen problem, due to the industrialization of livestock farming, the idea underwent a revival.

During World War II, researchers and developers stressed the importance of leaf protein concentrate for providing the population with sufficient protein because of food-supply shortages in Europe. After the occupation of France by the Germans in 1940, Great Britain in particular, was cut off from the food supply on the continent. Thus, the United Kingdom enforced large-scale developments and put priority on nutrition by use of green-plant proteins.

All large-scale developments revealed technical problems and were not very profitable, and development was stopped because of the American-British Land Lease Agreement in 1941. Nevertheless, young Pirie, Scientist at the Rothamsted Experimental Station in Hertfordshire, UK, was able to accomplish important pioneering work for later industrial production of leaf protein [15–17].

In the sixties development of production plants utilizing green leaves began again. Five main reasons can be identified for the relaunch of leaf protein plants. First, forecasts suggested a lack of protein-rich products worldwide. Second, the industrial livestock farming which was developing demanded standardized and metered feeding. Third, the interest of the industrialized world in the nutritional problems of the developing countries was increasing. Fourth, the member states of the Warsaw Pact wanted to separate themselves from the world market and generated their own supply of food and feed protein. Finally, the rising cost of energy (the later oil price shock) focused interest on extraction of leaf protein as alternative to other means of green forage conservation.

The first modern industrial process for leaf protein extraction was called the Rothamsted process, developed by Pirie. The procedure based on heat coagulation of green plant juice at 70 °C, resulted in leaf protein concentrates with 60%

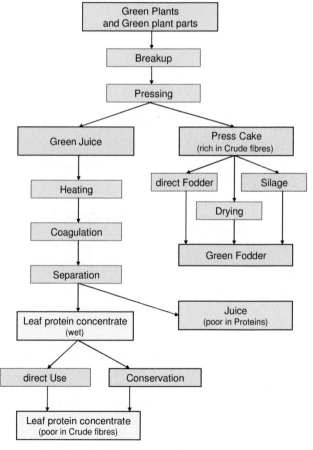

Fig. 12.1 Flow chart of the fractionation of green plant parts for extraction of leaf protein concentrate.

protein content and a lipid content of 20 to 25% (lipid–protein concentrate) [4, 18]. Later, processes were developed which were based on heat coagulation at 80 °C [19, 20]. Finally, procedures based on two-step heating of the green press juice enabled fractionated extraction of proteins, leading to products of different composition [21, 22].

The basic fractionation process is the same for all concepts, as shown in Fig. 12.1.

Delays between harvesting in the field and processing in the factory should be reduced to a minimum. After grinding and crushing in mills the green matter is pressed. Wet fractionation (pressing) leads to two fractions – the press cake and the press juice. The press cake is rich in crude fiber and the press juice contains proteins, water-soluble sugars (WSC), ash and other interesting substances, for example lutein.

The developments mentioned above resulted throughout the seventies in market-leading technologies such as the Proxan procedure and the Alfaprox procedure, which are used for generation of protein–xanthophyll concentrates, including utilization of the by-products, although predominantly in agriculture [14, 23].

12.2.3
First Production of Leaf Dyes

Chlorophylls, often termed the "pigments of life", are green colored macrocyclic pigments which are the primary photosynthetic pigments in nature. The term *chlorophyll*, coined by Berzelius in 1838, is derived from Greek roots and indicates the green of leaves [24]. In fact, as green pigments they are responsible for the primary biochemical energy generation in nature and give the only indications of life on earth visible from outer space. Reduction of the chlorophyll (leaf green) gives the xanthophylls (leaf yellow) and carotenes that are not dissolved and remain in the leaf, resulting in showy yellow and orange tinges. The red color pigments are derived from anthocyan, created by metabolic alteration of the leaves [25].

Although scientists had previously studied the green plant pigment it was only in 1913 that the first significant research on its structure, separation, and properties was reported. This work, which won the 1915 Nobel Prize for the German chemist Willstätter, serves as the basis for subsequent production of chlorophyll [26, 27].

In the United States, commercial production of chlorophyll and carotene by extraction from alfalfa leaf meal has conducted since 1930 [28, 29]. Chlorophyll, in various forms, was reported to be present in 1000 products that consumed 10 000 pounds of the green material per month in 1952, with a market value of 50 Million USD [30]. For example, Strong, Cobb and Company obtained 0.5 ton of chlorophyll per day from alfalfa in 1952. The water-soluble chlorophyll, or chlorophyllin, found use as a deodorizing agent in toothpastes, soaps, mouthwashes, shampoos, chewing gums, candies, deodorants, and pharmaceuticals [31].

Since 1990 chlorophyll has also been used for conversion of light energy into electric energy. Electrochemical solar cells, e.g. the Graetzel cell a TiO_2–chlorophyll-SnO_2 solar cell, use organic dyes (not a semiconductor material), for example the leaf dye chlorophyll, for absorption of light [32].

12.3
Green Biorefinery Raw Materials

12.3.1
Raw Materials

The major raw material of green biorefineries is "green biomass", including the large group of green plant materials (green grass from meadows, willow, extensive willow management, other natural resources), wild fruit and crops, alfalfa and clover, and immature cereals and plant shoots. The green plant material contains complex natural and valuable materials in the form of carbohydrates, proteins, fibers, fragrances, dyes, fats, hormones, amino acids, enzymes, and other important substances [5, 7, 33, 34].

Ecologically friendly agriculture is based on primary production by photosynthesis in green plants during the whole growth season. During a vegetation period successive harvest and re-growth of one and the same crop can give a maximum yield of dry matter and protein per area. Green grasses and immature cereals are excellent for this purpose. Especially, grasses can be grown on most types of soil in most types of climate, on both normal agricultural land and marginal land. Thus C3 species in temperate climates can yield up to 20 tonnes of dry matter and 4 tons of protein per ha (hectare $= 10\,000$ m^2) per year whereas C4 species in tropical climates can produce 80 tonnes of dry matter and 6 tonnes of protein [33, 34].

The yield of dry matter and protein from grass and the quality of the leaf protein concentrate (LPC) obtained is affected by the type of photosynthesis [35]. Leaf anatomy and cell structure are different for the two types of plant adapted to different climates. The C4 species have a more efficient carbon dioxide fixation mechanism and are grown on soils poor in nitrogen. Thus C4 species have a very high dry-matter production per soil area, but have a low protein content of the dry matter. The C3 species lose fixed carbon dioxide by a process called photorespiration. Thus C3 plants produce less dry matter per unit area. In C3 species more leaf cells are rich in protein (FI protein/rubisco protein). Therefore, a relatively high proportion of the dry matter of C3 species consists of protein. Subsequently, LPC from C3 species is rich in protein. Both temperate grass species, including green cereals [34, 35] and tropical grasses [36], have been investigated for LPC production (Table 12.1).

The second important raw material source is the green harvesting residue material from agricultural cultivated crops. In particular the vegetables of importance are those with green foliage. This includes, e.g., not insignificant

Table 12.1 Grasses and green cereals investigated for green
crop fractionation [34, 35].

Avena sativa	*Holcus lanatus*	*Pennisetum purpureum*
Bromus arvensis	*Hordeum vulgare*	*Phalaris arundinacea*
Cynodon dactylon	*Lolium multiflorum*	*Secale cereale*
Dactylis glomerata	*Lolium perenne*	*Tricum aestivum*
Festuca arundinaceae	*Paspalum dilitatum*	*Zea mays*
Festuca pratensis		

amounts of sugar beet leaves (sugar beet for the sugar industry), hemp scrapes
and leaves (hemp for fiber production), residues from flax processing, and residues from the fresh vegetable production.

Further potential refinery raw materials are the little standardized juice-rich
waste biomass. This should contain moisture and mainly natural and valuable
materials or have a substantial conversion grade. According to coupling effects
of material and energy use, the constitution can strongly vary. Such waste biomass is not yet standardized, but is a renewable natural waste resource that
must be managed. Such biomass can be residues from plant production (mixed
and ripe harvest residuals), potato juice, hydroxycarboxylic acid-rich waste as silage seepage, juices from the canned food industry, or residues from the sugar
industry or animal production.

The fourth large group is the little standardized dried biomass and waste biomass. These often contain a large amount of plant cellulose and will therefore
be supplied as raw material to press-cake-using production lines. This can be residual straw, hay, and all kinds of dried foliage (e.g. maize hay). Residues from
in-plant waste paper and wood, e.g. for energy production or cardboard production, are also included in this category. This group also includes modern concepts of dry crop fractionation, for example immature cereals [37].

It should be mentioned that transitions between raw material types will and
should be fluid [38].

12.3.2
Availability of Grassland Feedstocks for Large-scale Green Biorefineries

In Europe, grassland amounts to about 45 Mio ha, which is approximately 35%
of the arable land (basis: 15 member states without new member states). A
large part of this grassland is regarded as absolute grassland habitat which cannot legally be converted into plain arable land. Based on an average yield of
10 tons dry matter per ha per year, however, the European grassland produces
about 450 Mio tons dry matter each year [39]. The main purpose of grassland
cultivation is still the production of forage for animal farming. The use of grassland for feed production is dropping, because limitation of production quotas
and the increasing efficiency of animal breeding (especially dairy farming) is
leading a decrease in livestock numbers. Other uses for grassland must there-

Table 12.2 Production of green pellets or powder in Europe.

Country	Amount dry matter (t a^{-1})	Country	Amount dry matter (t a^{-1})
Germany	320 000	The Netherlands	214 300
Austria	1 292	Ireland	5 337
Belgium	3 600	Italy	704 000
Denmark	170 868	Portugal	3 734
Spain	2 100 678	Great Britain	56 539
Finland	1 518	Sweden	11 571
France	1 398 445	Czech Republic	29 158
Greece	48 848	**Europe**	**5 069 888**

fore be found, for example the supply of raw material for the bio-industry. This trend is apparent throughout Europe [40].

Because of its ability to fix nitrogen from the air and enrich the soil with this element, alfalfa is the most important forage crop in the world, cultivated on approximately 32 million hectares. The plant contains the protein rubisco as approximately 20% of the total dry matter [41].

Green forage drying plants, especially, offer a very good possibility for use in biorefinery systems. These plants can be seen as agro–industrial knots in grassland farming. More than 300 green forage drying plants are used to produce over 5 Mio tons of dried pellets and powder (Table 12.2) [42].

In the USA the *Alfalfa New Products Initiative* (ANPI) has the objective of extending the cultivation and utilization of alfalfa. The ANPI consists of five states: North Dakota, South Dakota, Minnesota, Wisconsin, and Michigan. Prominent technology in this context is dehydration and fractionation (dry or wet) [43].

12.3.3
Key Components of Green and Forage Grasses

The research literature on forage grasses is mainly concerned with their nutritive aspects as fodder grass, hay, or silage. From a biochemical perspective the composition of forage grasses is well described. Thus, a comprehensive inventory of forage grass chemical/material constituents is available in the literature. The components can be conveniently categorized according to their location within the grass, either as a cell wall constituent or as a component within the cell.

12.3.3.1 Structural Cell Wall Constituents
Cell wall constituents comprise structural polysaccharides (hemicellulose, cellulose), lignin, and pectin substances. The qualitative and quantitative composition of constituents within the cell walls varies during the growing season.

Hemicellulose, Cellulose, and Lignin The hemicellulose, cellulose, lignin, and crude fiber content of fresh herbage, hay, and silage from meadow grasses has been compared [44]. The crude fiber content of grass harvested as fresh herbage was 24.0–35.5% of the dry matter (DM). The crude fiber content increased with delay in harvesting and was higher in hay and silage than in the fresh herbage. The combined total hemicellulose, cellulose, and lignin content was twice that of crude fiber in grasses. During ensiling of grasses the hemicellulose content was reduced by an average of 3–11%, the cellulose remained unchanged, and the lignin content increased by 23%.

With advancing maturity, the concentrations of cellulose, hemicellulose, and lignin, in grasses increase. In general, the digestibility of cellulose decreases during the growing season; this commonly attributes to an increasing lack of accessibility of the polymer to be attacked by microorganisms [45]. This variation should be considered when assessing grasses as feedstock for industrial processes, particularly when a decision to harvest a forage grass specifically for its fiber content must be made.

Chemical composition and digestibility were studied in vivo and in vitro [45]. The main finding was that although the grass species studied had similar gross chemical composition, the digestibility varied substantially at comparable stages of maturity. Thus a rapid decrease in digestibility was observed between the two first cuts whereas only small changes were observed between the two times of harvesting the re-growth. Although digestibility in this study was studied with reference to ruminants, variation in this property may become significant when considering the use of grass as an industrial fermentation feedstock, for example xylitol or lactic acid production.

The more digestible rye grasses have two to three times more $(1 \rightarrow 4)$-linked D-xylose units without branch points at the O-2 and O-3 positions, the proportions of those branch points being substantially reduced. The changes were greater in the early cut samples [46].

Similarly, it has been noted that re-growth has a lower nutritional value than the first cut at a comparable stage of growth. *Dactylis glomerata* and *Lolium perenne* were cut 1 to 3 times and analyzed chemically. The material from the first cutting had the highest total digestible nutrient content, 55.96%. Protein utilization value was lowest in the third cut grass [47]. The amounts of D-galactose and other carbohydrates were much lower in the re-growth [48].

Åman and Lindgren studied [49] the change in the chemical composition and degradability of six grasses including *Festuca pratensis*, *Festuca arundinacea*, and *Dactylis glomerata* which were harvested at two stages of maturity in both the first and second cuts. The results are shown in Tables 12.3 and 12.4.

Composition studies have also been driven by recognition of the effect of covalent binding between the cell wall polymers on utilization of the cell wall as a nutrient source.

Morrison investigated [45] variations in the hemicellulose and lignin composition of grasses over the growing season. It is known that these two cell components are covalently bonded and it is believed that the lignin has a substantial

Table 12.3 Composition of grasses harvested at early first cut and late first cut (% of DM of unextracted material, sugar residues given as anhydrosugars).

	Dactylis glomerata	*Festuca pratensis*	*Festuca arundinacea*
Early first cut			
80% Ethanol extract	31.5	29.2	28.2
Crude protein	16.6	14.2	14.3
Polysaccharides	37.5	38.8	40.5
Rhamnose	0.1	0.1	0.1
Arabinose	2.6	2.6	2.8
Xylose	11.2	10.6	13.1
Mannose	0.2	0.1	0.2
Galactose	1.4	1.0	0.9
Glucose	19.1	21.3	20.0
Uronic acids	2.9	3.1	3.4
Glu/Xyl + Ara	1.4	1.6	1.3
Klason lignin	7.7	10.3	9.1
Ash	10.0	10.2	10.0
NDF	51.4	55.4	55.4
ADF	28.5	31.4	30.8
Permanganate lignin	4.2	5.2	4.8
Residual organic matter			
in vitro	12.1	15.8	16.5
in vivo	25.8	22.8	27.1
Leaf percent	48.0	41.0	42.0
Late first cut			
80% Ethanol extract	28.1	24.9	26.6
Crude protein	10.6	9.8	9.8
Polysaccharides	44.2	48.3	44.9
Rhamnose	0.1	0.1	0.1
Arabinose	2.8	3.1	2.5
Xylose	12.1	15.5	14.4
Mannose	0.2	0.2	0.2
Galactose	0.8	0.9	0.9
Glucose	25.3	25.4	22.9
Uronic acids	3.0	3.1	4.0
Glu/Xyl + Ara	1.7	1.4	1.4
Klason lignin	13.2	13.8	15.0
Ash	8.6	8.5	8.5
NDF	57.9	62.3	62.4
ADF	32.6	35.6	34.3
Permanganate lignin	6.0	6.2	5.7
Residual organic matter			
in vitro	21.1	24.6	28.9
in vivo	31.8	32.2	35.7
Leaf percent	17.0	34.0	25.0

Table 12.4 Composition of grasses harvested at early second
cut and late second cut (% of DM of unextracted material,
sugar residues given as anhydrosugars).

	Dactylis glomerata	*Festuca pratensis*	*Festuca arundinacea*
Early second cut			
80% Ethanol Extract	22.2	22.7	25.6
Crude Protein	9.9	10.0	10.0
Polysaccharides	47.2	44.8	44.1
Rhamnose	0.1	0.2	0.2
Arabinose	3.2	3.2	3.1
Xylose	11.9	10.2	12.5
Mannose	0.2	0.2	0.2
Galactose	1.2	1.5	1.1
Glucose	26.3	26.2	24.0
Uronic acids	4.2	3.2	3.1
Glu/Xyl + Ara	1.7	2.0	1.5
Klason lignin	13.1	13.8	13.8
Ash	9.7	11.5	10.9
NDF	65.1	60.5	61.2
ADF	40.0	37.0	34.0
Permanganate lignin	8.3	5.4	5.0
Residual organic matter			
in vitro	20.5	19.4	18.4
in vivo	30.9	28.4	29.2
Leaf percent	55.0	73.0	77.0
Late second cut			
80% Ethanol Extract	24.3	22.0	24.8
Crude Protein	9.0	8.7	9.7
Polysaccharides	45.8	46.9	43.3
Rhamnose	0.3	0.2	0.1
Arabinose	2.9	3.2	2.9
Xylose	10.5	11.8	11.2
Mannose	0.2	0.4	0.2
Galactose	1.2	1.7	1.3
Glucose	26.7	26.4	23.4
Uronic acids	4.0	3.3	4.2
Glu/Xyl + Ara	2.0	1.8	1.7
Klason lignin	16.0	19.0	12.9
Ash	9.8	10.6	11.5
NDF	63.5	62.3	60.6
ADF	41.2	39.2	34.7
Permanganate lignin	8.6	7.4	5.7
Residual organic matter			
in vitro	19.1	19.9	16.8
in vivo	32.9	29.6	30.1
Leaf percent	68.0	81.0	77.0

effect on the digestibility of the hemicellulose moiety. In this study, ten varieties of temperate grass were studied by harvesting at five stages of maturity, taking only a first cut. The lignin and hemicellulose content were measured, with the hemicellulose being further fractionated into linear and branched hemicellulose by iodine treatment. The hemicelluloses were analyzed for the neutral sugars L-arabinose, D-xylose, D-galactose and D-glucose. The results are shown in Table 12.5.

Lignin–carbohydrate complexes from *Lolium perenne* contained high proportions of D-glucose residues (ca 50%). Leaf tissue complexes had the highest D-glucose content, whereas stem and leaf sheath were very similar. The other neutral sugar residues present in these complexes were mainly L-arabinose and D-xylose. The polysaccharide components of the lignin-hemicellulose complexes contained mainly D-xylose (63–77%) and L-arabinose (19–28%) [50].

Forage grass lignin was more extensively solubilized by acid detergent than forage legume lignin. Forage plant lignins were characterized by guaiacyl–syringyl lignin with *p*-hydroxyphenylpropane units. The number of ferulic acid cross-linkages in the cell wall matrices of forage grasses increased with plant maturation [51].

Two classes of phenolic–carbohydrate complexes were purified from the water-soluble products obtained from digestion of *Lolium perenne* cell walls with a cellulase preparation [52]. They contained D-glucose, D-xylose, L-arabinose, D- galactose, and D-mannose in the ratios 3.6:10:6.3:1.4:2.3 and 5.3:10:3.0:1.1:2.1, respectively. The complexes were based on $(1 \rightarrow 4)$-β-D-xylan chains to which were attached residues of L-arabinofuranose and D-galactopyranose. Mixed linkage $(1 \rightarrow 3),(1 \rightarrow 4)$-$\beta$-D-glucan chains also seemed to be integral components of these complexes.

The principle outcomes of these studies were:

1. The quantities of hemicellulose increased with increasing maturity with the increase being larger in stem tissue compared with leaf tissue. For example, the hemicellulose content of *Lolium perenne* leaf tissue increased from 7.6 to

Table 12.5 Hemicellulose concentrations (g kg^{-1} DM) in the leaf and stem tissue of forage grasses.

	Leaf					Stem				
Cut no.	1	2	3	4	5	1	2	3	4	5
Lolium perenne S24	83	114		162		101	133		244	
Lolium perenne Reveille	79	104		140		97	136		211	
Lolium perenne S23	76	120	167	183	211	99	137	204	228	291
Lolium perenne Barpastra	78	111	153	180	199	89	136	183	194	272
Festuca pratensis	113	159		202		147	177		270	
Festuca arundinacea S170	124	172		194		162	201		193	

21.1% of dry matter over the study period. The D-xylose content of the linear hemicellulose increased concomitantly from 69 to 85%.

2. The hemicellulose content of stem tissue increased from 9.9 to 29.1% with the linear hemicellulose increasing from 74 to 91%.
3. The linearity of hemicelluloses tended to increase with crop age.
4. Higher lignin content was associated with hemicellulose of a higher linear : branched ratio.
5. Hemicellulose also had higher D-xylose : L-arabinose ratios.

In summary:
1. Time of harvesting has a significant effect on the sugar composition.
2. Hemicellulose sugars increase during the growth season.
3. Stem tissue contains greater amounts of hemicellulose (xylans) than leaf tissue.
4. Digestibility of grasses decreases with age, which may affect yields of fermentation-derived products such as xylitol and lactic acid.

Although, overall, at higher maturity, the absolute quantities of potentially fermentable sugars (e.g. D-xylose, present as hemicellulose) are greater, their accessibility to fermentation media may be reduced.

Pectin Substances Extraction of mesophyll cell walls from the leaves of *Lolium perenne* afforded 25 mg of a uronic acid polymer per gram of material [53]. The polymer was identified as a 1,4-linked homogalacturonan, essentially free from neutral sugar residues, with a low degree of acetylation (3.6%) and methyl esterification (3.3%). Thus, the pectin was similar to the pectins of dicotyledons but the amounts found were substantially lower than in most dicotyledonous plants. On that basis there seems little scope for industrial end uses of forage grass pectins.

12.3.3.2 **Cell Contents**
The cell contents of forage grasses contain sugars, fructans, amino acids, proteins, silica, alkanes, starches, minerals, nucleic acids, lipids, and alkaloids. Protein and sugars are the most abundant components. The concentration of nonstructural carbohydrates in leaves and stems is highest in winter for *Lolium perenne* – 13% of dry matter. Seasonal variations in element concentration are small [54]. *Festuca pratensis* and *Dactylis glomerata* are characterized by high cell wall contents.

Sugars D-Glucose, D-fructose, D-sucrose, and fructans are the main nonstructural carbohydrates in *Lolium perenne* tissues [55]. The D-glucose, D-fructose, D-sucrose, and D-xylose, D-mannitol, D-sorbitol, glycerol, and D-maltose content of *Dactylis glomerata*, *Lolium perenne*, and *Festuca pratensis* cut three times on different dates without interim harvesting have been recorded [56]. The results are reported in Table 12.6. Significant findings were:

Table 12.6 Changes in water-soluble carbohydrate content and mono- and disaccharide content (% on dry matter basis) of *Lolium perenne* and *Festuca pratensis*.

Species	Monosaccharides			Sugar alcohol			Disaccharides		Mono+ Dis-acch.	WSC
	Glc	Fru	Xyl	Mann	Sorb	Glyc	Sucr	Malt		
Lolium perenne										
June 6	3.11	5.43	0.00	0.05	0.05	0.24	0.15	0.10	9.12	27.0
June 21	3.82	4.62	0.05	0.00	0.00	0.24	0.14	0.14	9.02	16.1
July 6	2.89	3.92	0.08	0.04	0.04	0.20	0.12	0.16	7.45	18.1
Aug 6	4.36	6.25	0.26	0.13	0.00	0.46	0.26	0.26	11.98	9.2
Aug 21	2.43	5.10	0.23	0.08	0.00	0.32	0.00	0.16	8.32	9.8
Sep 3	1.46	1.87	0.11	0.00	0.00	0.19	0.11	0.08	3.83	7.8
Sep 30	5.00	7.47	0.14	0.07	0.00	0.40	0.27	0.20	13.53	16.0
Festuca pratensis										
June 6	2.38	4.91	0.00	0.00	0.00	0.24	1.42	0.10	9.04	13.8
June 21	2.93	3.48	0.00	0.00	0.00	0.19	0.12	0.12	6.85	9.0
July 6	2.13	3.33	0.07	0.00	0.00	0.18	0.00	0.21	5.95	12.5
Aug 6	2.07	3.30	0.15	0.25	0.00	0.20	0.30	0.40	6.66	4.9
Aug 21	1.74	2.8 1	0.07	0.07	0.00	0.34	0.00	0.20	5.22	7.6
Sep 3	1.53	0.47	1.80	0.19	0.12	0.19	0.19	0.27	4.78	6.6
Sep 30	4.56	6.56	0.13	0.13	0.06	0.44	0.19	0.19	12.25	10.3

Glc: D-glucose; Fru: D-fructose; Xyl: D-xylose; Mann: D-mannitol; Sorb: D-sorbitol; Glyc: glycerol; Sucr: D-sucrose; Malt: D-maltose; Mono+disacch: monosaccharides+disaccharides; WSC: water-soluble carbohydrate

- *Lolium perenne* contained the most water-soluble carbohydrate (27%) in the early season, compared with *Festuca pratensis* (13.8%).
- This figure decreased steadily through the growing season to 7.8% in early September although it increased to 16% at the end of the month.
- *Lolium perenne* also contained the most xylose (0.26%) in mid-season.
- In *Lolium perenne*, glucose levels peaked in early August and again in late September. Although xylose levels similarly peaked in early August, there was no corresponding peak in late September. Similar trends were observed for *Festuca pratensis*.

In analogous work, Fales and colleagues [57] reported results for stems of *Festuca arundinacea*. The stems were extracted with 95% ethanol and water to afford D-glucose, D-fructose, D-sucrose, and fructans. The fructan extract was hydrolyzed with sulfuric acid and shown to contain D-glucose and D-fructose. A hemicellulose fraction was hydrolyzed and found to contain D-xylose, L-arabinose and small amounts of D-glucose.

Fructans In grasses, fructan reserves are mobilized from vegetative plant parts during seasonal growth, after defoliation during grazing. In expanding leaves, fructans are accumulated in cells of the elongation zone [58]. Fructan structures have been characterized in *Lolium perenne* as belonging to essentially three series: the inulin series, the inulin neoseries, and the levan neoseries [59]. *Festuca arundinacea* contains an inulin and neokestose based series of oligosaccharides [60].

Fructans are an important class of carbohydrate of substantial biotechnological importance [61]. First, they are a potential source of D-fructose, for which there is a growing market in the food industry as a sweetener. The use of fructans has been reviewed by Fuchs [62]. Fructans are mainly used in the food sector. More pertinently, fructans could be chemical feedstocks from which a variety of chemicals can be produced. Hydrolysis to D-fructose and subsequent dehydration leads to hydroxymethyl furfural which, like lactic acid, is regarded as key chemical intermediate for chemistry based on renewable raw materials. Similarly, hydrolysis of inulin to D-fructose followed by catalytic hydrogenation yields D-mannitol/D-sorbitol mixtures from which D-mannitol can be easily crystallized. D-Mannitol, like xylitol, is a valuable, non-cariogenic low-calorie sweetener. Other chemicals that could be derived from fructans include ethanol, other organic solvents, and chemicals such as furans [63].

Inulin is the best known sub-class of the fructans. Inulin is colorless and odorless, and has a pleasant slightly sweet taste; it is moderately soluble in water and acts as a gel-forming agent at concentrations $> 30\%$; it is also a foam stabilizer and texturing agent. Its calorific value is 4 kJ g^{-1}, but it acts as dietary fiber. It suppresses putrefying bacteria and selectively supports bifidobacteria and lactobacilli in the colon. In food applications its main functions are to replace fat and sugar, to enrich with dietary fiber, to activate bifidobacteria, and to reduce cariogenicity. It is classified as a foodstuff [64].

Amino Acids The amino acid composition of *Festuca pratensis*, *Dactylis glomerata* and *Lolium perenne* has been studied. There were no significant differences between the species. As the grasses aged, amounts of aspartic acid, glutamic acid, alanine, tyrosine, and phenylalanine decreased and amounts of threonine, serine, and proline increased. Lysine, histidine, arginine, glycine, valine, methionine, isoleucine, and leucine did not change with plant age nor did the total amino acid content [65].

In amino acid analysis of six crops and the corresponding juice, the amino acid composition of the juice deviated only slightly from that of the crop but the amounts of glutamic acid and aspartic acids were somewhat higher and correspondingly the amounts of other amino acids, particularly arginine, glycine, alanine, tyrosine, and phenylalanine were somewhat lower [66].

Degradation of protein and amino acids in juice extracted from ryegrass can be reduced by adding hydrochloric acid. For complete preservation, the pH must be less than 3. Heating to 80 °C also has a preservative effect [67].

Proteins   Leaf protein concentrate is obtained by green crop fractionation. The acceptability of leaf protein concentrate in the human diet has been discussed by McDougall [68]. Lesnitski has also advocated [69] the manufacture of high protein feeds from green mass for partial replacement of, for example, soybean protein and dried skim milk.

Silica   In comparison with elements commonly associated with the nutrition of higher plants, silicon has received relatively little attention. Biogenic amorphous silica (BAS) is a natural constituent of living matter. In some plants some of the BAS occurs externally as pointed or irregularly shaped fibers, and these have been implicated as human toxicants [70]. Silica deposits commonly called phytoliths occur in cell walls, cell lumens or in extracellular locations. Silicification occurs in roots and shoots, including leaves, culms, and in grasses, most heavily in the inflorescence. Biogenic silica structures provide support and protection [71].

Grasses are heavy accumulators, but substantial variation occurs between and within species. Deposition is heaviest in inflorescence bracts [72]. Silica has been detected in the leaf mesophyll of *Lolium multiflorum* at an estimated concentration of 1–2%. Samples were also subjected to a range of techniques for removal of organic matter, to confirm the presence of silica throughout the cell walls [73]. In *Lolium perenne*, only the epidermal cell walls of the leaf edges and the trichomes contained silica [74]. The *Lolium perenne* variety Fortis, which has some resistance to stem borer, had many silica bodies between the veins of the leaf sheath [75].

The silica content of each of four cuts of 3 *Dactylis glomerata*, 4 *Festuca pratensis*, 5 *Lolium perenne*, 5 *Lolium multiflorum* are reported by Puffe and colleagues [76]. Silica content is lower in legumes than in grasses.

Alkanes   The total *n*-alkane (C_{27}–C_{35}) content of *Dactylis glomerata*, *Lolium multiflorum*, and *Lolium perenne* was found to be 143, 681, and 531 mg kg^{-1} dry matter, respectively. The concentrations of C_{29} and C_{31} were always highest [77]. These levels do not seem to be high enough for commercial exploitation.

Starch   The starch content of forage grasses is low – a maximum of 3% starch is accumulated in field-grown grasses. Cocksfoot contains more starch than *Lolium perenne* or *Lolium multiflorum* [78]. This low level rules out industrial use of forage grass starches.

Minerals   The dry matter of extracted juice of *Lolium perenne* has a high mineral content [66] that may be exploitable as plant fertilizer.

Alkaloids   Perloline, perlolidine, and loline are alkaloids of the *Lolium* spp. The toxicity of lolium species is because of to a symbiotic fungal infection of the plants [79].

Antifreeze Protein   A plant antifreeze protein from *Lolium perenne* has been reported [80]. Present in organisms enduring freezing environments, antifreeze proteins have the ability to inhibit damaging ice-crystal growth. The macromolecular antifreeze protein present in *Lolium perenne* has superior ice recrystallization inhibition activity compared with fish and insect antifreeze proteins [81].

12.4
Green Biorefinery Concept

12.4.1
Fundamentals and Status Quo

Green biorefineries are complex systems based on ecological technology for comprehensive (holistic), substantial, and energy utilization of renewable resources and natural materials in the form of green and waste biomass from focused sustainable regional land utilization. Such green biomass is, e.g., grass from cultivation of permanent grassland, fallow land cultivation, nature reserves, or green crops, for example alfalfa, clover, and immature cereals from extensive land cultivation. Thus, green plants are a natural chemical factory and food plant. Careful wet fractionation technology is used as a first step (primary refinery) to isolate the substances in their native form. Thus, the green crop (or humid organic waste goods) is separated into a fiber-rich press cake (PC) and a nutrient-rich green juice (GJ). Besides, cellulose and starch, the press cake contains valuable dyes and pigments, crude drugs, and other organic substances. The green juice contains proteins, free amino acids, organic acids, dyes, enzymes, hormones, minerals, high quality crude drugs, and other organic substances. By use of this biotechnology, ecotechnology, and "soft" and "green" chemistry, these valuable materials can be isolated in their natural form or, by mild careful conversion, can be utilized economically [7].

Activity in the green biorefinery field is increasing and developing into an independent aspect of the large field of biomass technology. Raw material and technological aspects of this system are particularly characterized by consideration of sustainability criteria and incorporation of technology from regional and rural living and business (sustainable economy, sustainable agriculture, and sustainable regional development).

The term "green biorefinery" is, on the one hand, used for model processes but, on the other hand, also used for an entire program. To "refine" is originally French (raffiner) and means "to improve something, to purify". A refinery is, by definition, a technical facility for purification, separation, and refining of materials and products. "Green" in the field of plants means, simultaneously, high concentrations of chlorophyll, nutrients, and water, "bio" is Greek (bios) and means "live", something biological and natural. Programmatically, the green biorefinery stands for technology (refinery) formed by imitation of nature (biologically) with the target being soft and sustainable [7].

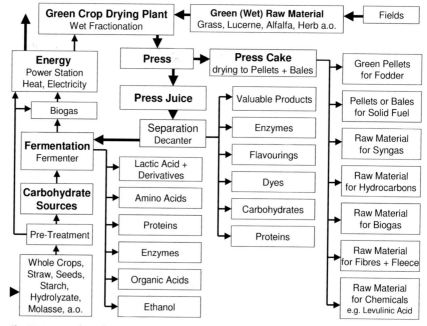

Fig. 12.2 Green biorefinery combined with a green crop-drying plant. Concept of the Havelland biorefinery, Selbelang, State of Brandenburg, Germany [82, 83].

In principle, the primary conversion technology is set up on the basis of the water content of the different raw materials [84]. It is reasonable to use mechanical pressing for green nature-wet biomass in the first step. Traditionally green crop fractionation was regarded as providing edible protein for humans. Fractionation separates the crop into pressed matter, which can be used to feed ruminants, and leaf protein concentrate (LPC) that can be eaten directly by humans [15–17, 68]. Different choppers and shredders, e.g. hammer-mills and different presses, e.g. screw-presses, roller-presses, and piston-presses, are used as technical equipment for fractionation of green biomass [85–88]. The literature also mentions the separation of proteins [89, 90]. The company "France Luzerne" has realized a process for separation of proteins on an industrial scale. The resources, mainly alfalfa, are treated by four main process steps:

- pressing,
- heat coagulation,
- centrifugation, and
- drying.

The technical specifications of the product and, especially, its high xanthophyll content make it very useful in poultry farming for egg yolk and broilers (Table 12.7) [91].

Table 12.7 Industrial production of PX (protein–xanthophylls) and their specification [91].

Product	Production year	Quantity	Specification
PX 1	1977	1300 T	50% crude protein and 1.000 ppm of total xanthophylls
PX 1	1980	6200 T	50% crude protein and 1.000 ppm of total xanthophylls
PX Super	1997	13000 T	52% crude protein and 1.250 ppm of total xanthophylls

12.4.2
Wet Fractionation and Primary Refinery

The special first feature of the green biorefinery is the wet fractionation of green biomass (Fig. 12.3 A).

This is also called first fractionation step or primary refinery step. (It includes, for example, the harvest, fractionation, conservation, and storage of the primary fraction.) Here, fresh harvest and waste goods are treated. Thus, the plant compounds are mostly unadulterated; the green goods should, in any case, be treated immediately, however. This processing step, usually performed by means of an industrial press, produces a fiber-rich, water-insoluble, solid material, press cake (PC), and a nutrient-rich green juice (GJ) or brown juice (BJ). The wet fractionation is based on soft separation of water-soluble and water-insoluble components of the green biomass.

The silage wet-fractionation is a form of the primary refinery technology (Fig. 12.3 C). The green goods are conserved by organic acids or fermentation processes before treatment by the procedure shown. Treatment of silage from green resources has many advantages (decentralized raw material preparation, simple and low price conservation and storage, reasonable whole year operation of the biorefinery, etc.) [92]. The end products of silage are different from that of the substances in the green juice, because silage fermentation degrades the cell walls and modifies or converts substances because of the biotechnological processes involved.

The so called "decomposition" methods are the third category of primary refinery technology (Fig. 12.3 B). "Decomposition" methods are mainly applied to the humid or dry whole plant. The processes work with enzymatic, fermentative, hydrolytic, chemical, thermal, or combined thermal and fractionation methods. The strength (depth of operation) of the decomposition varies, and ranges from low (enzymatic, fermentative) to high intensity (chemical, hydrolytic). For every step classification is needed to check if it belongs to green biorefinery technology. A high single yield of products can be achieved if the complete plant decomposition occurs at the primary refinery step (e.g. saccharification, which increases the total amount of sugars in the raw charge). But these procedures reduce the level of native product diversity. Nevertheless decomposition methods have been regarded as feasible technologically and economically. This is also true for the secondary prod-

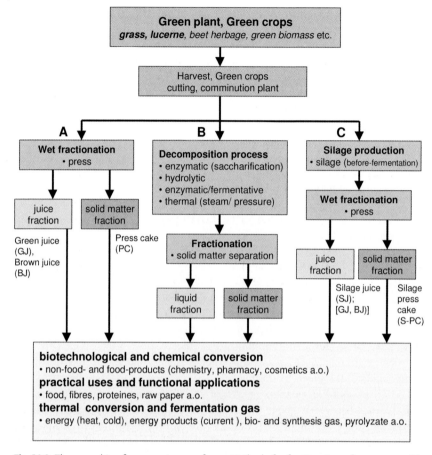

Fig. 12.3 The green biorefinery – primary refinery. Methods for fractionation of green crops [7].

uct lines. Problems with the green biorefinery system may be solved by further development of new biotechnological decomposition methods.

All primary fractionations after the secondary refinery steps contain processes for substantial and energy utilization of the fractionation products. The kind and number of the secondary fractionation steps are determined by the composition and energy potential of the input green biomass and waste biomass, the type of technology, and the marketability of potential products of the refinery.

The company Avebe operates a pilot plant at Veendam (The Netherlands) and has formed a consortium with other partners to explore the potential of grass to supply a range of fiber, protein, and nutraceutical products. The current pilot plant processes 3 tons of fresh grass per hour. Depending on the outcome, a full-scale (200 tons per hour, 50 000 tons per year) factory may be commissioned. The intended full-scale plant requires 1000 ha per annum of mixed grass sources harvested from a radius of up to 50 km [93].

The concept of the Havelland biorefinery, Selbelang, State of Brandenburg, Germany is the fractionation of 25 000 tons of fresh green biomass per year, in its first stage of expansion, and the production of proteins and fermentation medium from green juice. Production of feed, tech-paper, and chlorophyll from press cake [94] (Fig. 12.2) will also be established.

The *Austrian-Concept* is based on a decentralized system to take into account small scale agriculture. The system is, however, built around grass silage fermentation and the production of lactic acid, amino acids (hydrolyzed proteins), and fiber [92].

The problem of storage of fresh green biomass must be solved, i.e. green biomass must be preserved such that it is available for longer periods of time to enable continuous year-round operation of the plant.

The development of sustainable green biorefinery systems requires a combination of central and decentralized/localized units, i.e. large-scale conversion and processing plants that take advantage of economies of scale must be combined with smaller and localized units as close to biomass feedstock as possible, resulting in improving rural economies and reducing the environmental impact of transportation [95].

12.5
Processes and Products

The kind and number of products from a green biorefinery is nearly unlimited, if the fractal character of the biosynthesis and biochemistry of green plant materials is considered [96]. Characterization of a plant by a new analytical method usually discovers, in addition to the main components, innumerable new side products. Not all substances have been discovered and technologically obtained from natural products even from plants with great trading importance, e.g. alfalfa [97]. For the green biorefinery the main products, side-products and impurities are of interest [98]. Economic aspects reduce the diversity of products of interest, however. Soft technology such as biotechnology is used to reduce the complex molecules of natural materials. Nevertheless, the scientific field of ecotechnology develops new methods, preferring a reduction of technological strength (depth of operation). This can be done by using, e.g., biodiversity before molecular modification or applying less intensive methods, etc. [99].

12.5.1
The Juice Fraction

12.5.1.1 Green Juice
In the (especially) freshly pressed (Fig. 12.3 A) green juice (GJ) we can find proteins, lipids, glycoproteins, lectins, sugars, free amino acids, dyes (carotenes), hormones, enzymes, minerals, and other materials. The GJ can be fractionated by heat, treatment with organic and inorganic acids, acid anaerobic fermenta-

tion, centrifugation, and gel filtration into a leaf nutrient concentrate (LNC) and a brown juice (BJ). The LNC consists of a mixture of chloroplast and other organell membranes plus denatured soluble plant-cell proteins. The composition of a LNC is: true protein (60–70%); lipid (especially palmitic acid, linoleic acid, and linolenic acid) (20–30%), starch (5–10%), ash (1–10%), carotenoide/polyene dyes: β-carotene (1–2 g kg^{-1}), and xanthophyll [6, 100]. The LNC is mainly used for nonruminant feed to enhance the color (red β-carotene, or lutein) of chicken skin or egg yolk. It also produces tender meat in chickens, ducks, and pigs. Feeding pigs with LNC results in pork with an increased content of healthy oleic and linoleic fatty acids in the fat [101].

Sugars (in Particular Glucose, Fructose, and Fructans) GJ and BJ contains valuable special sugars and have highly valuable and sometimes expensive applications. Other sugars in GJ are erythrose, rhamnose, xylose, galactose, mannose, mannitol, maltose, and derivatives, for example myoinositol and glycerin. Before these compounds are fermented they are studied with regard to their potential characterization, and isolation [98, 102].

Dyes and Vitamins Green leaf nutrient concentrate (GLNC) enriched in β-carotene may have anti-cancer effects. β-Carotene (provitamin A) and xanthophyll are used in cosmetic drugs and as food, textiles, and toy-coloring agents (see also chlorophyll) [28, 29, 31]. Green juice contains further vitamins, for example vitamin B1, vitamin B2, and vitamin E [103].

Fatty Acids GLNC is also rich in oleic and linoleic fatty acids, especially palmitic acid, linoleic acid, and linolenic acid. The lipids provide good health value. The lipids can be separated by steam distillation. They are also of interest to the cosmetic industry [100].

Crude Drugs/Ingredients Because the BJ contains specific secondary plant substances, for example saponins and nicotine, these can be separated from the juice for pharmacological or pesticide purposes (isolation is described elsewhere [97]).

Proteins The proteins in the green juice can be fractionated by advanced technology, in a second step, into a green leaf nutrient concentrate GLNC. The main protein is the enzyme ribulose-1,5-bisphosphate carboxylase/oxygenase, also known as fraction-I (F-I) protein (rubisco EC 4.1.1.39). In alfalfa leaves proteins account for 30 to 70% of total nitrogen, depending on the physiological stage or genotype [106]. Rubisco has a molecular weight (MW) between 500000 and 600000 Daltons and is composed of eight large and eight small subunits with MW of approximately 55000 and 12500, respectively. The sedimentation coefficient is close to 18.5 S. Rubisco has a compact, tightly folded three-dimensional structure typical of globular proteins. Because of its amino acid composition Rubisco is mildly acidic and is negatively charged at neutral pH (isoelectric

Table 12.8 Comparison of the amino acid composition of the different protein fractions of lucerne [113, 114], according to [124].

Protein	Amino acids (parts per thousand, by weight)				
	Hydrophilic (H)	Charged	Apolar (A)	Small	H/A
Rubisco	414	289	285	180	1.45
White protein	421	303	272	183	1.55
Green protein	432	286	268	180	1.61
Soluble protein	491	333	239	143	2.10
Oligomeric soluble protein	451	310	275	166	1.70
Membranous protein	427	288	299	169	1.40

Hydrophilic: Asp + Glu + Ser + Thr + Arg + Lys + His
Charged: Asp + Glu + Arg + Lys
Apolar: Val + Ile + Leu + Phe + Met
Small: Gly + Ala

point pH 4.4–4.7) [107]. It also has a relatively high average hydrophobic value of 1275 cal/residue, calculated according to Bigelow [108]. Native Rubisco from alfalfa contains 90 sulfhydryl groups, of which eight are "free" (one per protomer), 36 are exposed after denaturation by SDS, and 46 are involved in the formation of disulfide bonds within the Rubisco subunits [109]. The denaturation temperature of alfalfa rubisco varies between 70 (pH 7.5) and 61 °C (pH 10.3) [110]. More details about Rubisco are available in reviews [106, 111].

Fraction-II protein consists of a mixture of proteins originating from the chloroplasts and cytoplasm with molecular weights from 10 000 to 300 000 Daltons and sedimentation constants from 4 S to 10 S [112]. On the basis of amino acid composition, Rubisco and the green and white fraction of leaf proteins are regarded as hydrophobic (Table 12.8).

The F I protein can be used in medical diets to enhance recovery from brain damage, where a high calorie/high protein diet is needed. People with kidney problems can easily digest F I protein with no negative effects on body metabolism. Both F I and F II proteins are advocated for solid foods and drinks as a supplement. The nutritive value and functional properties of LNC and white leaf protein isolated for incorporation in human diets have been reviewed [68, 69, 115–118].

12.5.2
GJ Drinks/Alternative Life

Young green cereal leaves are used for production of health food grass juices and cosmetics. Dried, finely ground, and resolved young leaves are used as "green tea" and added to health-food drinks [119, 120]. Those familiar with folk medicine also know much about the effects of wild mixed grasses, herbs, and herb teas [97].

12.5.2.1 **Silage Juice**

To facilitate continuous year-round operation of a green biorefinery it may be very reasonable to introduce common agricultural technology. For that reason the concept involves not only processing of directly cut grass, but also of silage, which can be prepared in the growing season and stored in a silo. Silage is the product formed when grass or other material of sufficiently high moisture content (grass optimum of 28 to 35% dry matter; maize 25–30% dry matter) liable to spoilage by aerobic microorganisms is stored anaerobically. It is formed by the process referred to as ensilage which occurs in a vessel or structure called a silo. Normally during ensilage the fodder undergoes acid fermentation in which bacteria produce lactic, acetic, and butyric acids from sugars present in the raw material. The net result is a reduction in pH (to approximately pH 4 to 4.5) which prevents the growth of spoilage microorganisms, most of which are intolerant of acid conditions [121].

Table 12.9 Physicochemical characteristics of grass silage juice [123].

Property	Value
Conductivity (20.5 °C)	35.8 mS
pH (20.5 °C)	4.04
Dry matter	13.6%
Color	Dark brown
Cations (g L^{-1})	
K$^+$	15.63
Na$^+$	0.15
NH^{4+}	1.22
Ca^{2+}	1.78
Mg^{2+}	0.50
Anions (g L^{-1})	
Lactate	37.54
Acetate	2.08
Cl$^-$	6.41
NO$_3^-$	2.13
PO$_4^{3-}$	4.38
SO$_4^{2-}$	2.55
Sugars (g L^{-1})	
Glucose	8.88
Fructose	14.99
Saccharose	5.36
Arabinose	1.72
Xylose	1.44
Galactose	2.86
Mannitol	3.09
Amino acid	26.13

The silage juice (Fig. 12.3 C) contains a relatively high concentration of lactic acid, amino acids, sugars, and inorganic salts. Protein and peptide degradation occurs during ensiling. In silage juices only 5 to 10% of the crude proteins (organic nitrogen compounds) are peptides >1.2 kD (~15 amino acids). At least 18 amino acids are found in the juice with a total amino acid content of 26.13 g L^{-1}. Among the most important are alanine, leucine, lysine, GABA (γ-aminobutyric acid), aspartic acid, and isoleucine (all in the L form) [122, 123] (Table 12.9).

12.5.3
Ingredients and Specialities

12.5.3.1 Proteins/Polysaccharides
The polysaccharide and protein components of *Festuca* spp cell walls have been transformed into emulsifiers by extraction and treatment with xylan-hydrolyzing enzyme preparations. The emulsifiers are useful, for example, for food, cosmetics, pharmaceuticals, and industrial chemicals applications [125].

12.5.3.2 Cholesterol Mediation
It has been demonstrated that polysaccharide–lignin complexes from fodder grasses are active sorbents of cholic acid, a metabolite of cholesterol [126]. Equations have been derived for calculating the sorption of cholic acid by the grass material. The equations can be used to construct dietary fiber with the desired properties, for example for cholesterol metabolism in humans and animals.

12.5.3.3 Antifeedants
Festuca arundinacea and *Lolium perenne* can become infected with fungal endophytes (*Neotyphodium* spp). The symbiosis between plant and fungus leads to the synthesis of alkaloids that have been shown to be either toxic or act as feeding detergents against insect pests. Alkaloid production/accumulation in *Festuca arundinacea* and *Lolium perenne* is enhanced by reduced mowing frequency [132]. Such alkaloids may have a role as insecticides for agrochemical use [104, 105] or in the clinic as a result of their pharmacology [79].

12.5.3.4 Silica
A process has been described for manufacture of high-purity amorphous silica from biogenic materials [127]. Rice hulls are given as the example. The hulls are finely divided, screened, subjected to a surfactant wash, rinsed, and soaked in water to accelerate and enhance penetration of an oxidizing solution. The oxidizing solution removes organic compounds, and volatile impurities are removed by heated oxidation to leave silica. The remaining silica may be rinsed with water, acid solution, or other solution to remove even trace impurities. At

the end of the process, a fine white amorphous silica of extremely high purity is produced.

12.5.3.5 Silicon Carbide

Rye grass has been proposed as a raw material for the production of polytypically pure β-silicon carbide in an economically effective and ecologically compatible procedure. When the particle size of starting raw material is defined then the particle size of the developing silicon carbide is also controlled [128]. Silicon carbide has many industrial applications and is a valuable chemical used for cutting, grinding, and polishing applications. Silicon carbide is also used in the electronics industry in hostile environments where its ability to function in high-temperature, high-radiation conditions overcomes the limitations of conventional silicon-based systems. It is used as a component of blue and violet light-emitting diodes.

12.5.3.6 Filter Aids

Highly purified biogenic silica has an intricate and diatomaceous SiO_2 structure and a high-SiO_2 specific volume. These products are extremely bright and can be used in filtration processes [129]. In one example the adsorbent has been used for the removal of proteins in chillproofing of beer [130].

12.5.3.7 Zeolites

Artificial zeolites are manufactured by heating a mixture of grass husks and plants with aqueous alkali solutions to elute silicic components. These are mixed with aluminum-enriching agents and treated under heat and pressure. The zeolites have high cation-exchange properties and are be useful as fertilizers [131].

12.5.4
The Press-Cake (Fiber) Fraction

The products and product groups described below are technologically possible after fractionation in accordance with Fig. 12.3 A and C. Use of the PC as feed (silage, bale press food, green pellets) is well known [133]. Furthermore, extraction of plant dyes (chlorophyll, carotenes, xanthophyll) [25, 28] and applications in the food and candle industry [31], in environmental analysis [134] or, after refining, in cosmetics, medicine, biochemistry [135], electronics (nematic liquid crystals) [136], and photovoltaics (organic dyes [32]) have also been described in the literature.

Because of the structural similarity of chlorophyll and blood hemoglobin one can expect interesting developments in the field of plant dyes and colorants. The resulting fraction will, substantially, be thermally treated analogous to unex-

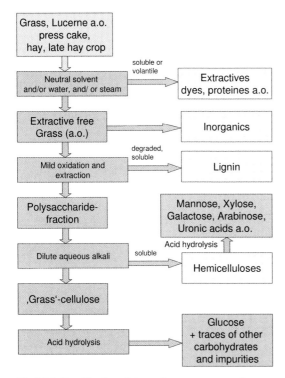

Fig. 12.4 Classification of the major components of grass press cake, hay, and late hay crop (by analogy with Ref. [143]).

tracted PC. The suitability (and applicability) as feed depends mainly on the corresponding extraction compounds and has to be tested.

The PC fraction can be separated by analogy with wood raw materials into its main components (Fig. 12.4). On the one hand, this green plant fractionation does not seem to make much economic sense today (because of wood competition). There are, on the other hand, interesting applications for special vegetable celluloses, hemicelluloses, and lignin. The "green plant" polyoses (hemicelluloses) are nutrient-physiologically valuable [137]. Furthermore, they can be used (similarly to plant rubber) as protecting colloids, emulsifiers in cosmetics, thickeners in the food industry [138a], adhesives, additives in the pulp and paper industry, stabilizers for environmentally friendly inks and dyes [138b], or as thickeners for crude oil drilling [139].

Lignin is one component of press cake. Isolated lignin can be used as a dispersant in the food industry, as stabilizer for foams and bitumen, or as an environmental friendly adhesive [140–142].

12.5.4.1 **Fibers**

Non-wood fibers have been used to manufacture all kinds of paper, including printing, writing, and packaging. Such feedstock is expected to play an important role in improving the sustainability of the pulp and paper industry [144], by enabling more rational utilization of forest resources. Non-wood fiber pulps can be used effectively in combination with recycled papers, improving many of their attributes and enabling overall cost reduction because of a decrease in the use of starch [145].

Semi-chemical Pulping The process starts with atmospheric alkali cooking in a continuous digester [145]. The semi-chemical pulp obtained is washed, refined, screened, and sent to the paper mill for corrugated paper manufacture. From the black liquor obtained in the pulping process, lignin is initially recovered by precipitation then given a post-treatment to improve its filterability. Most of the silica remains with the filtrate and the resulting lignin cake is high in purity and contains less than 1% silica and less than 3.5% sugars. Lignin sales increase overall mill revenues and lead to a possible reduction of the minimum plant scale required for economic operation. The filtrate after lignin recovery can be processed in a biological treatment plant. Alternatively, oxygen-based wet oxidation of the filtrate can be used to generate energy and green liquor. From the latter, a precipitate that typically accounts for 70–90% of the silica in the wet-oxidation feed can be filtered, effectively purging silica from the cycle. The filtered green liquor can be made caustic to generate white liquor for re-use in pulping. A study of the pulping characteristics and mineral composition of 16 field crops grown in Finland showed that the most suitable species for alkali cooking were the grass and cereal crops, which gave the highest pulp yields and the lowest amounts of rejects. On the basis of the test results, *Festuca arundinacea*, *Festuca pratensis*, reed canary grass, and spring barley were selected for further study [146]. Further work selected *Festuca arundinacea* and reed canary grass as worthwhile candidates [147].

Steam Explosion Steam explosion of ryegrass straw has been reported in a patent application to yield separate portions of usable straw pulp and a usable aqueous by-product comprising lignins and hemicellulose. The pulp was blended with Kraft pulp and old corrugated containers to make linerboard [148].

Mechanical Pulping A recent Chinese patent describes the production of non-polluting grass pulp and a method for reclaiming its by-product [149]. Grass is processed into refined grass chip and refined grass residue, the refined grass chips are treated by soaking with water, softening, washing, and pulping to produce high-quality grass pulp, and the refined grass residue is mixed with an additive containing functional preparation (organic selenium, organic calcium) and carrier (refined grass powder) to produce a high-quality fiber feed.

Downstream Processing of the Grass Fiber Fraction (PC) The biorefinery primary process generates a fibrous press cake (Fig. 12.3 A and C). This fraction can either be further processed while wet – by applying technology used in the pulp und paper industry – or it can be dried. After mechanical fractionation grass and silage press cake particles are typically less than 3 cm in length. The structure of grass stems and leaves is mostly eliminated and the bulk has a fibrous appearance.

Basic Properties of Grass Fibers Sfiligoj et al. [150] evaluated the fundamental physical properties of press cake fibers (from Ryegrass (*Lolium hybridum*), wheat (*Triticum aestivum L.*), red clover (*Trifolium pratense*), and lucerne (*Medicago sativa L.*) after mechanical separation. Investigation involved isolation of elementary fibers or fiber bundles from the press cake fraction using chemical or biological retting. For the resulting samples density, size, and strain-stress-behavior were analyzed in wet conditions (Table 12.10).

There are no significant differences between mechanical properties of fiber bundles of different origin (green or ensiled grass). For the press cake of trefoil, ryegrass and alfalfa tenacity values of stem fiber bundles were measured in the range 11.4 to 21.4 cN/tex, leaf fiber bundles reached 6.8 to 13.1 cN/tex [150]. The geometrical properties (length and diameter) of press cake fibers were similar to those of soft wood fibers and the mechanical properties (e.g. tenacity and elongation) of elementary fibers were comparable with those of bast fibers (jute, hemp). Grass fibers, especially the dry fibers, have poor bending strength and are characterized by brittleness. They are, therefore, used for non-woven textiles, preferably for technical applications. Chemical analysis of different press cake fractions gave the average results (% dry matter content): ∼5.8–7.6% cellulose, 14.7–28.7% hemicellulose, and 27.5–31.6% lignin. Crude fiber was 29.1–32.9% and crude ash 6.3–9.1%. These values are for the first cut of grass and may alter for later harvests.

Table 12.10 Basic properties of grass fibers from press cake – green and ensiled.

Property	Unit	Measured value
Fiber content, stem	[%]	20.2–39.5
Fiber content, leaves	[%]	6.9–10.2
Fiber length, stem [a]	[mm]	0.8–3.2
Fiber length, leaves [a]	[mm]	0.6–1.3
Fiber diameter	[µm]	15–18
Linear density [b]	[dte x]	12–105
Tenacity	[cN/tex]	6–21 [c]
Elongation	[%]	1–6

[a] Elementary fibers
[b] Fiber bundles (technical fiber)
[c] Coir 15 cN/tex; jute 23–31 cN/tex; hemp 29–47 cN/tex

Products From Grass Fiber (PC) Generally speaking, the grass and silage fibers fraction of the green biorefinery may be used as raw material for:
- insulation material (mats, boards, loose fill material)
- building panels (fiber and chip boards)
- products used in horticulture and landscaping (mulch fleece, erosion-control, peat substitution)
- bio-composites
- packaging material
- pore forming additives (e.g. brick and tile industry)
- gypsum boards
- pulp and paper [151]
- thermoplastics [156].

Paper and Cardboard Paper has been manufactured from PC of lucerne [152, 153] and from reed canary grass, wild mix grass, and Cock's foot [7, 154]. It has also been shown that the quality of grass cardboards is the same or even better (for the paper re-working industry) than analog waste paper and that they are also less expensive [7, 155].

Thermoplastics Adhesive films have been produced from grass fiber by preparation of alkali cellulose and then film-forming. The adhesive film can be used as agricultural mulching film or packing material [156]. Grass fiber has been proposed as a component of a biodegradable protein/starch-based thermoplastic composition. The grass fibers function as reinforcement filler. The composition is processed by conventional methods, for example extrusion and injection molding, into packaging material or articles that are low density and have high compressive strength and tensile strength and good resilience [157].

12.5.4.2 Chemicals

It is reasonable to combine the primary refining of green biomass with fermentation processes for production of chemicals. This assumption is based on the high water content of the raw material and the occurrence of many different substances in green biomass, important for biotechnological processes. Green juice, brown juice, and silage juice (Fig. 12.3 A and C) contain all the necessary macroelements (minerals, peptides, amino acids, sugar) for making fermentation products [103, 123, 158–160, 168, 170]. After enrichment with further sources of carbohydrates (sugars from lignocellulosic feedstock, for example press cake) it should be possible to produce a variety of biotechnologically basic chemicals [7]. Chemicals which provide two or three functional groups and can be integrated into the product trees of the chemical industry are of most interest [162, 163]. An assortment of industrial biotechnologically produced chemicals are:
- (C_2) chemicals such as ethanol [160, 161, 166, 167] and acetic acid,
- (C_3) chemicals such as lactic acid [48, 159, 164, 165], acetone [167], and 1,3-propanediol [171],

- (C$_4$) chemicals such as *n*-butanol [167],
- (C$_5$) chemicals such as itaconic acid [171], and
- (C$_6$) chemicals such as lysine [158, 168, 170].

Products from lactic acid include, e.g., polylactic acid and ethyl lactate [83, 164, 172]. The biotechnological production of polyhydroxybutyrate from switchgrass is currently in a stage of industrial development, and chemical or combined chemical/biotechnological decomposition of lignocellulosic press cake or switchgrass can be used to produce basic chemicals [169].

Basic chemicals which can be used as precursors in genealogical trees are furfural [174] and xylitol [175, 176] from the hemicellulose line and hydroxymethylfurfural [177] and levulinic acid [178] from the cellulose line. Esparto grass is a particularly important source of xylitol [179], and grasses with a high concentration of fructan, for example *Lolium perenne* are a source of hydroxymethylfurfural. The same is true of chicory roots [180].

12.5.4.3 Residue Utilization

Green juice, brown juice, and silage juice can be used as bio-fertilizer (soil bioactivators) to return to the soil the macro and micro mineral nutrients which were removed by harvesting the green crop [101]. The low-molecular-mass substances in this juice are quickly transformed into methane in fermentation units [183, 184]. This has been developed a production process for biogas, heat, and electricity in a combined green biorefinery–animal-breeding complex [7, 94]. Silage residues have been used as sources of natural chelates to improve the ecological and economical balance of leaching techniques for remediation of metal-polluted soils. Silage effluent containing a variety of aliphatic carboxylic acids, sugar acids, and amino acids has been used to remove approximately 75% of the cadmium and more than 50% of the copper and zinc from contaminated soils [181]. A trial led to the conclusion that biomass residues have potential to serve as extractants in remediation techniques.

Porous carbon fibers have been obtained from cut grass by baking in an oven in a roped form for formation of coiled carbonized fibers. The porous carbon fibers are useful for sound absorbers, adsorbents, purification materials, and radio wave absorbers [182]. The press cake has also been used as a medium for growing mushrooms, as a mulch/green crop enhancer, and as a fertilizer [34].

12.6
Green Biorefinery – Economic and Ecological Aspects

Plant biomass is the only foreseeable sustainable source of organic fuels, chemicals, and other materials. A variety of forms of biomass, notably many ligno-cellulosic feedstocks, are potentially available on a large scale and are cost-competitive with low-cost petroleum whether considered on a mass or energy basis, in terms of price defined on a purchase or net basis for both current and projected mature technologies, or on a transfer basis for mature technology [185]. Green plant biomass and lignocellulosic feedstocks are the dominant source of feedstocks for biotechnological processes for production of chemicals and materials [7, 158, 162, 163, 173]. The development of integrated technology for conversion of biomass is essential for the economic and ecological production of products. The biomass industry or bio-industry produces basis chemicals such as ethanol (15 Mio tons per year), amino acids (1.5 Mio tons a year of which L-lysine amounts to 500 000 tons per year [186]), and lactic acid (200 000 tons per year). The target of a biorefinery is to establish a combination of a biomass–feedstock mix with a process and product mix [162, 163]. A life cycle assessment (LCA) is available for production of polylactic acid (capacity 140 000 tons per year) [187]. In total assessment of the utilization of biomass one must consider that plant cultivation must fulfill economic and ecological criteria. Agriculture both creates pressure on the environment and plays an important role in maintaining many cultural landscapes and semi-natural habitats [188]. Green crops, especially, are available in large quantities. Additionally, grassland can be cultivated sustainably [92]. European grassland experiments have shown that species-rich grassland cultivation has both ecological and economic advantages. With plant diversity grassland is more productive and protects the soil against nitrate leaching.

Seventy-one species have been examined, of which 29 had significant influence on productivity. In particular, *Trifolium pratense* has an important function with regard to productivity. On sites where this species occurs more than 50% of the total biomass has been used. Legumes, like clover and herbs, also play an important role, as do fast-growing grasses [189]. An initial assessment of the concept of a green biorefinery was performed by S. Schidler et al. for the Austrian system approach [190]. An Austria-wide concept for use of biomass and cultivable land for renewable resources has yet to be developed; the same is true for Europe [191]. The size of such plants depends on the rural structures of the different regions. Concepts with more decentralized units would have a size of about 35 000 tons raw material per year [192] and central plants could have sizes of approximately 300 000 to 600 000 tons per year [174].

The synthetic method used for modeling biorefinery systems [192] is based on combinatorial acceleration of separable concave programming developed by Nagy et al. [193].

Table 12.11 Cost calculation for production of grass in comparison to straw, including intermediate storage [195].

Raw material	Yield t DM/ha	Work			
		Person-h ha^{-1}	Person-h t^{-1} DM	Euro ha^{-1}	Euro t^{-1} DM
Late cut Grass	5.0	4.46	0.89	297	60
Straw	2.1	1.58	0.75	77	36

Cost calculation for raw materials in the green biorefinery are based on the supply of agricultural products. For late-cut grass and straw the costs of cultivation, harvest, and intermediate storage have been calculated for Germany (Table 12.11 [194]).

Currently, the costs are US $ 30 per ton for corn stover or straw [196]. The prices for green pellets are also available and range from 80 € per ton in Germany to 160 € per ton in Sweden [42]. Production of pellets from silage has been calculated to be approximately 110 to 155 Euro per ton in Austria [190].

12.7
Outlook and Perspectives

Technology and research challenges associated with converting plant biomass into commodity products must be considered in relation to green biomass in combination with lignocellulosic biomass [196] (converting biomass into reactive intermediates) and product diversification (converting reactive intermediates into useful products). After isolation of the valuable products (chlorophyll, carotenoids) biomass precursors such as carbohydrates and proteins must be considered. Their isolation as functional products and their biotechnological or chemical conversion into derivatives such as *O*-chemicals and *N*-chemicals must be included in the development of the relevant technologies. Biotechnological conversion methods must be integrated into the concepts of utilization of nature – wet biomass. It is necessary to establish green biorefinery demonstration plants which are best suited for the different regional rural structures of grassland agriculture and the cultural landscape.

Acknowledgment

The authors thank Michael Mandl and Niv Graf, Joanneum Research, Graz, Austria, for investigations silage fibers, and Werner Koschuh, University of Natural Resources and Applied Life Sciences, Vienna, for investigations of silage juice.

References

1 The Bible – Old Testament, First Book Moses, Genesis 4.2

2 Roulle, H. M.; *J. Med. Chirurg. Pharm.*, **40** (1773) 59–67

3 Schwenke, K. D.; Leaf Proteins in the history of Protein research. *Ernährungsforschung*, **37** (1993) 1–11 (germ.)

4 Pirie, N. W.; Leaf protein as human food. *Science*, **152** (1966) 1701–1705.

5 Pirie, N. W. (ed.). Leaf Protein: its agronomy, preparation, quality and use. IBP Handbook 20 [Blackwell, Oxford, **1971**]

6 Pirie, N. W.; Leaf protein: a beneficiary of tribulation. Nature, **253** (1975) 239–241

7 Kamm, B.; Kamm, M.; The green biorefinery – Principles, Technologies and Products, 2nd International Symposium Green Biorefinery, October, 13–14, 1999, SUSTAIN, Verein zur Koordination von

Forschung über Nachhaltigkeit (Hrsg.), Feldbach, Austria, **1999**, S. 46–69

8 Pheloung, P.; Brady, C. J. J. Sci. Food Agric., **30** (1979) 246–250

9 Schwenke, K. D.; Leaf proteins, *Ernährungsforschung*, **28** (1983) 125–129 (germ.)

10 Douillard, R.; Porcheron, A.; Lola, M.; Guy, P.; Genier, G.; *Agronomie*, **10** (1991) 273–284

11 Hari, V.; *Anal. Biochem.*, **113** (1981) 332–335

12 Hirano, H.; *Phytochemistry*, **21** (1982) 1513–1518

13 Slade, R. E.; Birkinshaw, J. H. (ICI); Improvement in or related to the utilization of grass and other green crops. *Brit. Pat.* **BP 511,525** (1939)

14 Ullmanns –Encyklopedie der technischen Chemie; Proteine., 4. Aufl. Bd. 19 [Verlag Chemie, Weinheim, Florida Basel]

15 Pirie, N. W.; *Chemy Ind.*, **61** (1942) 45

16 Pirie, N. W.; *Nature*, **149** (1942) 251

17 Tilley, J. M. A.; Raymond, W. F.; *Herb. Abstr.*, **27** (1957) 235

18 Davys, M. N. G.; Pirie, N. W.; Batch production of protein from leaves. *J. Agric. Eng. Res.*, **8** (1963) 70–73.

19 Kohler, G. O.; Knuckles, B. E.; Edible protein from leaves. *Food Technol.*, **31** (1977) 191–195

20 Telek, L.; Graham, H. D.; Leaf protein concentrates. [AVI Publishing Comp., Westport, Connecticut, **1983**]

21 Defremery, D.; Miller, R. E.; Edwards, R. H.; Knuckles, B. E.; Bickoff, E. M.; Kohler, G. O.; Centrifugal separation of white and green protein fractions from alfalfa juice following controlled heating. *J. Agric. Food Chem.*, **21** (1973) 886–889.

22 Edwards, R. H.; Miller, R. E.; Defremery, D.; Knuckles, B. E.; Bickoff, E. M.; Kohler, G. O.; Pilot plant production of an edible white fraction leaf protein concentrate from alfalfa. *J. Agric Food Chem.*, **23** (1975) 620–626.

23 Knuckles, B. E.; Bickoff, E. M.; Kohler, G. O.; *J. Agric. Food Chem.*, **20** (1972) 1055

24 Krasnovsky, A. A.; Jr. *Photosynth. Res.*, **76** (2003) 389–403.

25 Senge, O. M.; Richter, J.; Adding Color to Green Chemistry? An Overview on Fundamentals and Potential of Chlorophylls. In this book, **2005**

26 Willstätter, R.; Stoll, A.; Untersuchungen über Chlorophyll. Methoden und Ergebnisse. [Verlag Julius Springer, Berlin, **1913**]

27 Willstätter, R.; Stoll, A.; Investigations on Chlorophyll [Science Press, Lancaster Pa., **1928**] transl. from [28]

28 Schertz, F. M.; Isolation of Chlorophyll, Carotene and Xanthophyll by improved methods, *Ind. Eng. Chem.*, **30** (1938) 1073–1075

29 Shearon, W. H.; Gee, O. F.; *Ind. Eng. Chem.*, **41** (1949) 218–226

30 Stenerson, H.; *Chem. Eng. News*, **30** (1952) 2040

31 Judah, M. A.; Burdick, E. M.; Carroll, R. G.; Chlorophyll by solvent extraction. Ind. Eng. Chem., **46** (1954) 2262–2271

32 Graetzel, M.; Liska, P.; "Photoelectrochemical Cells and Process for Making Same", US Patent 5,084,365 (**1992**)

33 Carlsson, R.; An ecological better adapted agriculture. Wet-fractionation of biomass as green crops, macro-alga, and tuber crops, Proc. 2nd Int. Conf. Leaf Protein Res., Nagoya, Japan, **1985**, pp. 93–100

34 Carlsson, R.; Status quo of the utilization of green biomass, In: The Green biorefinery, Kamm B, Kamm M, Soyez K (eds); The Green Biorefinery, Concept of technology, 1st International Symposium Green Biorefinery, Oct. 1997, Neuruppin, Society of ecological technology and system analysis, Berlin, **1998**, 39–45

35 Carlsson, R.; A tentative list of plant for commercial production of leaf protein concentrates, Proc. 3rd Int. Leaf Protein Res. Conf., Pisa–Perugia–Viterbo, Italy, **1989**, 350–353

36 Telek, L.; Graham, H. D. (Eds.) Leaf protein concentrates, AVI Publ., Co., Inc., Westport, Conn., USA, **1983**, 81–116

37 Coombs, J.; Hall, K.; The potential of cereals as industrial raw materials: Legal technical, commercial considerations. In: Cereals – Novel Uses and processes [G. M. Campbell, C. Webb and S. L. McKee (eds.), Plenum, New York, **1997**] 1–12.

38 Kamm, M. et al., Product family trees: Lignocellulose – Hemicellulose and Cel-

lulose based chemical products, In this book, **2005**

39 Statistisches Jahrbuch über Ernährung, Landwirtschaft und Forsten, Ed.: Bundesministerium für Ernährung, Landwirtschaft und Forsten), Landwirtschaftsverlag GmbH, Münster, Germany, **2004**

40 Pickert, J.; Grassland Economy in Germany – Potentials for Green Biorefinery, In: biorefinica 2004, Proceedings and Papers, October, 27–28, Osnabrück, Eds.: Kamm, B.; Hempel, M.; Kamm, M; biopos e.V., Teltow **2004**, p. 26, ISBN 3-00-015166-4

41 http://europa.eu.int/comm/research/infocentre/export/0331e_374.html

42 Production of dry-crop in Europe: CIDE-Comision Intersyndicale des Déhydrateurs Européen, **2004/2005**, Brussels

43 http://www.hayconference.com; http://www.auri.org/research/alfproce.htm

44 Jagiello, R. and Wojcik, S. A.; Comparison of the contents of hemicellose, cellulose, lignin and crude fibre in fresh herbage, hay and silage from meadow grasses and lucerne. *Annales Universitatis Mariae Curie-Sklodowska, E*, **31**, (1976), 525–535.

45 Morrison, I. M.; Changes in lignin and hemicellulose concentrations of ten varieties of temperate grasses with increasing maturity. *Grass and Forage Science*, **35**, (1980) 287–293.

46 Gordon, A. H., Lomax, J. A. and Chesson, A. Glycosidic linkages of legume, grass and cereal straw cell walls before and after extensive degradation by rumen microorganisms. *Journal of the Science of Food and Agriculture*, **34**, (1983) 1341–1350.

47 Kolarski, D., Koljajić, V., Koljajić, V., Popović, J. and Popović, Z.; Potential biological value of some roughages. *Krmiva*, **32**, (1990) 101–106.

48 Seyfarth, W., Knabe, O. and Arnold, H. Changes in the carbohydrate fractions of grasses during growth and effects on fermentability. *Proceedings of the 13th International Grassland Congress. Sectional Papers, Sections 8-9-10* (**1977**) pp 238–243.

49 Åman, P. and Lindgren E. Chemical composition and in vitro degradability of individual chemical constituents of six Swedish grasses harvested at different stages of maturity. *Swedish Journal of Agricultural Research*, **13**, (1983) 221–227.

50 Morrison, I. M. Lignin-carbohydrate complexes from Lolium perenne. *Phytochemistry*, **13**, (1974) 1231–1235.

51 Kondo, T.; Chemical and physical studies on characteristics of forage lignins. *Bulletin of the Tohuku National Agricultural Experiment Station*, **85**, (1993)103–214.

52 Tanner, G. R. and Morrison, I. M.; Phenolic-carbohydrate complexes in the cell walls of Lolium perenne. *Phytochemistry*, **22**, (1983) 2133–2139.

53 Chesson, A., Gordon, A. H. and Scobbie, L.; Pectic polysaccharides of mesophyll cell walls of perennial ryegrass leaves. *Phytochemistry*, **38**, (1995) 579–583.

54 Thom, E. R., Sheath, G. W. and Bryant, A. M. Seasonal variations in total nonstructural carbohydrate and major element levels in perennial ryegrass and paspalum in a mixed pasture. *New Zealand Journal of Agricultural Research*, **32**, (1989) 157–235.

55 Prud'homme, M. P., Gonzalez, B., Billard, J. P. and Boucaud, J.; Carbohydrate content, fructan and sucrose enzyme activities in roots, stubble and leaves of ryegrass (Lolium perenne L.) as affected by source/sink modification after cutting. *Journal of Plant Physiology*, **210**, (1992) 282–291.

56 Masuko, T., Kodama, I., Uematsu, H., Kuboi, S., Maeda, Y. and Yamanaka, Y. Changes in mono and disaccharide contents of temperate grass cut at three stages of growth in Hokkaido. *Nippon Sochi Gakkaishi*, **40**, (1994) 230–233.

57 Fales, S. L., Holt, D. A., Lechtenberg, V. L., Johnson, K., Ladisch, M. R. and Anderson, A. Fractionation of forage grass carbohydrates using liquid (water) chromatography. *Agronomy Journal*, **74**, (1982) 1074–1077.

58 Simpson, R. J. and Bonnett, G. D. (1993). Fructan exohydrolase from grasses. *New Phytologist*, **123**, (1982) 453–469.

59 Pavis, N., Chatterton, N. J., Harrison, P. A., Baumgartner, S., Praznik, W., Boucaud, J. and Prud'homme, M. P.; Structure of fructans in roots and leaf tissues of Lolium perenne. *New Phytologist*, **150**, (2001) 83–95.

60 Spollen, W. G.; Fructan composition and physiological roles in wheat, tall fescue, and timothy. *Dissertation Abstracts International B, Sciences and Engineering*, **51**, (1990) 523.

61 Azis, B. H., Chin, B., Deacon, M. P., Harding, S. E. and Pavlov, G. M.; Size and shape of inulin in dimethyl sulphoxide solution. *Carbohydrate Polymers*, **38**, (1999) 231–234.

62 Fuchs, A., In M. Suzuki and N. J. Chatterton, *Science and technology of fructans*. N. J. Boca Raton, Florida: CRC Press, p. 319 (**1993**).

63 Pontis, H. G.; Fructans. *Methods in Plant Biochemistry*, **2**, (1990) 353–369.

64 Teeuwen, H., Thoné, M. and Vandorpe, J.; Inulin – From traditional food source to an all-round raw material. *ZFL, Internationale Zeitschrift für Lebensmittel-Technik, Marketing, Verpackung und Analytik*, **43**, (1992) 732, 734, 737–738.

65 Mela, T. and Rand, H.; Amino acid composition of timothy, meadow fescue, cocksfoot and perennial ryegrass at two levels of nitrogen fertilisation and at successive cuttings. *Annales Agriculturae Fenniae*, **18**, (1979) 246–251.

66 Pedersen, E. J. N., Witt, N. and Mortensen, J.; Fractionation of green crops with expression of juice and preservation of pressed crop and juice. 3. Relationship between chemical composition of the crop and that of the juice. *Tidsskrift for Planteavl*, **88**, (1984) 25–36.

67 Pedersen, E. J. N., Witt, N., Mortensen, J. and Soerensen, C. Fractionation of green crops and preservation of pressed crop and juice. 2. Preservation of juice. *Tidsskrift for Planteavl*, **85**, (1981) 13–30.

68 McDougall, V. D. Support energy and green crop fractionation in the United Kingdom. *Agricultural Systems*, **5**, (1980) 251–266.

69 Lesnitski, V. R. High-protein feeds from green mass. *Kormoproizvodstvo*, **1/2**, (1997) 61–62.

70 Rabovsky, J. Biogenic amorphous silica. *Scandinavian Journal of Work, Environment and Health*, **21** (1995) 108–110.

71 Sangster, A. G., Hodson, M. B. and Tubb, H. J.; Silicon deposits in higher plants. *Studies in Plant Science*, **8**, (2001)85–113.

72 Parry, D., Hodson, M. J. and Sangster, A. G.; Some recent advances in studies of silicon in higher plants. *Philosophical Transactions of the Royal Society of London, B*, **304**, (1984) 537–549.

73 Dinsdale, D., Gordon, A. H. and George, S.; Silica in mesophyll cell walls of Italian ryegrass (Lolium multiflorum Lam. Cv. RvP). *Annals of Botany*, **44**, (1979) 73–77.

74 Bode, E., Kozik, S., Kunz, U. and Lehmann, H.; Comparative electron microscopic studies for the localization of silica in leaves of two different grass species. *Deutsche Tierärztliche Wochenschrift*, **101**, (1994) 367–372.

75 Moore, D.; The distribution of silica bodies in leaf sheaths of two perennial ryegrass cultivars differing in their susceptibility to attack by dipterous stemborers. *Grass and Forage Science*, **39**, (1984) 205–208.

76 Puffe, D., Morgner, F. and Zerr, W.; Investigations on the contents of different constituents in important forage plants. 2. Mineral and silicic acid contents. *Wirtschaftseigene Futter*, **30**, (1984) 52–70.

77 Malossini, F., Piasentier, E. and Bovolenta, S.; n-Alkane content of some forages. *Journal of the Science of Food and Agriculture*, **53**, (1990) 405–409.

78 Jones, D. I. H. and Hayward, M. V.; Starches in forages. *UK, Welsh Plant Breeding Station: Report for 1977*, (**1990**) 109–110.

79 Rizk, A. F. M. and Hussiney, H. A.; Chemistry and toxicity of Lolium species. In A. F. M. Rizk, *Poisonous plant contamination of edible plants* (pp. 95–106), (**1991**) Boca Raton: CRC Press Inc.

80 Sidebottom, C., Buckley, S., Pudney, P., Twigg, S., Jarman, C., Holt, C., Telford, J., McArthur, A., Worrall, D., Hubbard, R. and Lillford, P. Heat-stable antifreeze protein from grass. *Nature*, **406** (2000) 256.

81 Kuiper, M. J., Davies, P. L. and Walker, V. K. A theoretical model of a plant antifreeze protein from Lolium perenne. *Biophysical Journal*, **81**, (2001) 3560–3565.

82 Kamm, B.; Kamm, M.; Principles of biorefineries, Appl. Microbiol. Biotechn. **64** (2004) 137–145

83 Kamm, B.; Kamm, M.; Biorefinery-Systems. Chem. Biochem. Eng. Q., **18** (2004) 1–6

84 Okkerse, C.; v. Bekkum, H.; From fossil to green, Green Chemistry, **1** (2) 1999, 111

85 Heier, W.; Das Fraktionieren von Gras, In: Grundlagen der Landtechnik, **33** (1983) 2

86 Sundberg, M.; Mekanisk avvattning av vallföder – En litteraturöversikt (Mechanical dewatering of forage crops – a litteratur review); Jordbrukstekniska institutes, Rapport **134**, Uppsala, 1991

87 Kasper, G. J.; Fractioning of grass and lucerne. *Landbouwmechanisatie*, **49**, (1998) 47–48.

88 Kaczmarek, J.; Lange, B.; Ohm, H.-D.; Investigation for fractionation of biorefinery-raw material, In: The Green biorefinery, Kamm B, Kamm M, Soyez K (eds) The Green Biorefinery, Concept of technology, 1st International Symposium Green Biorefinery, Oct. 1997, Neuruppin, Society of ecological technology and system analysis, Berlin, **1998**, 126–130

89 Bruhn, H. D.; Straub, R. J.; Koegel, R. G.; A systems approach to the production of plant protein concentrate; Proceedings of the International Grain and Forage Harvesting Conference, **1978**, (Ed.) American Society of Agricultural Engineers

90 Kamo, M. and Nakagawasai, H.; Studies on the development of effective grass utilization techniques. 1. The separation and concentration of leaf protein from grass juice by centrifuging. *Bulletin of the National Grassland Research Institute, Japan*, **31**, (1985) 81–92.

91 France Luzerne Alfalis – Dossier PX. France Luzerne, **2000**.

92 (a) Kromus, S.; Wachter, B.; Koschuh, W.; Mandl, M.; Krotschek, C.; Narodoslawsky, M.; The green biorefinery Austria – Development of an Integrated System for Green Biomass Utilization, Chem Biochem Eng Q 18 (1) (2004) 13–19; (b) Kromus, S.; Die Grüne Bioraffinerie Österreich – Entwicklung eines integrierten Systems zur Nutzung von Grünlandbiomasse. Dissertation, 2002, TU Graz (German).

93 (a) Ketelaars, J. J. M. H., Bio-raffinage van natuurgras, Netherland, **2001**, www.precisievoeding.nl/projecten/ p07_10316.htm; (b) Hulst, A. Bio-refinery of grass and other raw materials from vegetable sources and product applications; GreenTech 2002, Amsterdam, 24–26 April, **2002**: Abstract book, p. 37; http://www.ienica.net/greentech/ hulst.ppt

94 Kamm, B.; et al Green biorefinery Brandenburg, Article to development of products and of technologies and assessment. Brandenburg. Umweltber. 8, (2000) 260–269.

95 Biomass R&D, Technical Advisory Committee, Roadmap for Biomass Technology in the United States, Dec. **2002**, Washington D.C., www.bioproducts-bioenergy.gov/pdfs/FinalBiomassRoadmap.pdf, 30

96 (a) Peitgen, H.-O., Richter, P. H.; The beauty of fractals [Berlin, **1986**], (b) Mandelbrot, B.; Die fraktale Geometrie der Natur [Basel, **1987**]

97 Hagers Handbuch der pharmazeutischen Praxis (Hagers handbook of pharmaceutical practice) band 1–5, chemicals and drugs, band 1–5 [W. Kern et al. (eds), Springer Verlag, Berlin, Heidelberg, New York, **1972–78**] (a) bd 1, p. 732–736; (b) bd 2, lipides

98 Starke, I., Holzberger, A., Kamm, B., Kleinpeter, E.; Qualitative and quantitative analysis of carbohydrates in green juices (wild mix grass and alfalfa) from a green biorefinery by gas chromatography/ mass spectrometry, Fresenius J. Anal. Chem., **367**, (2000) 65–72

99 Moser, A.; (ed); Eco-tech The technical Development [Verlag TU Graz, Austria, **1997**]

100 Schwenke, K. D.; Eiweisquellen der Zukunft [Aulis-Verlag Deubner, Köln, **1985**, ISBN 3-7614-0858-7] pp. 82.

101 Carlsson R.; Food and Non-food uses of immature cereals. In: Cereals – Novel Uses and processes [G. M. Campbell, C. Webb and S. L. McKee (eds.), Plenum, New York], (1997) 159–167.

102 Kirk, R. E.; Othmer, D. F. (ed.).; Encyclopedia of chemical technology [John Wiley and Sons, New York, **1994**].

103 Keller, K.; Technology for two-steps conservation of green biomass, In: The Green biorefinery, Kamm B, Kamm M, Soyez K (eds); The Green Biorefinery, Concept of technology, 1st International Symposium Green Biorefinery, Oct. 1997, Neuruppin, Society of ecological technology and system analysis, Berlin, **1998**, 120–125

104 Simmonds, M. S. J.; Molecular- and chemo-systematics: do they have a role in agrochemical discovery? *Crop Protection*, 19, (2000) 591–596.

105 Wang, Y. R. and Li, Q.; Investigation and evaluation of native plant resources in Loess Plateau of Gansu Province. In J. Z. Ren, *Proceedings of the International Conference on Farming Systems on the Loess Plateau of China* (1992) (pp. 246–250). Lanzhou: Gansu Science and Technology Press

106 Douillard, R., de Mathan, O.; Leaf protein for food use: potential of Rubisco. In New and developing sources of food proteins (Ed. Hudson BJF), Publisher Chapman and Hall, London, UK, (1994) 307–342.

107 Bahr, J. T., Bourque, D. P., Smith, H. J.; Solubility properties of fraction I proteins of maize, cotton, spinach, and tobacco. J. Agric. Food. Chem. **25** (1977) 783–789.

108 Bigelow, C. C. On the average hydrophobicity of proteins and the relation between it and protein structure. J. Theor. Biol. **16** (1967) 187–211.

109 Hood, L. L.; Cheng S. G.; Koch, U.; Brunner, J. R.; Alfalfa proteins: Isolation and partial characterization of the major component – fraction I protein. J Food Sci **46** (1981) 1843–1850.

110 Burova, T. V.; Soshinskii, A. A.; Danilenko, A. N.; Antonov, YuA; Grinberg, Vya; Tolstoguzov, V.B.; Conformation stability of ribulose diphosphate carboxylase of alfalfa green leaves according to the data of differential scanning microcalorimetry, Biofizika **34** (1989) 545–549.

111 Barbeau, W. E.; Kinsella, J. E.; Ribulose bisphosphate carboxylase/oxygenase (Rubisco) from green leaves – potential as a food protein, Food. Rev. Int. **41** (1988) 93–127.

112 Jones, W. T., Mangan, J. L. Large-scale isolation of fraction 1 leaf protein (18S) from lucerne (Medicago sativa L). J. Agr. Sci. **86** (1976) 495–501.

113 Hatch, F. T., Bruce, A. L.; Amino acid composition of soluble and membranous lipoproteins. Nature **218** (1968) 1166–1168.

114 Douillard, R.; Biochemical and physicochemical properties of leaf proteins. In Proteines Veg, Publisher Tech. Doc. Lavoisier, Paris, France, (1985) 211–244.

115 Betschart, A. A.; The incorporation of leaf protein concentrates and isolates in human diets, In "Green Crop Fractionation" [Ed. R. J. Wilkins (ed.) The British Grassland Society, c/o Grassland Research Institute, Hurley, Maidenhead, SL6 5LR, UK, **1977**] pp. 83–96.

116 Carlsson, R.; White leaf protein products for human consumption. A global review on plants and processing methods. In "Tobacco Protein Utilization Perspectives", Proc. Round Table Conf. At 1st Int. Congr. Food and Health [(P. Fantozzi (ed.), CNR/Italian National Res. Council, Special Project IPBR, Subproject L. EEC Agrimed Project, **1985**] pp. 125–145

117 Kung, S. D.; Saunders, J. A.; Tso, T. C.; Vaughan, D. A.; Womack, M.; Staples, R. C.; Beechers, G. R.; Tobacco as a potential food sources and smoke material: Nutritional evaluation of tobacco leaf protein. *J. Food Sci.*, **45** (1980) 320–332, 327.

118 Linnemann, A. R. and Dijkstra, D. S. Toward sustainable production of protein-rich foods: appraisal of eight crops for Western Europe. Part 1. Analysis of the primary links of the production chain. *Critical Reviews in Food Science and Nutrition*, **42** (2002) 377–401.

119 Wolfrum, C.; Wheat grass – The power in the green Juice [Gräfe und Unzer Verlag GmbH, München, **1998**, ISBN: 3-7742-4072-8] (German)

120 Gaynor, M. L. and Hickey, G. P.; Green nutritional powder composition containing natural food and herbal products. *US Patent Application 5904924* **(1999)**.

121 Messman, M. A., Weiss, W. P., and Koch, M. E.; Changes in total and individual protein during drying, ensiling and ruminal fermentation of forages. J. Dairy Sci. **77** (1994) 492–500.

122 Koschuh, W., Povoden, G., Vu Hong, T., Kromus, S., Kulbe, K. D., Novalin, S., Krotscheck, C.; Production of leaf protein concentrate from ryegrass (*Lolium perenne×multiflorum*) and alfalfa (*Medicago sativa subsp. Sativa*). Comparison between heat coagulation/centrifugation and ultrafiltration. Desalination **163** (2004) 253–259.

123 Vu Hong, T., Koschuh, W., Kulbe, K. D., Kromus, S., Krotscheck, C., Novalin, S. Desalination of high salt content mixture by two-stage electrodialysis as the first step of separating valuable substances from grass silage. Desalination **162** (2004) 343–353

124 Kamm, B.; Kamm, M.; Scherze, I.; Muschiolik, G.; Bindrich, U.; Biobased polymers by chemical valorization of biomass components, In: Vasile, C.; Zaikov (Eds.) Polymer reactions and properties, Publishing House Nova Science – New York (in press)

125 Oyama, K., Kobayashi, T., Imazato, Y.; Kumasawa, Y.; Polysaccharides from fescue plant cell walls, emulsifiers containing them, and method for emulsification. *Japanese Patent Application*, 10237107 (**1998**).

126 Cherno, N. K., Adamovskaya, K. D. and Lobotskaya, L. L.; Polysaccharide–lignin complexes of raw materials not traditional for the food industry, and their properties. *Khimiya Drevesiny*, **3** (1991) 95–98.

127 Shipley, L. W. Manufacture of high purity amorphous silica from biogenic material. *US Patent Application*, 6406678 (**2002**).

128 Noeske, R. and Horn, I. Procedure for the production of silicon carbide from renewable raw materials. *German Patent Application*, 10020626 (**2001**).

129 Shiuh, J. C., Palm, S. K., Nyamekye, G. A., Smith, T. R., Taniguchi, J. D. and Wang, Q. Highly purified biogenic silica product and its preparation. *European Patent Application*, 758560 (**1997**).

130 Palm, S. K., Smith, T. R., Shiuh, J. C. and Roulston, J. S.; Filterable composite adsorbents with adsorptive and filterable components as filter aids suitable for beer chillproofing. *PCT International Application*, 9830324 (**1998**).

131 Itsumi, A., Sakagami, E.; Manufacture of artificial zeolites from grass. *Japanese Patent Application*, 2001323109 (**2001**).

132 Salminen, S. O. and Grewal, P. S.; Does decreased mowing frequency enhance alkaloid production in endophytic tall fescue and perennial ryegrass? *Journal of Chemical Ecology*, **28** (2002) 939–950.

133 Fechner, M.; Grassland economy in Brandenburg. In: Proceedings of the 1st. Int. Symposium on Green Biorefinery, Neuruppin, Germany 1997 [K. Soyez, B. Kamm, M. Kamm (eds.), Berlin, Germany, **1998**, ISBN 3-929672-06-5] (German) 47–52

134 Wantanabe, T.; Fujishima, A.; Honda, K.; Dye-sensitive electrodes. In: Energy Resour. Photochem. Cat. [M. Grätzel (ed.), Academic Press, **1983**] 359

135 Cohen, B. S., et al.; J. Agric. Food Chem. **32** (1984) 516

136 Leblanc, R. M., et al.; *Photobiochem. Photobiophys.* **7** (1984) 41

137 Girio, F. M. F. Development of xylo-oligosaccharides and xylitol for use in pharmaceutical and food industries (XYLOPHONE) (**1997**) *FAIR-CT97-3811.*

138 Aspinall (ed.); The polysaccharides. Vol. 2 [Academic Press, New York, **1983**] (a) p. 98–193, (b) p. 411–490

139 Davidson (ed.); Handbook of Water soluble Gums and Resins. [McGraw-Hill, New York, **1980**]

140 Perl (ed.); The Chemistry of Lignin [Dekker, New York, **1967**]

141 Crawford (ed.); Lignin Biodegradation and Transformation. [John Wiley and Sons, New York, **1981**]

142 Hofrichter, M.; Steinbüchel, A.; (ed.) Biopolymers: Lignin, humic substances and coal; **2001**, Wiley-VCH, ISBN 3-527-30220-4

143 Nay, W. H. and Fuller, W. S.; Method for processing straw into pulp and animal feed byproduct and paper product

therefrom. *PCT International Application*, (**1999**), WO9918285.

144 Sonnenfeld, D.A.; Logging vs recycling: Problems in the industrial ecology of pulp manufacture in south-east Asia. *Greener Management International*, **22** (1998) 108–122.

145 Lora, J.H. and Escudero, E. Soda pulping of agricultural fibres for boardmaking applications. *Paper Technology*, **41** (2000) 37–42.

146 Pahkala, K.A., Mela, T.J.N. and Laamanen, L.; Pulping characteristics and mineral composition of 23field crops cultivated in Finland. In J.F. Kennedy, G.O. Phillips and P.A. Williams, *The Chemistry and Processing of Wood and Plant Fibrous Materials [Cellucon '94]* (1996) (pp. 119–125). Cambridge: Woodhead.

147 Saijonkari-Pahkala, K.; Non-wood plants as raw material for pulp and paper. *Agricultural and Food Science in Finland*, **10**, (2001) 1–101.

148 Janes, R.L.; In: The pulping of wood. 2nd edn, vol 1 [R.G. MacDonald (ed), McGraw-Hill, New York, **1969**] p. 34

149 Fan, W., Xu, J., Guo, Y. and Xing. Q. Production of nonpolluting grass pulp and method for reclaiming its by-product. *Chinese Patent Application*, (**2001**) 1298984.

150 Sfiligoj Smole, M.; Kleinschek, K.S.; Kreze, T.; Strnad, S.; Mandl M.; Wachter, B.; Physical properties of grass fibers; Chem. Biochem. Eng. Q. (CABEQ) **18**(1) (2004): 47–53

151 Bartl, A.; Mihalyi, B.; Marini, I.; Applications of renewable fibrous materials; Chem. Biochem. Eng. Q. (CABEQ) **18**(1) (2004): 21–28

152 Holm-Christensen; The dehydration plant as producer for the cellulose industry. Proc. Dry-Crops 89, 4th Int. Green Crop Drying Congr., Cambridge [Agra Europe Ltd., London, UK, **1989**] pp. 91–94

153 Carlsson, R.; Pressed crop for possible production of paper crop. Proc. 4th Int. Conf. Leaf Protein Res., New Zealand–Australia **1993**, pp. 69–74

154 Fechner, M.; Hertwig, F.; Paper made of grass very much in the future. *Neue Landwirtschaft*, **11** (1994) 29–31 (in German)

155 Hille, C.; Prenacell-process, UVER GmbH, Germany, **1999**

156 Jiang, Z., Zang, W. and Feng, S.; Production of grass fiber adhesive film. *Chinese Patent Application*, 1235735 (**1997**).

157 Wang, S.H.; Biodegradable protein/ starch-based thermoplastic composition. *PCT International Application*, 9956556 (**1999**).

158 Thomsen, M.H.; Bech, D.; Kiel, P.; Manufacturing of Stabilised Brown Juice for L-lysine Production – from University Lab Scale over Pilot Scale to Industrial Scale, Chem. Biochem. Eng. Q. (CABEQ) **18**(1) (2004) 37–46

159 Kamm, B.; Neue Ansätze in der Organischen Synthesechemie – Verknüpfung von biologischer und chemischer Stoffwandlung am Beispiel der Biorafinerie-Grundprodukte Milchsäure und Carnitin, Habilitationsschrift, University of Potsdam, Germany, **2004** (German)

160 Grass, S.; Hansen, S.; Sieber, M.; Müller, P.H.; Production of Ethanol, Protein concentrate, and Technical Fibres from Clover/Grass; In: Proceedings of the fourth biomass conference of Americas, Biomass, A Growths Opportunity in Green Energy and Value added Products, Vol. 1, Overend, R.P.; Chornet, E. (ed.); Elsevier Science Ltd., **1999**, 911–914, ISBN 008 0430198

161 Dale, B.E.; Biomass Refining, protein and ethanol from alfalfa. Ind. Eng Product Research and Development, **22** (1983) 446

162 Werpy, T.; Petersen, G.; (eds.); Top Value Chemicals under the refinery concept: A Phase II Study [US Department of Energy, Office of scientific and technical information], **2004**, No.: DOE/GO-102004-1992, www.osti.gov/ bridge

163 Kamm, B.; Kamm, M.; Gruber, P.R.; Kromus, S.; Biorefinery-Systems – An Overview; The Role of biotechnology, In this book, **2005**

164 Gruber, P.R.; Henton, D.E.; Starr, J.; Polylactic acid from Renewable Resources, In this book, **2005**

165 Neureiter, M.; Danner, H.; Madzingaidzo, L.; Miyafuji, H.; Thomasser, C.; Bvochora, J.; Bamusi, S.; Braun, R.; Lignocellulose Feedstocks for the production of lactic acid, Chem. Biochem. Eng. Q. (CABEQ) **18**(1) (2004) 55–63

166 McGrath, D.; Italian ryegrass as a source of fermentable sugars and protein feedstuff. Luxembourg: Commission of the European Communities, (1990).

167 Quereshi, N. and Blaschek, H. P.; ABE production from corn: a recent economic evaluation. *Journal of Industrial Microbiology and Biotechnology*, **27**, (2001) 292–297.

168 Starke, I.; Kamm, B.; Kleinpeter, E.; Separation, identification and quantification of amino acids in L-lysine fermentation potato juices by gas chromatography/ mass spectrometry, *Fresenius J. Anal. Chem.*, **371** (2001) 380–384

169 Kamm, B.; Kamm, M.; Schmidt, M.; Starke, I.; Kleinpeter, E.; Chemical and biochemical generation of carbohydrates from lignocellulose-feedstock (*Lupinus nootkatensis*), Quantification of glucose, Chemosphere (in press)

170 Kiel, P.; Thomsen, M. H.; Andersen, M.; Plant Juice in the Biorefinery – Use of plant juice as fermentation medium, In this book

171 Vorlop, K. D.; Willke, Th.; Prüße, U.; Biocatalytic and catalytic routes for the production of bulk and fine chemicals from renewable resources, In this book

172 Datta, R.; Tsai, S.-P.; Lactic acid Production and potential uses: A Technology and Economics Assessment. In: Fuels and chemicals from biomass, B. C. Sara, J. Woodward (ed.), ACS Symposium series, ISSN 0097-6156666, ACS, Washington D. C., **1997**, pp. 224–236

173 Tullo, A.; Renewable Materials, Two Pacts May Help Spur Biomass Plastics; Chemical and Engineering News, March 28, **2005**, www.CEN-ONLINE.org

174 Van Dyne, D. L.; Blasé, M. G.; Clements, L. D.; A Strategy for returning agriculture and rural America to long-term full employment using biomass refineries. In: J. Janeck (ed.) Perspectives on new crops and new uses. ASHS Press, Alexandria, VA, USA, **1999**, 114–123

175 Jiang, Z., Chen, R. and Wu, P.; Hydrogenation of xylose to xylitol in trickle-bed reactor. *Riyong Huaxue Gongye*, **6**, (1998) 6–8.

176 Nigam, P. and Singh, D.; Processes for fermentative production of xylitol – a sugar substitute. *Process Biochemistry*, **30**, (1995) 124–124.

177 Bhatt, S. and Shukla, R. P. HMF – a new route to industrial chemicals from sugars. *Taiwan Sugar*, **48**, (2001) 4–15.

178 Elliott, D. C.; Fitzpatrick, S. W.; Bozell, J. J.; Jarnefeld, J. L.; Bilski, R. J.; Moens, L.; Frye, Jr. J. G.; Wang, Y.; Neuenschwander, G. G.; Production of levulinic acid and use as a platform chemical for derived products; In: Proceedings of the fourth biomass conference of Americas, Biomass, A Growths Opportunity in Green Energy and Value added Products, Vol. 1, Overend, R. P.; Chornet, E. (ed.); Elsevier Science Ltd., **1999**, 911–914, ISBN 008 0430198

179 Rothschild, Z., Silva, H. C., Braga, G. L., Carlomagno, D. N., Prado, I. M. R., de Carvalho, R., Polizello, A. C. M. and Spadaro, A. C. C.; Xylitol a non-cariogenic sugar obtained from grasses of the genus Aristida and related species. *Arquivos de Biologica e Tecnologia*, **34**, (1991) 61–71.

180 de Baynast, R. and Renard, C.; Processes for extraction and transformation of products with high fructose content from chicory roots (*Cichorium intybus*). *Comptes Rendus de l'Académie d'Agriculture de France*, **80**, (1994) 31–46.

181 Fischer, K., Bipp, H.-P., Riemschneider, P., Leidmann, P., Bienek, D. and Kettrup, A.; Utilization of biomass residues for the remediation of metal-polluted soils. *Environmental Science and Technology*, **32**, (1998) 2154–2231.

182 Kato, H.; Porous carbon fibers from plant waste materials manufactured by baking the waste materials in an oven in the roped form for formation of coiled carbonized fibers and reuse of plant waste materials therefor. *Japanese Patent Application*, 2000303266 (**2000**).

183 Linke, B.; Schelle, H.; Anaerobe Ver-
fahren zur Reststoffbehandlung, In:
The Green biorefinery, Kamm B,
Kamm M, Soyez K (eds) The Green
Biorefinery, Concept of technology, 1st
International Symposium Green Biorefinery, Oct. 1997, Neuruppin, Society
of ecological technology and system
analysis, Berlin, (1998) 196–207

184 Verstrate, W.; Debeer, D.; Pena, M.; Let-
tinga, G.; Lens, P.; Anaerobic Bioprocessing of Organic Wastes, World Journal of Microbiology and Biotechnology,
12 (1996) 221–223

185 Fowler, P.A.; McLaughlin, A.R.; Hall,
L.M.; The potential industrial uses of
forage grasses including miscanthus;
BioComposites Centre, University of
Wales, Bangor, Gwynedd 2003;
www.nnfcc.co.uk/library/reports/
download.cfm?id=60

186 Elements, Degussa Science Newsletter
7 (2005) 35

187 Vink, E.T.H.; Rabago, K.R.; Glassner,
D.A.; Gruber, P.R.; Applications of life
cycle assessment to NatureWorks polylactide (PLA) production, Polymer degradation and stability 80 (2003) 403–
419

188 IEEP, Contribution to the background
study agriculture, The Institute for European Environmental Policy, 2004.

189 Hector, A.; et al.; Plant Diversity and
Productivity Experiments in European
Grasslands, Science, 286 (1999) 1123–
1127

190 (a) Schidler, S., Technikfolgenabschät-
zung der Grünen Bioraffinerie, Teil I:
Endbericht, Institut für Technikfolgen-
Abschätzung, Österreichische Akademie der Wissenschaften, 2003; Schidler, S., Adensam, H., Hofmann, R.,

Kromus, S., Will, M., 2003, Technikfolgen-Abschätzung der Grünen Bioraffinerie, Teil II: Materialsammlung, Institut für Technikfolgen-Abschätzung,
Österreichische Akademie der Wissenschaften, 2003 (German)

191 Narodoslawsky, M.; Kromus, S.; Development of decentral green biorefinery
in Austria; In: biorefinica 2004, Proceedings and Papers, October, 27–28,
Osnabrück, Eds.: Kamm, B.; Hempel,
M.; Kamm, M; biopos e.V., Teltow
2004, p. 24; ISBN 3-00-015166-4

192 Halasz L., G. Povoden, M. Narodo-
slawsky: *Process Synthesis for Renewable
Resources*, presented at the PRES 03,
Hamilton, Canada, 2003

193 Nagy, A.B., F. Friedler, and L.T. Fan,
Combinatorial Acceleration of Separ-
able Concave Programming for Process
Synthesis, presented at the AIChE An-
nual Meeting, Miami Beach, FL, USA,
November 15–20, 1998.

194 Fechner, M.; Hertwig, F.; Nachwach-
sende Rohstoffe auch vom Grünland,
Neue Landwirtschaft 11, (1994) 29–31

195 Dale, B.; Encyclopedia of physical
sciences and technology, vol 2, 3rd
edn. McGraw-Hill, New York, 2002,
pp. 141–157

196 (a) Lynd, L.R., Wyman, C.E. and Gerngross, T.U.; Biocommodity engineering. *Biotechnology Progress*, 15, (1999)
777–793. (b) Lynd, L.R.; Biomass Processing in Response to sustainability
and Security Challenges – A Vision for
What is possible, In: biorefinica 2004,
Proceedings and Papers, October, 27–
28, Osnabrück, Eds.: Kamm, B.; Hempel, M.; Kamm, M.; biopos e.V., Teltow
2004, p. 20; ISBN 3-00-015166-4

13
Plant Juice in the Biorefinery –
Use of Plant Juice as Fermentation Medium

Mette Hedegaard Thomsen, Margrethe Andersen, and Pauli Kiel

13.1
Introduction

Biotechnological utilization of waste and residues from agriculture and the agricultural industry has been the common goal for AgroFerm A/S and University of Southern Denmark. The concept of the green biorefinery has been described elsewhere [8]. Additionally, much experimental work has been performed on realizing these ideas for industrial purposes. This paper describes the possibility of using brown juice from the green crop-drying industry and potato juice from the potato starch industry as raw materials in Danish lactic acid production, as a basis for the production of bio-based polylactate to be used as packaging materials for fruit and vegetables. One single green crop-drying factory producing 50 000 tons of fodder pellets a year has enough brown juice to supply a 6 000 ton lactic acid factory with fermentation medium, and a 50 000 ton potato starch factory produces enough potato juice to supply a 35 000 ton lactic acid factory.

13.2
Historical Outline

Since 1997 work has been performed on a research project on the production and testing of bio-based packaging materials for food. The work has been performed as co-operation between The Technical University of Denmark, The Danish Technological Institute, The Royal Danish Veterinary and Agricultural University, Risø National Laboratory, The University of Aarhus, and The University of Southern Denmark. Bio-based materials are defined as materials originating from agricultural sources, i.e. produced from renewable and biological raw materials. The advantages of such materials are that they are CO_2-neutral and biodegradable.

Biorefineries – Industrial Processes and Products. Status Quo and Future Directions. Vol. 1
Edited by Birgit Kamm, Patrick R. Gruber, Michael Kamm
Copyright © 2006 WILEY-VCH Verlag GmbH & Co. KGaA, Weinheim
ISBN: 3-527-31027-4

13.3
Biobased Poly(lactic Acid)

Poly(lactic acid) (PLA) is a bio-based, biodegradable polymer with much potential as a material for food packaging because of its mechanical properties. Because it is a moisture and gas barrier and can be used to produce flexible water-resistant films, PLA is suitable for packaging of respiring fruit and vegetables and for liquid food applications, e.g. juice. PLA can be used [1, 2] as a pure product or it can be used in combination with other polymers. It may contain natural extracts/components e.g. lignin and waxes acting as preservatives or antioxidants preventing oxidation-sensitive products from deteriorating [3].

For PLA to compete with conventional packaging materials it must be produced from cheap raw materials and by feasible processes. Our objective in this collaborative research project was to find the cheapest and most suitable raw materials for Danish production of lactic acid for polylactate production.

13.3.1
Fermentation Processes

PLA is produced by polymerization of lactic acid. Lactic acid can be produced by chemical synthesis or by a fermentation process. Fermentation is a process whereby carbohydrates such as sucrose, glucose, fructose, or lactose are converted by microorganisms into a desired product. Most residues from the agricultural industry contain such carbohydrates either free or bound in long chains of polysaccharides. Molasses – a waste product from sugar beet production – contains saccharose; whey – a waste product from cheese making – contains lactose; potato waste – from the potato starch or French fries industry – contains starch, which can be metabolized by certain strains of microorganisms or hydrolyzed to glucose. Straw contains cellulose and hemicelluloses. Cellulose can be hydrolyzed to glucose and hemicelluloses can be hydrolyzed to xylose, which also can be metabolized by some strains. Green and brown juice from the green crop-drying industry contains several types of carbohydrate and other nutrients. Some of the waste products are available free, others can be purchased at very favorable prices and could be used as cheap raw materials in feasible production of PLA.

13.3.2
The Green Biorefinery

In the green biorefinery, jointly described by the University of Southern Denmark and AgroFerm A/S, crops are converted by means of mechanical and biotechnological methods into useful materials such as food and feed products and additives, and into materials and organic chemical compounds and bio-energy. The crops used in the green biorefinery are crops that give a high yield, fit in with normal crop rotation, absorb large amounts of organic fertilizers, are robust and require a minimum of pesticides.

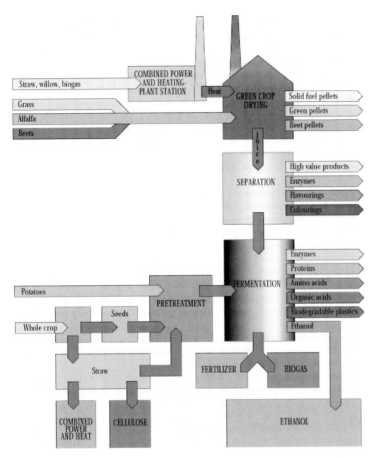

Fig. 13.1 The principles of the green biorefinery.

The crops are separated in a liquid fraction – the juice containing the soluble compounds and the press cake containing particles and insoluble high-molecular-weight compounds. Vitamins, colors, enzymes, and other phytochemicals can be isolated directly from the juice or press cake. The press cake can be used as animal feed or, after drying, as solid fuel.

After extraction of the high-value compounds from the juice, it can be used as a substrate for fermentation [4]. The fermentation products can be any organic compounds, for example enzymes, antibiotics, biodegradable plastics, organic acids, alcohols and amino acids.

13.3.3
Lactic Acid Fermentation

Lactic acid fermentation is normally performed by lactic acid bacteria. Lactic acid bacteria comprise several genera with similar physiology, metabolism, and nutritional needs. A primary similarity is that they all produce lactic acid as a major or sole end product and that they do not use oxygen in their metabolism (anaerobes). Nutritionally, lactic acid bacteria are extremely fastidious. A medium that will support their growth must contain many growth factors such as amino acids, peptides, nucleic acid derivatives, vitamins, salts, and fatty acids or fatty acid esters. When all these nutrients are present in the fermentation medium, lactic acid bacteria will convert carbohydrates to lactic acid.

13.3.4
Brown Juice as a Fermentation Medium

The green crop-drying industry in Denmark uses Italian rye grass, clover, and alfalfa as raw materials for production of green pellets. Approximately 300 000 tons of green pellets are produced in Denmark each year. The green crop-drying industry solves its energy-economical problems by pressing the green crop before drying. The by-product produced, green juice, typically has a dry-matter content of 3 to 8%. At some factories the green biomass is heated to 80 °C by steam before pressing, this causes the plant cells to burst and the protein to coagulate. The by-product produced is called brown juice. Typically brown juice has a dry-matter content of 4 to 8%. Approximately 200 000 m^3 of brown juice is produced each year in Denmark. Although the green and brown juice are spread on the fields as fertilizer, pollution of ground water, particularly with nitrate, in the late autumn has led to stringent regulations on the use of plant juice as a fertilizer. In Denmark plant juice can be spread on green fields only in the autumn and not in the period between October 1st and February 1st [5]. The problem with the plant juice can be solved by storing the juice in large lagoons from October 1st. Because storage can easily result in foul-smelling waste products, we have studied other possibilities.

It is common knowledge that grass and almost all kinds of crop decay if stored inappropriately, but it can be conserved by ensiling either by a spontaneous process in which the microorganisms present in the crops convert the carbohydrates to acid, or by adding a culture of lactic acid bacteria. Therefore the obvious solution is to use the brown juice as a fermentation medium for lactic acid fermentation [6].

13.4
Materials and Methods

13.4.1
Analytical Methods

13.4.1.1 Sugar Analysis

Sugar analysis was performed by HPLC using a Bio-Rad IG Carbo C pre-column and a Bio-Rad Aminex HPX-87C column. Before HPLC analysis samples were subjected to ion exchange through a cation-exchange column (Amberlite CG-120) and an anion-exchange column (Dowex 1(4)).

13.4.1.2 Analysis of Organic Acids

Analysis of organic acids by HPLC was performed using a Bio-Rad Aminex HPX-87H column. Before analysis of organic acids by HPLC, samples were subjected to ion exchange through a cation-exchange column (Amberlite IR-120) and an anion-exchange column (DEAE Sephadex A-25).

13.4.1.3 Analysis of Minerals

Cations, anions and trace minerals were kindly analyzed by the central laboratory of the Danish Co-operative Farm Supply, DLG, using EU-approved methods.

13.4.1.4 Analysis of Vitamins

Vitamins are analyzed by use of Bacto Assey Methods (Difco Manual, 11th edn, 1998).

13.4.1.5 Analysis of Amino Acids

Analysis of free amino acids was performed by EU-approved method 98/64 1EC.

13.4.1.6 Analysis of Protein

Nitrogen (N) analysis was performed by the Kjeldahl method and crude protein was calculated as $N \times 6.25$.

13.4.2
Fed Batch Fermentation of Brown Juice with Lb. salivarius BC 1001

A 2-L continuously stirred tank reactor containing 1.5 L fresh (non-heat treated) brown juice (2% DM) was used for the fed-batch experiment. The bioreactor was equipped with a Mettler Toledo pH meter, heat sensor (pT100, MJK automation) and a heating element (50 W, 220 V), to keep pH and temperature constant. pH was controlled automatically by addition of 4 m NaOH by a peristaltic pump, the computer program used for control and regulation of pH and temperature was Genesis 4.2.

Growth of the strain was followed by measurement of the dry cell mass. This was achieved by centrifuging samples and washing twice with saline water (0.9%) before drying the samples in an oven at 190 °C overnight. During fermentation 2% glucose (40% solution) was added successively.

13.4.3
Pilot Scale Continuous Fermentation with Lb. salivarius BC 1001

The pilot scale experiment with continuous lactic acid fermentation of brown juice was performed at the green crop-drying factory – Dangrønt Products, Ringkøbing, Denmark. The brown juice produced from the pressing of the crops was cooled to 30 to 40 °C and fed into an 8 m³ tank and the tank was inoculated with 4 m³ bacterial culture (*Lb. salivarius* BC 1001). Fermentation was initiated as batch fermentation, and after the pH in the tank had dropped to approximately 4.5, substrate flow was started. The initial flow rate was 3.5 m³ h⁻¹. The acidified BJ was led to a sedimentation tank from where the supernatant was pumped to a storage/buffer tank before evaporation to approximately 40% DM.

13.4.4
Study of Potato Juice Quality During Aerobic and Anaerobic Storage

Experiments were performed to investigate the quality of potato juice stored under aerobic and anaerobic conditions. The investigations were carried out in plastic containers with a volume of 25 L. The containers were filled with 10 L fresh potato juice from the Karup, Denmark, potato starch factory. For anaerobic storage the surface was covered with 1 to 2 cm corn oil. Containers were kept at a temperature between 15 and 20 °C.

13.5
Brown Juice

13.5.1
Chemical Composition

The chemical composition of the green and brown juice was analyzed to investigate the suitability of the brown juice as fermentation medium. The average composition of evaporated fresh brown juice determined from 42 different batches collected from June 9th 1998 to November 11th 2000 is shown in Table 13.1.

Table 13.1 Average composition of evaporated fresh brown juice determined from 42 different batches of brown juice collected from June 9th 1998 to November 11th 2000, and the calculated composition of average fresh brown juice with a dry-matter content of 4%.

Component	Average evaporated fresh brown juice					Average fresh brown juice
	Content (g kg^{-1} DM)	Maximum	Minimum	St. dev. (%)	Content (g L^{-1})	Content (g L^{-1}) (Calculated)
DM (%)	32.4	52.6	14.7	28.0		4.0
Density (kg L^{-1})	1.2	1.3	1.1	4.0		
pH	5.2	5.9	3.9	9.0		
Sugar						
Glucose	75.7	149.7	27.7	34.4	28.3	3.5
Fructose	104.5	168.1	60.2	25.6	39.0	4.8
Sucrose	50.1	123.1	4.4	57.6	18.7	2.3
Free sugars	229.7	355.7	96.4	26.7	85.8	10.6
Fructan	92.2	224.7	6.8	58.5	34.4	4.3
1-Ketose	9.1	29.0	0.0	67.5	3.4	0.4
Total	325.7	573.4	169.1	31.6	121.7	15.0
Acids						
Citric acid	17.5	27.4	6.5	28.0	6.5	0.8
Malic acid	24.0	50.2	0.0	41.5	9.0	1.1
Malonic acid	13.1	24.8	0.0	40.3	4.9	0.6
Succinic acid	13.2	22.9	1.7	37.5	4.9	0.6
Lactic acid	33.1	103.6	0.0	65.8	12.4	1.5
Acetic acid	17.8	42.9	0.0	62.9	6.7	0.8
Total	118.8	271.8	65.1	48.9	44.4	5.5
Cations						
Calcium	10.6	17.2	5.4	29.6	4.0	0.5
Magnesium	5.2	8.3	3.0	25.5	1.9	0.2
Sodium	9.5	16.8	4.6	40.4	3.5	0.4
Potassium	73.5	112.5	27.3	35.4	27.4	3.4
Ammonium	5.9	17.9	1.4	54.6	2.2	0.3
Total	98.7	149.9	28.3	31.1	36.9	4.6
Anions						
Phosphate	29.4	39.4	17.7	18.1	11.0	1.4
Chloride	52.8	83.1	28.5	24.8	19.7	2.4
Nitrate	5.2	14.7	0.0	88.2	2.0	0.2
Total	83.1	115.2	49.7	19.8	31.1	3.8
Trace-minerals						
Cobber	0.013	0.020	0.000	33.2	0.005	0.001
Zinc	0.106	0.216	0.048	46.6	0.040	0.005
Manganese	0.077	0.156	0.017	42.3	0.029	0.004
Iron	0.392	1.023	0.126	47.4	0.146	0.018
Total	0.585	1.277	0.289	37.4	0.219	0.027

Table 13.1 (continued)

Component	Average evaporated fresh brown juice					Average fresh brown juice Content (g L⁻¹) (Calculated)
	Content (g kg⁻¹ DM)	Maximum	Minimum	St. dev. (%)	Content (g L⁻¹)	
Vitamins						
Pantothenic acid	0.060	0.101	0.035	27.139	0.023	0.003
Niacin	0.133	0.190	0.068	17.676	0.050	0.006
Thiamin	0.015	0.028	0.011	23.158	0.006	0.001
Total	0.209	0.276	0.154	14.865	0.078	0.010
Amino acids						
Lysine	5.0	7.2	3.2	17.5	1.9	0.2
Serine	6.3	12.1	4.2	25.8	2.4	0.3
Glutamine	17.2	27.2	2.9	24.8	6.4	0.8
Glycine	6.2	16.4	4.0	33.8	2.3	0.3
Alanine	13.1	21.8	8.3	20.5	4.9	0.6
Asparagine	20.9	51.7	10.3	42.1	7.8	1.0
Methionine	1.2	1.8	0.6	22.5	0.4	0.1
Cystine	1.3	1.9	0.8	24.0	0.5	0.1
Threonine	6.0	7.9	3.8	18.0	2.2	0.3
Valine	7.3	10.4	4.6	19.7	2.7	0.3
iso-Leucine	4.6	6.6	2.6	20.7	1.7	0.2
Leucine	7.0	9.6	4.2	20.7	2.6	0.3
Tyrosine	2.3	5.9	0.0	70.6	0.9	0.1
Phenylalanine	4.4	6.8	2.3	24.7	1.6	0.2
Histidine	2.9	5.0	0.5	28.1	1.1	0.1
Arginine	4.0	8.8	0.5	32.5	1.5	0.2
Total	124.0	19.1	167.5	20.7	46.3	5.7
Crude protein	203.0	279.1	133.2	18.3	75.9	9.4

Mono-, di-, and trisaccharides are called free carbohydrates because they can be metabolized by most lactic acid bacteria. Fructans (including 1-ketose) are polymeric carbohydrates consisting of variable numbers of fructose molecules and terminal sucrose. Fructans can be decomposed to free carbohydrates both by enzymes in the crops, fructan fructohydrolases, and by some strains of lactic acid bacteria, especially in the genera *Lactobacillus plantarum* and *Lactobacillus paracasei subspecies paracasei* [7]. The enzymes in the crops are activated after harvesting, carving, and pressing. Alfalfa does not contain fructans.

13.5.2
Seasonal Variations

Table 13.1 also shows the highest and the lowest value for a component found in the 42 different batches of brown juice and the standard deviation. For most compounds there are very high deviations between batches. The composition of

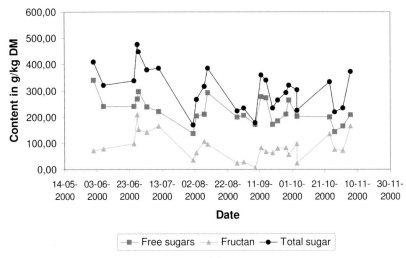

Fig. 13.2 Seasonal variation in free sugars and fructan in
different batches of brown juice harvested from June 1st to
November 6th 2000.

green crops is known to be influenced by many factors. These include climatic
influences such as light and night temperature, the fall of rain, management
practices, nitrogen application level, genotype, and relative proportions of leaf
and stem. The composition of the brown juice is further more influenced by
the type of crops harvested. Figure 13.2 shows the seasonal variation in free sugars and fructan in different batches of brown juice harvested from June 1st to
November 6th 2000.

The amount of free sugars in BJ has been found to vary between 135 and
340 g kg^{-1} DM and fructans between zero and 200 g kg^{-1} DM. The highest total
amount of carbohydrate was found at the beginning of the season in June and
lowest total amount of carbohydrate was found short periods in the beginning
of August and September when the fructan content, especially, drops dramatically. Because alfalfa contains no fructan and is harvested only in this period it
is likely that the drop is caused by a considerable increase in juice derived from
alfalfa in the mixed brown juice. A high content of organic acid in the BJ during this period indicates that some of the sugars are converted to organic acid
before pressing (Fig. 13.3).

Figures 13.4 and 13.5 shows the variation in minerals and amino acid/protein
in the brown juice.

The amounts of cations and anions in the brown juice seem to increase toward the end of the season whereas amounts of trace minerals are more stable.

The amount of amino acids and crude protein in the juice fluctuate throughout the harvesting season, but no great seasonal variations are found.

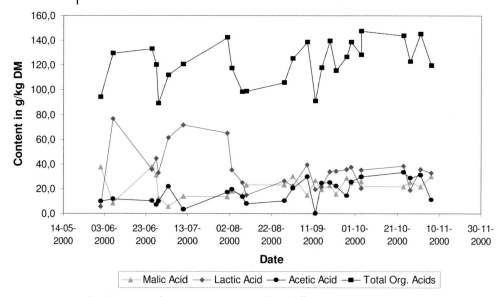

Fig. 13.3 Seasonal variation in organic acids in different
batches of brown juice harvested from June 1st to November
6th 2000.

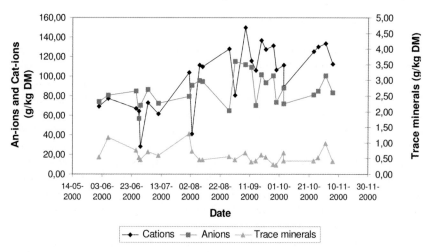

Fig. 13.4 Seasonal variation in minerals in different batches of
brown juice harvested from June 1st to November 6th 2000.

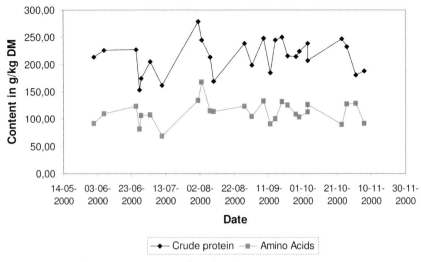

Fig. 13.5 Seasonal variation in amino acids and crude protein in different batches of brown juice harvested from June 1st to November 6th 2000.

13.5.3
Lactic Acid Fermentation of Brown Juice

Different lactic acid bacteria have been tested for their ability to utilize the most common carbohydrates. Several strains have been found suitable, but despite the fact that *Lactobacillus salivarius* is unable to metabolize fructan, it has been chosen for lactic acid fermentation of brown juice because of its high growth rate. This high growth rate makes *L. salivarius* BC 1001 robust and capable of competing with other microorganisms for an unsterile substrate [6]. By choosing a robust, fast-growing microorganism that can compete with unwanted microorganisms in the brown juice, sterilization of the substrate can be avoided. The brown juice contains both carbohydrates and amino acids, which in combination can form Maillard compounds during heat sterilization. This will cause a decrease in the nutrient-content and reduce the quality of the juice, because of the toxicity of some Maillard compounds.

Fermentation experiments with fresh non-heat-sterilized brown juice have shown that fructan is used in fermentations with *L. salivarius* even though this strain is unable to produce fructan-degrading enzymes. This is probably because of the activity of plant enzymes in the brown juice. Under monoseptic fermentation conditions fructan is not metabolized because enzymes in the juice are destroyed by heat sterilization [8].

Fed batch fermentation of fresh brown juice (2% DM) has shown that brown juice with only 2% DM contains enough nutrients in the substrate to achieve high lactic acid production. In this experiment the specific growth rate of *Lb.*

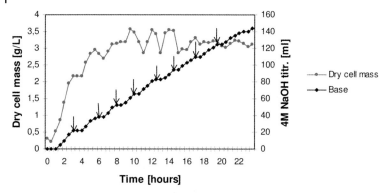

Fig. 13.6 Growth and titration curve for fed batch fermentation with *L. salivarius* BC 1001 in fresh non-heat-sterilized brown juice with 2% DM, to which glucose syrup, 40%, was added successively.

salivarius BC 1001 was 0.9 h^{-1} and a cell mass concentration of approximately 3 g L^{-1} was achieved (Fig. 13.6).

The composition of nutrients in the brown juice causes the growth of cell mass to stop at a certain concentration, whereupon the energy in the substrate is used exclusively for maintenance and production of lactic acid. This characteristic makes the brown juice suitable as a substrate for continuous lactic acid fermentation.

It has been shown that the growth rate of *L. salivarius* BC 1001 is higher in brown juice than in MRS-bouillon, which is a substrate commonly used for lactic acid fermentation [8].

13.5.4
The Green Crop-drying Industry as a Lactic Acid Producer

The green crop-drying industry in Denmark is located in Jutland. There are five factories with a total production of approximately 200 000 m³ green and brown juice 5% DM. It is shown in Fig. 13.6 that 2% DM is enough to achieve good conversion of carbohydrates to lactic acid. A single green crop-drying factory produces enough juice for lactic acid production of approximately 8000 tons per year if a carbohydrate source is added to achieve a lactic acid concentration of 8% in the fermentation broth.

Experiments with continuous lactic acid fermentation of brown juice have been performed at the green crop-drying factory: Dangrønt Products, Ringkøbing, Denmark. Figure 13.7 shows the process.

This pilot scale continuous lactic acid fermentation of brown juice was successful. The pH of brown juice was reduced to 4.7 and much of the sugar in the brown juice was converted to lactic acid. Table 13.2 shows the dry-matter content, density, and pH of the brown juice after the process. Table 13.3 shows results from analysis of the lactic acid fermented brown juice.

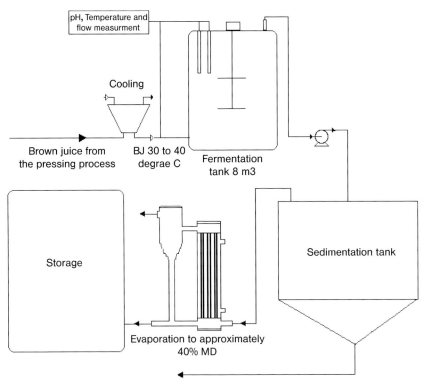

Fig. 13.7 The brown juice produced from the pressing of the crops was cooled to 35 °C±5 °C and fed into a 8 m³ tank. The tank was inoculated with 4 m³ bacterial culture (*Lb. salivarius* BC 1001). Fermentation was initiated as batch fermentation, and after pH in the tank had dropped to approxi- mately 4.5, substrate flow was started. The initial flow rate was 3.5 m³ h⁻¹. The acidified BJ was fed into a sedimentation tank, from where the supernatant was pumped to a storage/buffer tank before evaporation to approximately 40% DM.

Table 13.2 Dry matter, density, and pH of lactic acid ferment- ed and evaporated brown juice in pilot scale continuous fer- mentation at Dangrønt Products, Ringkøbing 16/10 2001.

Dry matter	Density (kg L^{-1})	pH
45.3	1.2	4.7

The analysis of the lactic acid fermented brown juice shows that efficient lac- tic acid fermentation has occurred. The amount of lactic acid produced is 280 g kg^{-1} DM, leaving only small amounts of sugar in the medium. The strain used for this fermentation (*Lb. salivarius* BC 1001) is a homofermentative strain, and only small amount of acetic acid and succinic acid is present in the fermen-

Table 13.3 Composition of lactic acid fermented and evaporated brown juice (45.3% DM) produced in pilot scale continuous fermentation at Dangrønt Products, Ringkøbing 16/10 2001.

Crude protein (g kg^{-1} DM)	Cations (g kg^{-1} DM)	Anions (g kg^{-1} DM)	Trace minerals (g kg^{-1} DM)	Free sugars (g kg^{-1} DM)	Fructan (g kg^{-1} DM)	Total sugars (g kg^{-1} DM)	Succinic-acid (g kg^{-1} DM)	Lactic-acid (g kg^{-1} DM)	Acetic-acid (g kg^{-1} DM)	Total org. acids (g kg^{-1} DM)	Amino acids (g kg^{-1} DM)
245.2	143.4	103.5	0.818	12.5	3.4	16.0	33.5	280.8	23.5	337.8	117.3

Crude protein (g L^{-1})	Cations (g L^{-1})	Anions (g L^{-1})	Trace minerals (g L^{-1})	Free sugars (g L^{-1})	Fructan (g L^{-1})	Total sugars (g L^{-1})	Succinic (g L^{-1})	Lactic (g L^{-1})	Acetic (g L^{-1})	Organic acids (g L^{-1})	Amino acids (g L^{-1})
132.0	77.2	55.7	0.440	6.8	1.8	8.6	18.0	151.2	12.7	181.9	63.2

tation product. Substantial amounts of nutrients (minerals and amino acids) remain in the brown juice after lactic acid fermentation, indicating that adding more carbohydrate could increase the yield of lactic acid. This would be necessary in the production of PLA to make the process feasible. This will be discussed in Section 13.7.

13.6
Potato Juice

13.6.1
Potato Juice as Fermentation Medium

At potato starch factories the potatoes are sorted, washed, and grated. After grating, the potato pulp is centrifuged and the starch, pulp, and potato juice are separated. Two waste products are produced: potato pulp and potato juice. The pulp is sold for animal feed and the juice is spread on fields as fertilizer. The potato starch industry thus faces the same problem as the green crop-drying industry – a waste product that must be stored in large lagoons from October 1st or be used for other purposes.

Experiments have been performed to investigate the quality of potato juice with regard to pH, lactic acid, and acetic acid formation, when stored under aerobic and anaerobic conditions. Figures 13.8 and 13.9 show the results of these experiments.

The figures show that aerobic and anaerobic storage of the juice causes a conspicuous drop in the pH of the juice within the first 7 days. This is because of lactic acid and acetic acid fermentation of the carbohydrates and some organic

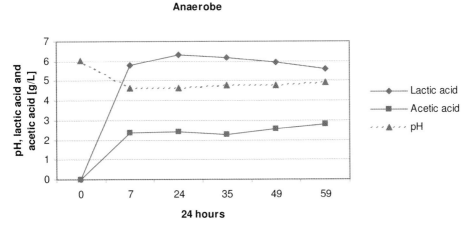

Fig. 13.8 pH, lactic acid and acetic acid during aerobic storage of potato juice at a temperature between 15 and 20 °C.

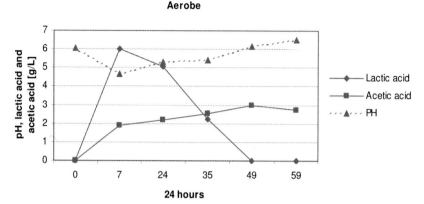

Aerobe

Fig. 13.9 pH, lactic acid and acetic acid during anaerobic storage of potato juice at a temperature between 15 and 20 °C.

acids in the potato juice by naturally occurring microorganisms in the juice. Further storage of the juice induces the pH level in the aerobic container to increase to over 6 whereas the pH in the anaerobic container remains stable at approximately 4.5. Accompanying this, a drop in lactic acid concentration and an increase in acetic acid concentration can be observed.

At Karup potato starch factory the potato juice is fermented by adding lactic acid bacteria and molasses to achieve a pH of approximately 4.5. Continuous fermentation is performed in a 6000 m³ tank before it is led to big lagoons (140 000 m³) where it is stored. During storage of the potato juice in the big lagoons it can be difficult to maintain a low pH for a long time, primarily because of access to air. A rise in pH provides good growth conditions for bacteria other than lactic acid bacteria, resulting in obnoxious smells. The results in Figs. 13.8 and 13.9 show that prevention of access to air by (anaerobically) covering of the lagoons could be a way of maintaining the quality of the potato juice and thus prevent obnoxious smells.

13.6.2
The Potato Starch Industry as Lactic Acid Producer

There are four potato starch factories in Denmark situated in Northern Jutland, Karup, Brande, and Toftlund, manufacturing a total of approximately 1 million tons of potatoes each year. This gives a total of approximately 200 000 tons of potato starch, 150 000 tons of potato pulp (12 to 13% DM) and between 1 and 1.5 million tons of potato juice (2 to 4% DM) depending on the production methods. At the factory in Karup 300 000 tons of potato juice (2% DM) are produced each year. On that basis Karup potato starch factory could produce approximately 35 000 tons of lactic acid a year if a sufficient amount of carbohydrate is added to the juice.

13.7
Carbohydrate Source

To profitably utilize brown juice from the green crop-drying industry or potato juice from the potato starch industry, a carbohydrate source must be added. The carbohydrate source could be another waste product from the agricultural industry such as molasses from beet sugar production, whey from the dairy industry, or soy meal extract from the production of soy protein. It could also be refined sugar (white sugar), hydrolyzed straw, or hydrolyzed cereal grains, e.g. wheat.

Wheat has advantages over other carbohydrate sources. Cereals, being much lower in moisture than molasses, are more energy intensive and have the advantage that they can be stored and transported easily. The sugar is in the form of starch and in addition cereal grains contain nutrients which can be separated easily from the grain and sold as lucrative by-products – bran, gluten, and A-

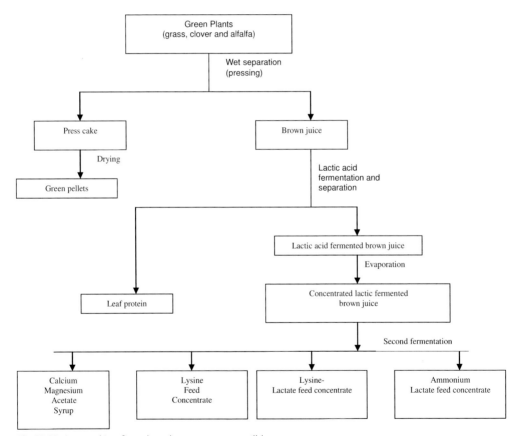

Fig. 13.10 A green biorefinery based on green crops will be able to produce products based on organic acids and amino acids made by fermentation [4].

starch. Gluten – a protein used in the baking industry – is the most profitable of these by-products.

Webb and Wang describe a process for utilization of wheat as a carbohydrate source for lactic acid fermentation in which gluten is separated from the grain before hydrolysis of the starch. The filamentous fungus *Aspergillus awamori* is capable of producing enzymes to break down the starch to glucose [9].

As shown in Fig. 13.10, there are many possibilities of producing fermentation products on the basis of on green crops and potatoes and thereby changing the green crop-drying factories and potato starch factories to green biorefineries.

13.8
Purification of Lactic Acid

The lactic acid must be recovered and purified from the fermentation broth. The classical method is the calcium lactate process in which the lactic acid is precipitated as calcium lactate and treated with sulfuric acid. The resulting calcium sulfate is separated from the lactic acid solution by filtration and the liquid is evaporated. The process gives residual amounts of gypsum, and waste gypsum disposal can be a problem.

The latest developments in lactic acid purification have been towards membrane processes such as ultrafiltration and electrodialysis. Other methods such as ion-exchange and solvent extraction involve heavy initial costs and operating costs; they are, therefore, not very suitable for low-cost production of lactic acid.

Electrodialysis is a membrane process in which the membranes allow passage only of either anions or cations (ion-exchange membranes), the driving force being potential difference. Because the membranes are easily fouled if the fermentation broth contains large impurities and particles, these are removed by ultrafiltration before electrodialysis. Problems with membrane processes arise if the fermentation broth contains large amounts of organic particles and inorganic ions such as calcium and magnesium, which damage the membrane.

Birgit and Michael Kamm use ultrafiltration, nanofiltration, and electrodialysis for purification of lactic acid from fermentation broth. They have developed a process whereby lactic acid is neutralized with piperazine, an amine that combined with two molecules of lactic acid makes piperazinium dilactate. The piperazinium dilactate can be converted to dilactid (a building block in the production of polylactate) without the production of undesired by-products. Birgit and Michael Kamm did not experience problems with fouling of the ultrafiltration membrane but some optimization of the nanofiltration and electrodialysis processes is still needed [10].

At the Technical University of Denmark a process has been developed in which the lactic acid is continuously removed and purified from the fermentation broth using various membrane processes (Donnan dialysis, electrodialysis with bi-polar membranes, and electrodialysis). In this process problems with fouling of the membranes are minimized or avoided [11].

13.9
Conclusion and Outlook

Waste products from the green crop-drying industry and the potato starch industry, brown juice and potato juice, contain all the nutrients necessary for lactic acid bacteria to convert carbohydrates to lactic acid. Brown juice 2% DM in a substrate contains enough nutrients to achieve good lactic acid production in continuous fermentation by addition of a carbohydrate source.

It is possible to use other cheap waste products from the agricultural industry, for example molasses or hydrolyzed straw, or purer products such as refined sugar or hydrolyzed starch, as a carbohydrate source. Hydrolyzed B-starch from wheat has several advantages compared with other carbohydrate sources. The most important is that the grain contains nutrients, for example bran, gluten and A-starch, which can be separated easily from the grain and sold as lucrative by-products.

At the Technical University of Denmark a very promising process has been developed for purification of lactic acid produced from agricultural waste products. This process can substantially reduce the cost of lactic acid production.

The experiments reported in this article show it is possible to produce lactic acid from brown juice or potato juice on an industrial scale using non-sterile brown juice or potato juice for fermentation. The fermented juice can be stored under anaerobic conditions and used as a substrate for all-year round production of lactic acid, lysine, and many other fermentation products.

Acknowledgments

This work was supported by the Danish Ministry of Food, Agriculture and Fisheries under the program "Increased Utilization of Renewable Resources for Industrial Non-food Purposes" (1997–2001). We thank Vagn Hundelbøll, Agro-Ferm A/S, and Jens Mikkelsen, the potato starch factory in Karup for the interesting co-operation.

References

1 Shogren, R., **1997**, Water Vapour Permeability of Biodegradable Polymers, *J. Environ. Polym. Degrad.* 5(2).

2 Weber, C.J., *Biobased Packaging Materials for the Food Industry Status and Perspectives – A European Concerted Action*, KVL Department of Dairy and Food Science, Frederiksberg, Denmark. Trio Design, Copenhagen

3 Petersen, K. et al., **1999**, Potential of Bio-based Materials for Food Packaging, *Trends Food Sci. Tech.* 10, 52–68.

4 Andersen, M., Kiel, P., **1999**, *Method for Treating Organic Waste Materials*, European Patent Application, 19 March 1999, WO 00156912.

5 The Danish Ministry of Environment and Energy's order no. 823 of 16 Sep-

tember 1996. Order of the use of waste products for agricultural purpose.

6 Thomsen, M. H., Bech, D., Kiel, P., **2004**, Manufacturing of Stabilized Brown Juice for L-lysine production – from University Lab Scale over Pilot Scale to Industrial Production. *Chem. Biochem. Eng. Q.* 18, 37–46.

7 Müller, M., Steller, J., **1995**, Comparative Studies of the Degradation of Grass Fructans and Inulin by Strains of *Lactobacillus paracasei* subsp. *paracasei* and *Lactobacillus plantarum. J. Appl. Bacteriol.* 78, 229–236.

8 Andersen, M., Kiel, P., **2000**, Integrated Utilisation of Green Biomass in the Green Biorefinery, *Ind. Crops Prod.* 11, 129–137.

9 Webb, C., Wang, R., **1997**, Development of a Generic Fermentation Feedstock from Whole Wheat Flour. In: Campel, G. M., Webb, C., McKee, S. L. (Eds) *Cereals: Novel Uses and Processes*, Plenum Press, New York, pp. 205–218.

10 Kamm, B., Kamm, M., Richter, K., Reimann, W., Siebert, A., **2000**, Formation of Aminium Lactates in Lactic Acid Fermentation. *Acta Biotechnol.* 20(3/4), 289–304.

11 Garde, A., Rype, J. U., Jonsson, G., **2000**, *A Method and Apparatus for Isolation of Ionic Species from a Liquid*. Not yet published patent. Application no. PA 2000 01862.

Part III
Biomass Production and Primary Biorefineries

Biorefineries – Industrial Processes and Products. Status Quo and Future Directions. Vol. 1
Edited by Birgit Kamm, Patrick R. Gruber, Michael Kamm
Copyright © 2006 WILEY-VCH Verlag GmbH & Co. KGaA, Weinheim
ISBN: 3-527-31027-4

14
Biomass Commercialization and Agriculture Residue Collection

James Hettenhaus

14.1
Introduction

In the next ten year biorefineries may be processing 100 million metric dry tons (dt) biomass annually for production of fuels and chemicals if a stretch goal set by the US Department of Energy is met [1–3]. Initially, feedstocks with no collection cost like paper mill sludge, bagasse, and rice hulls may be used to validate the conversion technology. They have no associated transport cost. Their quantities may also serve niche markets for high-value chemicals [4]. For larger markets like transportation fuels, their conversion is too small and costly to compete. The biorefining industry's growth is predicated mostly on corn stover, supplemented with straw and grasses with a delivered price of $30 to $35 dt^{-1} [5, 6]. The quantity and ready availability makes stover an early feedstock choice for initial biorefineries (Table 14.1), US Ag residue feedstock availability.

When the feedstock market is established with stover, other biomass feedstock, prairie grasses and energy crops, from wide geographic areas will emerge to supply biorefineries.

While great strides have been made in improving the conversion process, there remains much uncertainty regarding the feedstock supply. Economies of scale require a biorefinery size of 500 to 2000 dt feedstock per day. Supplying these large quantities raises major issues including:

Table 14.1 US Ag residue feedstock availability, metric dry tons (millions).

Corn stover	200
Cereal straw	70
Energy crops	74
Bagasse	6
Corn fiber	4
Rice hulls	1
Total dry tons	355

Biorefineries – Industrial Processes and Products. Status Quo and Future Directions. Vol. 1
Edited by Birgit Kamm, Patrick R. Gruber, Michael Kamm
Copyright © 2006 WILEY-VCH Verlag GmbH & Co. KGaA, Weinheim
ISBN: 3-527-31027-4

- agronomic systems for sustainable removal – maintaining soil quality;
- economic and environmental benefits for the farmer and other stakeholders;
- methods for improved feedstock collection, storage and transport; and
- infrastructure required for reliable feedstock supply.

More information is needed for the farmer to assess the opportunity for supplying the emerging biorefinery market for biomass feedstock. What is the value of the biomass to the soil and to the farmer? What cropping practice is needed for sustainable removal, balancing environmental and economic requirements? Previous studies of crop residue removal on soil quality are limited to small research plots that often do not align with current best practice. Although existing models provide guidelines for residue management to limit soil erosion, robust models that address soil quality and residue removal are just emerging.

Bulky crop residues are collected to meet small needs, mostly for local farm use–bales for animal bedding. There is negligible collection infrastructure to serve large markets like biorefineries. Sizable investment – $50 to $100 million – is probably needed in the supply systems for biomass harvesting, collection, storage and transport to supply a 1 million dt year^{-1} to a biorefinery [1]. Who will make these investments – the farmer, the potential processor, or a biomass supplier that aggregates individual growers? Current supply systems for grain like corn and wheat are highly evolved and efficient infrastructures and may provide valuable extensions. Existing grain elevators may serve as collection points for biomass.

Local conditions determine the potential feedstock quantities. Areas capable of providing large supplies have been identified – but like commercializing an idea, much work remains between *knowing* the location of promising biorefinery sites and reliably *supplying* them with economic, sustainable feedstock.

14.2
Historical Outline

Commercial ventures that require large quantities of crop residues have a mixed history of success. Collected material has found more use as co-products than those that remain in the field after harvest. For example, corn fiber is mixed with steepwater and sold as corn gluten feed with a nutrient value 1.1 times cracked corn for ruminant animals [8]. Bagasse has a long history and is discussed in Case Study 2.2. Small quantities like rice hulls offer little economic incentive to develop markets, therefore most remains to be disposed of, often by burning as a fuel or simply land applied [9].

For biomass left in the field – stover, straw and grasses – collection and transportation cost increases the economic hurdle. In areas of the world lacking trees, non wood fiber is pulped, producing quality papers [10]. They make a relatively poor animal feed because of low protein content [8] and their use as a fuel is limited by their composition, especially the low thermal content compared with coal and natural gas.

During the last decade the list of unsuccessful ventures using bagasse, grass, straw, and stover for particle board has grown by more than a dozen [11, 12]. This mixed record hinders enthusiasm among many growers and others to consider feedstock collection as a viable route for biomass commercialization.

14.2.1
Case Study: Harlan, Iowa Corn Stover Collection Project

The largest recent corn stover collection project was undertaken in Harlan, Iowa in 1996 by Great Lakes Chemical. Modern collection methods – self loading and unloading wagons and high speed, over the road tractors – were used to reduce feedstock cost for the production of furfural [13, 14]. The stover revenue to the farmer was $3 to $12 dt^{-1}, depending on the hauling distance (Table 14.2).

Total feedstock requirements were approximately 100000 dt per year. A collection center for approximately 50% of the total was constructed in Harlan, Iowa, USA, in 1996. The facility sampled and weighed all deliveries, then stacked bales for storage. During the year bales were removed from storage, milled, pelletized, and loaded into trailers and trucked 90 km to the furfural plant.

The first year was a learning experience for all. Meetings with local producers were held, and many showed interest in collecting stover for added income, and as a way to remove most of it so the soil would warm in the spring for seed germination without having to plow. The amount collected complied with soil erosion guidelines. But at the conclusion little stover was delivered. Great Lakes had left the collection with the farmers who mostly used their resources for harvesting the corn grain, not baling.

The second year Great Lakes employed contract balers and haulers, matching them up with the farmers and the result was an overwhelming collection success. More than 400 farmers committed 20000 ha of their corn fields. Thirty plus custom harvesters were contracted to perform the baling.

Self loading and unloading wagons pulled by high speed tractors were used for bale transport (Fig. 14.1). The bales were collected in the field – 17 round bales, approximately 9.5 dt – in less than 20 min. The wagon traveled at highway speeds, up to 90 km h^{-1}, en route to the collection center. At the collection center the load was weighed, sampled for moisture, and unloaded. In less than 10 min the driver was on the way to the next field.

Table 14.2 Corn stover pricing summary.

Revenue payments, dollars per dry ton (mkg)				
Radius, km	0–25	26–49	50–80	81–164
Producers revenue	$12.00	$9.05	$6.12	$3.19
Baler's revenue	$16.06	$16.06	$16.06	$16.06
Hauler's revenue	$6.71	$9.65	$12.58	$15.51
Total, delivered price	$34.76	$34.76	$34.76	$34.76

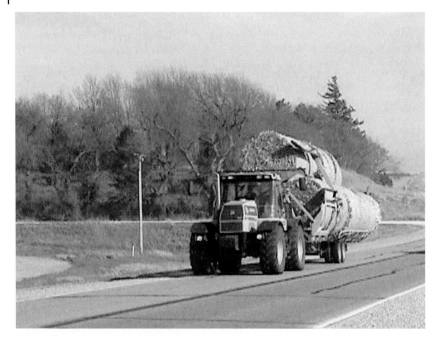

Fig. 14.1 Load-and-go wagon with high-speed tractor.

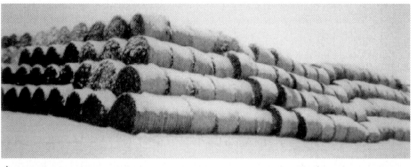

a)

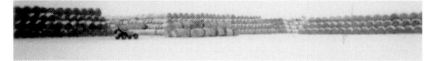

b)

Fig. 14. 2 Corn stover bale storage.

Start-up problems were mostly baler-related: working to achieve a dense bale, with a minimum 550 kg dry weight. Bales are often sold as a unit, not on a dry weight process. Low bale density made transporting a losing proposition. These difficulties were worked out and several weeks of productive baling occurred before the first blizzard on October 27. Afterward, the field conditions were too wet for baling. Approximately 12 000 ha were actually collected, because of the wet, unusually warm winter. The season ended with a waiting list of more than 40,000 ha, more than enough cropland to meet the total plant requirements IF weather permitted.

Meanwhile, the price of imported furfural dropped below the plant manufacturing cost, and the operation was bought out by another firm to make hydromulch. Economic, process, and product-quality problems slowed sales. Finally a bale fire destroyed most of their inventory, forcing a liquidation of their assets in 2002.

The major findings from the collection operation include the following [15]:
- Farmers are willing to sell excess stover when the economics fit.
- Collection practices have to meet farmers' requirements for success.
- Logistics are a major factor for successful collection.
- Contract operators are essential to meet the extra workload.
- Shortening the harvest window is essential to reduce collection risk due to weather.
- Bale storage is costly and adds no value.
- One-pass harvest, with the grain, can reduce cost and harvest risk.
- Bale fires are a serious hazard.

14.2.2
Case Study: Bagasse Storage – Dry or Wet?

Bagasse, the biomass remaining from sugar cane after the sucrose-containing juice has been extracted, has been used by the pulp and paper industry for more than a century [10]. It incurs no collection cost and competes favorably with wood pulp in a global market. The bagasse exits the mill with about 50% moisture. For stable storage it must be below 20% or above 60%.

In the early 1920s the sugar cane industry investigated ways to store bagasse for processing to particleboard and pulp. Particleboard processors preferred dry material. Pulp mills readily accepted wet material.

14.2.2.1 Dry Storage
Celotex produced insulation board, a dry process, and pursued ways to improve dry feedstock storage. Their effort resulted in using the heat from microbial fermentation to dry bales from 50% to less than 20% moisture [16]. The bales were sized and stacked to dissipate heat and acid fumes. Sheltered from the weather, bales kept for several years without serious deterioration (Figs. 14.3 and 14.4).

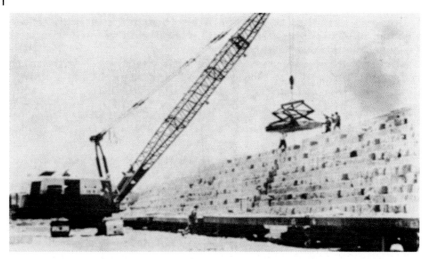

Fig. 14.3 Bale stacking, circa 1930.

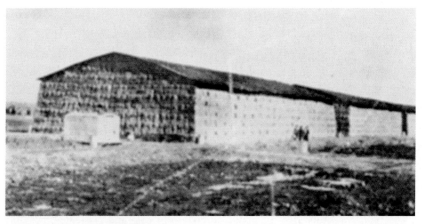

Fig. 14.4 Bale storage, 1930–1960.

Although this dry storage method was used for more than 40 years [17], a change to wet storage occurred in the 1960s because of increasing recognition of its advantages:
- The bales were relatively small, weighing 115 kg "as is".
- Mechanical handling was slow and costly.
- The bales had to be precisely stacked to vent fumes and dissipate heat.
- Procedures were labor-intensive.
- Several months were required to dry bales from 50 to 20% moisture.
- Fire loss and increasing fire insurance costs.

14.2.2.2 **Wet Storage**

Whereas Celotex pursued dry storage, other companies in the pulp and paper industry continued investigating wet storage, because pulping is a wet process. The results were more successful than dry storage. Wet storage of non-wood fibers was first commercialized by E. A. Ritter in 1950. Wet storage of bagasse has been in widespread use on a commercial scale since 1960 for both wet and dry downstream processes [18].

Figure 14.5 shows a typical collection area with a pile under construction in the foreground. Major studies on a commercial scale showed pulping the stored bagasse was superior to pulping dry bagasse and fresh, wet bagasse. The wet feedstock contained less solubles, required less chemical treatment, produced higher yields and had better processing characteristics compared with dry feedstock and fresh, wet bagasse [19]. In addition, wet feedstock stored for 6 months was superior to "green" bagasse, the fresh material from the current harvest in processing characteristics, with 80% less solubles and higher holocellulose composition. As a result, green bagasse is held over, for processing the following year [20]. Section 14.5.2 discusses storage further.

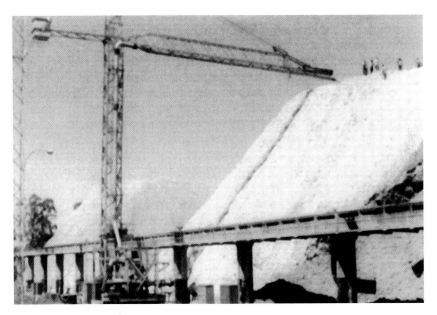

Fig. 14.5 Wet storage pile construction.

14.3
Biomass Value

Lacking large uses of crop residues, studies have not addressed the impact of removal of stover [21] and straw [22] on soil quality, although several implications can be drawn [23]. An environmental and economic balance is required for sufficient retention of residues to avoid erosion losses and maintain soil quality, while economically removing excess residue as biomass feedstocks. The impact of different levels of surface removal depends on local conditions and practices. Maintaining this balance is key for success.

14.3.1
Soil Quality

Agricultural residues provide a key role in maintaining soil quality. Surface cover is needed to prevent wind and water erosion, retain soil moisture, recycle nutrients from the plant back to the soil, and support assorted life. When residue is removed, reduced inputs from the residue to the soil can result in a negative flux from the soil and a loss of soil organic matter, SOM, and other nutrients leading to a breakdown of soil structure.

The amount of excess is a complex question. It depends on local factors like soil type, cropping practice, weather, and topography. For example, in some dry areas surface cover is required to retain moisture, mostly in western areas of the grain belt [24]. Further east, surface cover is given as a major reason for tilling, because the cover prevents the cold, wet soils from warming in the spring, delaying planting and reducing yield [25]. Recycling nutrients from the plant, especially P and K, back to the soil reduces the need for replacement. Conversely, in areas where manure is used, the P contained in the soil may already be too high, resulting in excessive run-off that contributes to algae formation in ponds and streams [26]. Surface cover provides shelter and food for many organisms – microbial and larger. Their contribution to the humic pool is important, but they also shelter destructive weed seeds, pests, and toxins that can harm the next crop [27].

Models are under development to better measure soil quality. For example, agricultural ecosystem models like Century, DayCent, and Cstore show some beneficial effects of removing residue while still meeting constraints of soil and wind erosion. Namely, nitrate leaching decreases tenfold in some situations and nitrous oxide emissions (a potent greenhouse gas) are also significantly reduced. These models can be used with actual field measurements for guidance in selecting among alternatives that best balance economic and environmental benefits [28]. Using field measurements with the soil conditioning index will show if the crop practice is correctly managing soil carbon and is recommended [29].

14.3.2
Farmer Value

Most farmers are forced to manage crop residues in place. Present markets are negligible for straw and corn stover. Less than 5% is used for animal bedding and feed, with the major portion used on the site and then recycled as soiled bedding or manure. Some growers have historically rented harvested corn fields for grazing, charging $12 to $25 ha^{-1}. This practice is declining as combines have become more efficient, lodging is less with Bt corn, and cattle ranching has grown more "factory-like" with heavy dependence on large feedlots.

If residue were removed, the phosphorus (P) and potassium (K) content in straw and stover will eventually need to be replaced. The composition is typically 0.1% P and 1% K, valued at $3.50 dt^{-1} [6]. The N fertilizer value is more complex, and depends on crop rotation and local conditions. Reduced field operations are estimated to reduce inputs $24 ha^{-1} for preparation of the seed bed [30].

Carbon credits are likely to add additional economic incentive for US farmers. Reducing tillage or no-till sequesters about 0.3 to 0.5 metric tons C equiv ha^{-1}. The increased soil carbon improves yields, and this benefit continues with each crop year. Eventually, over decades, soil carbon equilibrium is achieved. In the European Union, carbon is currently trading for about $35 per ton C equiv. A small, voluntary greenhouse gas trading market has been established for agricultural carbon sequestration as part of the Chicago Board of Trade, the Chicago Climate Exchange [31]. Recent efforts to move US policy in this direction call for a $26 per ton of C-equivalent credit that would fund renewable fuels research and development [32].

Reducing N fertilizer use is also possible, depending on crop rotation. Microbes desire a 10:1 ratio of C/N for breaking down residue. Because the C/N ratio of straw and stover is 40 to 70:1, 10 kg N fertilizer addition per ton of residue is typically recommended to avoid denitrification of the next crop. For 250 ha of 9 dt ha^{-1} corn (170 bu acre^{-1}), 30 to 40 tons of N fertilizer may be avoided. In addition to the out-of-pocket costs, environmental benefits include reducing N run-off to streams and groundwater, and reducing greenhouse gas – 0.17 to 3.5 tons of N_2O/100 tonnes applied – 5 to 100 tonnes C equiv ha^{-1} [33].

The economic benefit from selling stover to the farmer is summarized for three production yields – 6.9 dt ha^{-1}, 9.9 dt ha^{-1}, and 10.6 dt ha^{-1} (130, 170, and 200 bu acre^{-1}) in Table 14.3. More details are presented in Section 14.5. The example uses the following values:
- delivered sale price is $33 dt^{-1}
- moisture is 15% to adjust to dry basis
- harvest index of 0.5, a 1:1 ratio of grain to stover
- surface cover of 2.2 dt ha^{-1} left in the field,
- P and K fertilizer value of $3.50 dt^{-1} removed with the stover
- reduced field operations, $24 ha^{-1}
- no credit for carbon sequestration or other inputs like N fertilizer.

Table 14.3 Stover field value before transportation and collection cost, $ ha^{-1}.

Production case	1	2	3
Stover production, dt ha^{-1}, 1:1 ratio	6.9	9.1	10.7
Surface cover, 2.2 dt ha^{-1}, left in field	(2.2)	(2.2)	(2.2)
Stover sales, dt ha^{-1}	4.7	6.9	8.5
Stover revenue, $33 dt^{-1}	$155	$225	$278
P & K nutrient credit ($3.50 dt^{-1})	(16)	(24)	(29)
Reduced field operations, $24 ha^{-1}	24	24	24
Net value, bulk in field, $ ha^{-1}	$163	$226	$273

The net value in the field is $163 to $273 ha^{-1} before collection and transportation cost.

The net margin after Collection and transportation costs are determined is given for two examples – typical baled stover collection (Table 14.4), and one-pass collection (Table 14.5). Other costs like shrinkage or change in properties of the feedstock in storage, storage investment, and operation, and relative quality of final feedstock processed are not included in the examples. There is a large variation in these factors depending on the local situation.

Baled stover, Table 14.4, is trucked within a 50 km radius – an average 70 km round trip using high speed tractors and "load and go wagons" as in Harlan, IA. Baling and transport cost adds $25 dt^{-1}, leaving the farmer a net margin of $41 to $54 ha^{-1}. A minimum $50 ha^{-1} return is most often cited to raise grower interest [34, 35].

Table 14.4 Stover sale net to farmer, $ ha^{-1} W/custom bale and 50 km radius collection site.

Case	3.1	3.2	3.3
Net margin, bulk in field, $ ha^{-1}	$163	$226	$273
Less custom bale, $16.00 dt^{-1}	(75)	(109)	(135)
Hauling, 50 km radius, $9.9 dt^{-1}	(47)	(68)	(83)
Net margin to farmer after delivery, $ ha^{-1}	$41	$49	$54

Table 14.5 Sale net to farmer, $ ha^{-1}, W/one-pass harvest and 3–25 km radius collection sites.

Case	3.1	3.2	3.3
Net margin, bulk in field, $ ha^{-1}	$163	$226	$273
Less one-pass harvest, $40 ha^{-1}	(40)	(40)	(40)
Field to collection site, $6.00 dt^{-1}	(28)	(41)	(51)
Hauling, 50 km radius, $9.9 dt^{-1}	(35)	(51)	(63)
Net margin to farmer after delivery, $ ha^{-1}	$59	$93	$119

One pass collection of grain and stover, with stover trucked from field to one of three collection centers within a 25 km radius – 35 km average round trip, stored above 60% moisture, then transported via rail to the biorefinery – offers more opportunity to reduce cost and reduce harvest risk [36]. Even with higher transport cost, $13.50 vs $9.90 dt^{-1}, the farmer's net margin after delivery ranges from $59 to $119 ha^{-1} (Table 14.5). The difference is greatest for fields with high yields, with nearly twice the margin compared with baling.

One-pass harvest prototypes are under development, and further discussed in Section 14.5.

14.3.3
Processor Value

Carbohydrate feedstock is being seriously considered as an alternative to petroleum and natural gas feedstocks by the chemical and plastic materials industry. The escalating cost of fossil feedstocks and their pricing instability have contributed significantly to the industries low margins. Added environmental concerns, especially emissions that contribute to global warming have generally shrunk their market value.

Low cost fermentation sugars coupled with rapid advances in biotech tools offers these industries a potentially economic and sustainable feedstock for production of transportation fuels, chemicals, and materials. For example, E85 fuel, 85% ethanol in gasoline, reduces greenhouse gases by 64% compared with gasoline. The effective benefit is 170 kg C equiv mitigated per dt corn stover processed compared with regular gasoline [37].

Sourcing low-cost feedstock is a common critical success factor. Successful crop residue-processing plants wish to achieve an economy of scale well below the local feedstock supply limits to accommodate expansion. Most biorefineries plan to have a business model that offers the grower an option to participate in the value chain to help ensure a win–win business relationship. An example is corn growers who are also shareholders in dry mill plants now growing hybrids with traits that produce more liters of ethanol kg^{-1} corn. They have no grain yield drag and processing this corn adds value to their stake in the dry mill [35].

Sustainable supply is of prime importance to the processors. Environmental concerns are a major driver for the industry to move from fossil feedstocks. Assurances will be needed that the long-term effect on the soil quality is neutral or better to avoid the claim that removal of residues is depleting the soil of needed nutrients [35].

Feedstock pricing has a major effect. The National Renewable and Energy Laboratory uses $33 dt^{-1} delivered cost to the biorefinery in the base case of their process. The result is based on extensive experimentation, process modeling and industry peer reviews. A $5 dt^{-1} change in feedstock price affects ethanol 1¢ to 1.5¢ L^{-1}, depending on process yield [7].

Wet or dry feedstock can be processed, but if dry, some prefer bulk delivery of milled product to avoid the multi-million dollar investment in equipment and dust-explosion-proof installation [38].

Clean feedstock with consistent composition and properties are desired, but more information remains to be provided by the processors. Because dirt, inorganics and ash add to the processing cost, and higher cellulose and hemicellulose content can increase yields, feedstock pricing based on composition and ease of processing is expected to emerge, not paying just per dry ton. Rapid analytical methods for compositional analysis are under development and are expected to be validated and available for incorporating in a feedstock payment program [39].

14.4
Sustainable Removal

Removing residues from the soil depletes the amount available for replenishment for nutrients and increases the possibility of erosion. Compensating for this will probably require revising some present agronomic practices. For example, leaving anchored stubble, 20 cm or more above the crown may suffice in some areas to control erosion, especially with narrow planting rows, e.g. 40 cm compared with 80 cm, the most prevalent practice for corn rows. This and other contemplated needs are discussed in this section.

With a biorefinery, the excess is removed, processed into fuels – and "digested" by the autos – the CO_2 exits from the auto's exhaust, instead of being exuded from microbes in the field. The benefits are huge, BUT only when this is conducted in a sustainable manner by controlling erosion and maintaining soil quality, especially soil organic material (SOM).

14.4.1
Soil Organic Material

Tilling causes loss of SOM, an important measure of soil quality. If too much stover is removed or a cover crop is not planted that adds to the biomass, SOM can be depleted. SOM is more strongly affected by below-ground residues (i.e. roots), with above-ground residue contributing less to SOM formation. Studies at the National Soil Tilth Laboratory shows 80% or more of the surface material is lost as CO_2 within months, and three times the amount of SOM comes from roots compared with surface material [40].

The tillage effect on soil carbon loss after corn harvest is shown for various field operations in Fig. 14.6 [41].

The CO_2 flux emitted from the soil is shown for various cases over time. The amount of loss depends on the amount of disturbance – more exposure, more oxidation of the organic material and more lost soil carbon. The bottom line in the figure shows normal soil respiration as microbes and other organisms in the soil and on the soil surface emit CO_2 as they digest biomass carbohydrates and lignin. The top line shows the highest loss when plowing the soil – an initial burst of CO_2 occurs as the plow rips open the soil and the anaerobic soil environment is exposed to oxygen in the air.

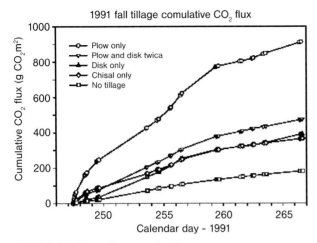

Fig. 14.6 Fall tillage effect on soil carbon.

No-till or reduced-till practices are needed to maintain soil organic material when stover is removed – if not, the carbon loss from tillage will deplete the soils' carbon pool, resulting in negative effects on soil quality, including aggregate instability, less water-holding capacity, and an associated drop in productivity.

14.4.2
Soil Erosion Control

Loss of topsoil remains a concern and continues to be a severe problem in many areas. Not only does much soil get lost in waterways, erosion also depletes soil fertility. The SOM is greatest in the topsoil, and up to 20% of the SOM is estimated to eventually be lost to the atmosphere as a result of cropping practices [42].

For adequate feedstock supply and efficient collection less tillage will be required to control erosion in addition to maintaining SOM. With present tillage practices all of the residue must remain in 60% the corn fields and 70% of the wheat fields to comply with USDA erosion control guidelines. The USDA guidelines are based on extensive studies that indicate all the residue should remain in fields with conventional till, i.e. less than 30% of the surface is covered. The guidelines are based on "tolerable" soil loss, a judgmental value [21].

Less tillage, referred to as mulch till, has more than 30% of the surface covered, allows some residue removal while no-till or ridge till permits most of the surface material to be removed. Ridge-till or strip till, involves tilling a strip through the field, clearing away the residue in a space adequate for planting and warming the soil in the seed area for early germination. The ridge is favored with furrow irrigation. Without the ridge, it is referred to as strip till.

For example, using the USDA water-erosion model, revised universal loss equation (RUSLE), and wind erosion equation (WEQ), the variation in required erosion cover for selected counties in the top corn-producing states – Illinois, Iowa, and Nebraska – are shown in Table 14.6. Wheat is included, because irrigated wheat yields enough to warrant straw collection in Peoria County, IL, Jasper County, IA, and Rock County, NE [43]. Unless wheat is irrigated, much of the wheat yield on dry land is below 2.2 dt ha^{-1}, negating any straw removal. Even with no till, economic quantities are difficult unless yields approach corn, 8 to 10 dt ha^{-1}.

The historic tillage practices for corn and wheat for the US are summarized in Tables 14.7 and 14.8. The values are based on a nationwide survey conducted by the Conservation Technology Information Center (CTIC) [44]. Table 14.7 shows about 20% of corn is no-tilled or ridge-tilled, enabling efficient collection.

More than 80% of farmers employ some form of tillage to manage surface residues, with 60% of corn fields conventionally tilled. This has become a larger task as yields have increased. In 1960, corn belt states averaged 3.6 tons ha^{-1}. In 2003 the yield had increased to 10.0 tons ha^{-1}.

Adapting to no-till corn will be easier in many areas when some of the stover is economically collected, especially in the northern parts of the corn belt where cold moist soils can delay germination in the spring. Each day delayed is 25 kg corn grain lost according to local lore. Most corn growers till for removing, i.e., burying, corn stover to induce spring soil warming.

Table 14.6 County-level stover and straw cover required for water and wind erosion.

State	County	Corn, dt ha^{-1}		Wheat, dt ha^{-1}	
		No-till	Mulch till	No-till	Mulch till
IL	McLean	1.1	2.2	NA	NA
IL	Peoria	2.1	4.6	NA	NA
IA	Grundy	1.6	2.7	NA	NA
IA	Jasper	2.8	6.7	NA	NA
NE	Rock	2.4	4.0	1.1	2.3
NE	Dawson	1.6	2.4	1.1	1.7

Table 14.7 Corn tillage practice, % total.

Year	1994	1996	1998	2000	2002
No till	18	17	16	18	19
Mulch	22	23	23	19	16
Ridge till	3	3	3	2	2
Conventional	60	60	61	63	64

Table 14.8 Wheat tillage practice, % total.

Year	1994	1996	1998	2000	2002
No till	5	7	9	10	11
Mulch	25	24	23	20	16
Conventional	69	69	68	70	73

For wheat, less than 10% of the acres are no-till (Table 14.8). Weed control of wheat is the primary reason for tillage. Changing to no-till wheat is slowly gaining favor, increasing from 5% in 1994 to 11% in 2002. But conventional till has increased 4% over the same period, despite higher fuel costs for field operations. Evidently, the new investment in no-till equipment, $70 000 to $150 000, coupled with low commodity prices is a significant obstacle to changing.

14.4.3
Cover Crops

Cover crops can offset the erosion effect from collecting residues by restoring the surface cover, reducing wind and water erosion. Cover crops can also improve soil quality: their additional biomass builds SOM, especially from their roots. Cover crops also choke out weeds and may retain N in its root system over the winter, thereby reducing N_2O emissions and nitrate leaching [45].

Cover crops require a higher level of management. Important factors for consideration include:
- Selecting appropriate cover crops to fit in the rotation to avoid allelopathic effects, inhibition of growth in one species of plants by chemicals produced by other species
- Planning to ensure enough growth occurs to provide the above benefits. Broadcast seeding may be used for the current crop to give it a timely start, and care must be taken not to hinder its growth during that crop's harvest
- Cover crop harvesting or killing growth needs to consider soil moisture conditions. It can deplete needed soil moisture in a dry spring, or if left to grow longer in a wet spring, deplete excess soil moisture
- Growth must be stopped for some cover crops like rye before it goes to seed or it will interfere with future cash crops.

Establishing local, credible test plots to investigate the impact of residue removal for various cropping practices is important to provide information to both the grower and the processor.

14.5
Innovative Methods for Collection, Storage and Transport

Most previous studies focus on collecting and baling dry material after the grain harvest. Grain is the cash crop and is at risk until safely collected and stored. Collecting, storing, and transporting bulky straw and stover is secondary. Additional field operations add cost and increase risk.

Straw is normally dry enough to bale, but corn stover must dry from 30–50% moisture to less than 20%. Feedstock drying and densification methods can reduce collection delays and increase density. These approaches may be appropriate when a dry, compacted material is desired for co-firing or for thermo-chemical processes. These operations increase cost to $50 dt^{-1} or more, however [46]. Densification inhibits wet processing and pellets need to be "reconstituted" by soaking in water to shorten digestion time for hydrolysis.

One-pass harvest of corn grain and stover, wet storage, and transport to the processor seem to be advantageous where wet feedstock is acceptable, as already shown in Tables 14.4 and 14.5. Custom bailing and transporting bales from the field to a processing point within a 50 km has a relative return of $41–$54 ha^{-1} depending on the production. One-pass harvest and transport to 3–25 km collection centers for storage and then supplying the processing plant from these sites is estimated to increase margins to $59–$119 ha^{-1}, a 44 to 118% improvement. The relative difference between custom baling and one-pass harvest with wet storage and transport for the farmer is shown in Table 14.9.

These cost comparisons are relative. Other costs like shrinkage or change in properties of the feedstock in storage, storage investment and operation, and relative quality of final feedstock processed are not included. There is a large variation in these factors depending on the local situation. These are addressed in the following sub-sections.

14.5.1
Collection

Collection choices are divided into two general categories, baling the residue following harvest or one-pass collection of both grain and residue.

Table 14.9 Farmers net margin, stover sale comparison.

Case	1	2	3
Stover yield, dt ha^{-1}	6.9	9.0	10.6
A. Custom bale net margin, $ ha^{-1}	$41	$49	$54
B. One-pass, bulk, net margin, $ ha^{-1}	$59	$93	$119
% Improvement	44%	92%	118%

14.5.1.1 Baling

Many studies have been made of baling biomass on a large scale. For straw, baling is an option. Cereal grains, like winter wheat, are grown in dryer areas and mature earlier than corn, enabling a longer harvest window. When cereal grain is ready to harvest, straw moisture is usually suitable for collection. In contrast, stover is typically too high in moisture, 30 to 50%. It must remain in the field to dry and be collected later. To speed drying, some flail the stalk. Raking is then required before baling, adding more cost, increasing the foreign matter, especially dirt, in the bales and compacting the soil. A wet harvest season can prevent its collection entirely, because of wet residue [13].

For industrial feedstock, baling only adds cost, $15 dt^{-1} or more at the field [30]. Bales also add cost at the processor for additional equipment and disposal of twine, wrap and foreign contamination [38].

14.5.1.2 One-pass Collection

Achieving the target of $33 dt^{-1} with adequate farmer margins will probably exclude baling. This can be achieved with many variations. There are more choices for separation, i.e. ear and stalk, grain-stalk-cob, remove leaves and husk, or just leaves. Prototypes for one-pass harvest of straw and stover are under development, adapting existing equipment and examining new designs.

One-pass systems have been compared with multi-pass alternatives for wheat [47] and stover [36, 48–50]. Results indicate one-pass harvest can deliver $33 dt^{-1} target price with $70 ha^{-1} or more margin to the farmer when the following conditions are met:

- 9.0 dt ha^{-1} (175 bu acre^{-1}) or more yield when 2.2 dt ha^{-1} or less cover maintains soil quality
- 50 km or less collection radius
- bulk delivery
- 400 hours (700 ha) or more utilization of stover collection equipment.

Table 14.10 summarizes the harvest cost as a function of harvester utilization and yield, adjusted for 4th Q 2004 fuel pricing [51].

The key stover collection equipment issue resolves around one question: "What does customer need?" For example:

- Corn with ear and stalk? Or grain and stover?
- Number of harvester take-offs: 1, 2 or 3?
  - Component separation? Which parts?
  - Size reduction? How much?
  - Other pre-processing?
- On-farm storage or at a collection site?

Local requirements will vary. In areas where soybeans and corn rotate, the needs are different from wheat and corn or other crop rotations. For wheat, stripper headers work well now, leaving a standing stalk that is clean and readily harvested.

Table 14.10 Collection cost for forage harvester.

Annual collection		Harvest cost per ha			Harvest price per dt		
ha	Hours 1.8 ha h^{-1}	Fixed cost	Direct cost	Total cost +15%	Case 4.1, 7 dt ha^{-1}	Case 4.2, 9 t ha^{-1}	Case 4.3, 11 dt ha^{-1}
250	140	$ 70	$ 28	$ 113	$ 9.60	$ 7.03	$ 5.86
500	281	$ 35	$ 28	$ 72	$ 6.20	$ 4.52	$ 3.76
1000	561	$ 18	$ 28	$ 52	$ 4.50	$ 3.26	$ 2.71
1500	842	$ 12	$ 28	$ 45	$ 3.90	$ 2.84	$ 2.36

Some areas may be satisfied with one take off, separating the grain and other components of the field. Others may desire to use existing equipment, but at the same speed, separating the grain from the stover in the field. One design offers three field separation possibilities as cobs offer commercial value as a carrier for herbicides and other chemicals, cat litter, and metal-polishing applications.

Development cost for a new design is $ 2 million or more for prototypes, with millions more required to bring to market. The definition of the customer's needs, regional differences, market size uncertainty and the cyclical economic performance of this industry makes significant up-front development beyond paper studies difficult to justify until the market for machine sales exist. Without subsidizing development, a "chicken and egg" dilemma exists.

14.5.2
Storage

Maintaining quality of feedstock in storage is a major concern. Stable storage is possible only when the material is dry, less than 20% moisture, or wet, greater than 60% moisture. In the US most industrial experience is with dry storage, mostly bales, and the associated need to keep dry and protect from fire. Pest infestations have not been noted with corn stover, but some report straw is more susceptible.

Wet storage of large quantities is also familiar for silage, fermented forage crops. Ensiling green sorghum and corn plants has been practiced for years as a means of preserving feedstock for ruminant animals. These crops are chopped and stored in bags, bunkers, or silos at 65% moisture. The storage life can extend to years, with losses less than 3%. In addition, in many tropical areas "Ritter" wet storage is practiced to supply pulp mills – 250 000 to 500 000 dt piles are built via circulating liquor, saturating the feedstock to 80% moisture. Residual sugar results in fermentation that drops the pH below 4, halting microbial activity. Less area is required; fire is eliminated when stored above 60% moisture. A comparison of dry bale and wet bulk storage is shown in Table 14.11.

Table 14.11 Dry and wet storage comparison [36].

Property	Dry (bales)	Wet storage
Dry density, lb ft^{-3}	7 to 10	12 to 14
Storage area	10×	1×
Storage loss	>10%	<5%
Foreign matter and soil nutrients	High	Low
Non-volatile solubles removal	Process residue	Storage liquor
Weather risk	Rain	Extreme cold
Fire hazard	High	None
Investment	Low to high	Medium to high
Storage quantity	Small, mostly farm use	Large, bagasse for pulp

14.5.2.1 Density

The dry density of bales is about half that of wet stored material, ranging between 112 kg m^3 for round bales to 160 kg m^{-3} for square bales. Wet storage density depends on the stack height, with 40 meters achieving 200 kg m^{-3} average pile density [52].

14.5.2.2 Storage Area

Square bales require about ten times the wet storage space because of bale stacking limits, access corridors, and a measure of fire protection. The total area required for 1 million dry tons is approximately 500 acres for square bales. With wet storage, a 333 000 dt pile requires 15 acres. For 1 million dt storage, just 3 piles or about 50 acres is needed. The equivalent land rent depends on the local situation, adding zero to $2 or more per dt.

14.5.2.3 Storage Loss

Bales are adversely affected by wet weather and without shelter can decompose and break apart. For 6″ dia × 5′ bales, 30% of the mass is in the outer 4 inches and 25% weight loss can easily occur in one season. Stored inside barns, both round and square bales had 14% weight loss over 10 months in eastern Canada [53].

For wet storage, the major losses are the 5 to 8% solubles removed during storage. Typical cellulose and hemicellulose losses reported by the pulp and paper industry are 1 to 3% [54]. Surface loss depends on the total surface exposed relative to the stored tons. The higher the pile, the smaller the exposed surface and the surface loss. While there may be aesthetic or zoning limits, wet storage piles height is limited by design considerations for pump head and recovery, varying between 30 and 40 m.

The lignin, pentosans, and holocellulose increased in proportion to decreases of the solubles in water, alcohol–benzene, and 1% caustic soda. The absolute quantity of lignin, pentosans, and holocellulose remained constant during the

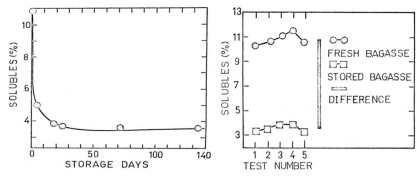

Fig. 14.7 Solubles removal in wet storage.

storage period. The loss in solubles during storage is shown in Fig. 14.7, declining from 10 to 3% within weeks, and fresh bagasse having 7% less solubles for the five trials.

The pentosans and holocellulose, which consists of the alpha-cellulose plus the hemicelluloses, continue to increase over a longer period (Figs. 14.8 and 14.9).

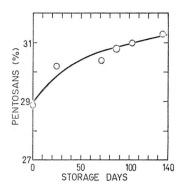

Fig. 14.8 Pentosan change in wet storage.

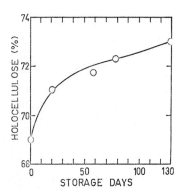

Fig. 14.9 Holocellulose change in wet storage.

14.5.2.4 Foreign Matter and Solubles

Bales contain soluble soil nutrients along with foreign material that can be dele-terious during storage and processing. Wet storage has proven to remove dirt, foreign matter and solubles over time. Removing the nutrients during storage, returning them to the fields is much preferable to processing the bales and dis-posing of the process ash. Fewer solubles in the wet feedstock, with the abso-lute values of holocellulose and pentosans unchanged, increases the plant capac-ity up to the distillation step: 7% removal opens up 7% more pretreatment, hydrolysis, and fermentation capacity.

14.5.2.5 Storage Investment

Storage investment cost must be investigated and evaluated as part of the sup-ply chain – from collection through the disposition cost of the residue and stor-age liquors. Investment can vary widely for both types of storage. An uncovered stack of round bales on the ground requires negligible investment. Sheltered bale storage investment can be high, depending on the degree of automation. Wet storage investment may consist of a conveyor for building the pile and a water spray system to raise the pile moisture to above 60%. A more elaborate system is shown in Fig. 14.5 can add $1 million or more.

Bale-storage systems were recently estimated for rice straw [55]. Short term, tarps were favored at a cost of $6 to $11 dt^{-1}. Longer term, pole barns are fa-vored, costing 50% less with the upfront investment. For a 1 million dt plant, the pole barn investment would range between $6 and $11 million.

At the plant, the bale unloading, interim storage and handling system de-signed for NREL's model has a $12.9 million capital cost, $2.94 dt^{-1}. The oper-ating cost is $2.62 dt^{-1} based on twelve operators, twenty-four hours a day, seven days a week, to handle the bales, adding a total of $5.56 dt^{-1} to the feed-stock cost [38]. Truck or rail car unloading of wet or dry bulk material can be automatic, with minimum additional plant labor.

14.5.3
Transport

Transport is divided into two components:
- harvest period for the annual crop, typically 20 to 40 days
- biorefinery supply requirements: 2000 to 3000 dt day^{-1}.

During harvest, existing resources are stretched just collecting and transporting the grain in the field while keeping the combines operating continuously. In-creasing the resources to accommodate up to 2.5 to 3 times that quantity from the filed is a serious increase.

14.5.3.1 Harvest Transport

Transportation distance from the field to a storage site during harvest needs to be short for truck requirements to remain manageable. Leaving the feedstock at the edge of the field or at multiple collection sites 20 to 30 km in diameter can reduce the trucking requirements, potentially reduce cost by better utilization of equipment, and reduce traffic congestion.

Delivering 1 million dt to one site during harvest cause much congestion. For a 20-h delivery day, 100 trucks per hour rumble past, in and out of the location. Sugar cane harvest approaches this, with deliveries to some mill sites reaching 22 000 dt day^{-1}, 1 000 or more truck deliveries.

In areas with high yields, three collection sites with a 25 km radius (200 000 ha) can supply 1.5 million dt assuming 30% of the land is harvested. The average round trip is 35 km for each site. Increasing to four sites further reduces congestion during harvest and shortens trips by 35%, to 23 km.

The simplest and most efficient logistics occur when the ear and stover are transported together, Weight and volume limits are met using standard trailer dimensions with the resulting bulk density. Baled or bulk stover loads generally reach a maximum volume before reaching the weight limit. Milling the stover or straw increases the bulk density, more closely approaching the maximum weight.

14.5.3.2 Biorefinery Supply

Because an annual feedstock supply, 1 million dt, is not expected to be stored on the biorefinery sites, reliable supply is required by the biorefinery throughout the year. Processors have indicated a minimum one to two week supply is desired on site, with deliveries made daily, 5 to 6 days per week. Truck transportation is most common. Other transportation modes previously considered include rail, pipelines, and dirigibles.

The viable transport options are truck and rail, and wet or dry feedstock. Truck transportation is most common. Rail is most efficient when prompt service is available. Pipelines are possible but, because of the high absorption of water by the fiber (80%), slurries of more than 96% water are desired – huge volumes that may require a 2nd pipeline for water return [56].

Truck Transport   Truck transport has long been favored for both wet and dry materials for short distances. Dry material is bulky and flammable. Flaming trailers in transit are a serious hazard, especially in populated areas. Depending on biomass density and local regulations, the dimensional limits for road transport may be exceeded before the weight limit is reached. Because trucking cost is based on distance, $1.00 to $1.50 km^{-1}, less than a full weight load results in higher cost. For example, round bale transport using load-and-go wagons was just 9 dt per trailer load, a transport cost twice that of a full load, normally 18.2 tons.

Wet material from storage can be passed through a dewatering press and reduced to 50% moisture before transporting. It is perishable with this moisture content and requires timely delivery. Full truck loads are readily achieved, but

50% water results in the same pay load as the load-and-go wagon. The water volume requires management.

Rail Transport   Rail shipments for short distances have become feasible as a result of improved practices, especially when shipments remain on the same line of a regional railroad. With multiple collection points along the rail line, the collection area for the biorefinery can be more than doubled. Moving a rail car 100 to 300 miles is $150 to $250 with little regard to weight [57]. The cost of rail transit was estimated to be $3.00 to $5.00 dt^{-1} for transporting feedstock several hundred miles. Modeling shows conversion costs drop 30% for a 4 million dt plant.

Rail shipment of dry material has the associated fire liability issue. The higher weight limits make wet feedstock shipments possible at lower cost. Maximum load per car is usually 114 tonnes, 91 tonnes net, to accommodate grain shipments.

Truck traffic increases with increased plant size while rail car shipments are more manageable. Assuming 50 car unit trains traveling at 50 km h^{-1} (off the main line), approximately 1.5 min is required for the train to pass a road crossing. In contrast, when the truck delivery is limited to just 10 hours each day and 6 days per week, the truck traffic *just from feedstock delivery* is 50 to 60 trucks in and out *every hour* for a 1 million dt plant. Storing 1/3 of the feedstock on site reduces the value accordingly, but the disruption is still substantial. Trucks are assumed to carry maximum loads (Table 14.12).

14.6
Establishing Feedstock Supply

At the present time in the US, the dairy herd feed lots in Jerome County Idaho purchase about 1 million dt of straw from the surrounding irrigated barley and wheat fields with yields often exceeding 10 dt grain ha^{-1}. Grower participation and infrastructure evolved over years. It is 20 times the largest corn stover collection effort in Harlan, IA. Establishing a reliable feedstock supply system requires substantial investment, planning and outreach to the growers and other stakeholders.

Table 14.12 Plant feedstock requirements. Rail and truck traffic volume, units day^{-1}.

Plant, dt (000)		Units day^{-1} (60 h week^{-1} truck delivery)			
Mode	Moisture	1000	2000	4000	6000
Rail cars	Up to 70%	70	143	275	418
Trucks	50%	308	608	1230	1850
Trucks	15%	240	396	960	1920

14.6.1
Infrastructure

In addition to the biorefinery investment, farmers and biomass suppliers will be faced with investment decisions in the range of $70 million or more for equipment, excluding feedstock storage facilities. The storage facilities could add on more millions.

14.6.1.1 **Infrastructure Investment**
For the participating grower, new cropping practices may require investment in seed drills for planting, modifying existing equipment for less tillage and possibly narrow rows, managing cover crops, all exclusive of harvesting. Based on CTIC tillage survey, at least 50% of farmers require new tillage equipment. The new equipment can range up to $150 000 per farmer. If half of conventional till farmers make a collection commitment, their investment exceeds $50 million.

Assuming a net margin of $10 dt^{-1}, the grower needs to sell 15 000 dt for a simple pay back, the equivalent of 1500 high-yielding ha. Even half this amount is a significant hurdle for the grower assuming they offer 200 to 400 ha each, 25 to 50% of their crop, the payback time on the new equipment is 4 to 8 years. Other benefits, such as improved yields, may shorten this time [41].

In addition another $20 million investment is required for approximately 100 collection units needed for the annual campaign based on Section 14.5.2 – estimating a unit and the peripheral cost is equivalent to silage harvesters, $200 000 each, operating 40 days, averaging 1.8 ha h^{-1} and 14 hours per day.

Collection sites may require additional investment in land, material handling equipment and year-round facilities to transfer the material to the biorefinery. Trucking during the harvest nearly triples to remove the stover along with the grain for one-pass harvest.

Because of feedstock transportation demands, additional investment may be required to improve roads and bridges, rail track, and crossing to meet the increased traffic – an additional 2.5 million km of truck traffic from field to the three collection sites, with more for delivery to the biorefinery, depending on the use of rail.

14.6.1.2 **Organization Infrastructure**
For a corn processor, procuring grain is as simple as a phone call to purchase feedstock. Standards for grain quality are in place. Delivery schedules are routine to establish. Payment is usually made to local grain elevators that in turn pay the growers. If needed, grain is readily obtained from more distant suppliers. None of this is in place for biomass.

To supply 1 million dt, commitments from 1000 to 2000 farmers totaling 200 000 ha is required to insure adequate feedstock. Enlisting them is a time-consuming task. One likely business model is to mimic the "grain elevator" model. Local growers already deal with them for their grain business [14]. Accounts are in place, and their managers are skilled in logistics issues. Feedstock from other areas could also be sourced.

14.7
Perspectives and Outlook

Industry segments are beginning to move toward carbohydrate feedstocks as alternatives to fossil fuels. With improved biotech tools their processing cost are becoming competitive with present methods of chemical synthesis. Price instability and higher prices of petroleum and natural gas, global warming policies, and higher liability insurance costs are accelerating interest in a move to more sustainable feedstocks.

Global warming is driving policies like the Kyoto agreement, adding economic incentives in the form of carbon credits. Liability insurance companies are considering the potential for claims from policy holder emissions as they set rates for corporate coverage – all positive activities for the rural economy.

Feedstock supply must be given significantly more attention if it is to serve as a sustainable platform for this industrial shift to have significance. Sourcing the feedstock quantity has a high risk without improved methods for delivery to the processor from the field. There are many areas for economic and environmental improvement before it enters the processing plant. The target price, $33 \, dt^{-1}$, seems achievable with one-pass harvest and bulk delivery of clean feedstock.

Farmers are the key determinate for supplying the feedstock. Improved agronomic systems with more crop removal can also maintain soil quality. A business model with an option for the grower to participate in the value chain is important, because the bulky biomass is inherently local. Partnering with the processor insures a win–win for both.

Short term, two to three years, dry feedstock is most likely to be chosen to supply biorefineries. Straw collection will be favored, because of to reduced supply risk compared to stover.

Mid term, four to seven years, the economic and environmental advantages of one-pass harvest and wet storage will be validated. Chemical, biochemical, and microbial treatments will emerge, improving the feedstock "processability" from the collection centers before delivery to biorefineries.

Long term, 2014 and beyond, other feedstocks – especially energy crops grown on marginal croplands – will emerge as the processing technology is more proven. Plant science will enhance the feedstock value and co-products from the biorefinery will become more significant in their economic impact on the product mix.

References

1 J. DiPardo, Outlook for Biomass Ethanol Production and Demand, DOE EIA, 2002,http://www.eia.doe.gov/oiaf/analysispaper/biomass.html

2 The Vision for Bioenergy and Biobased Products in the United States, October 2002, http://www.bioproducts-bioenergy.gov/pdfs/BioVision_03_Web.pdf

3 USDA National Agriculture Statistics Service

4 S.W. Fitzpatrick, Commercialization of the Biofine technology for levulinic acid production from paper sludge, DOE/CE/41178, April 2002 www.osti.gov/gpo/servlets/purl/771246-zVDe5D/native/

5 M.E. Walsh, R.L. Perlack, A. Turhollow, D. de la Torre Ugarte, D.A. Becker, R.L. Graham, S.E. Slinsky, and D.E. Ray, Biomass Feedstock Availability in the United States: 1999 State Level Analysis, January, 2000

6 Biobased Industrial Products: Priorities for Research and Commercialization, National Research Council, National Academy Press, Washington, D.C. 1999

7 A. Aden, A., M. Ruth, K. Ibsen, J. Jechura, K. Neeves, J. Sheehan, B. Wallace, L. Montague, A. Slayton, J. Lukas, Lignocellulosic Biomass to Ethanol Process Design and Economics Utilizing Co-Current Dilute Acid Prehydrolysis and Enzymatic Hydrolysis for Corn Stover, National Renewable Energy Laboratory, NREL/TP-510-324328, June 2002.

8 T. Klopfenstein (1996) Crop residue as an animal feed. p. 315–340. In: P. Unger (ed.), Managing agricultural residues. Lewis Pub., Boca Raton, FL

9 Cooperative Research Centre for Sustainable Rice Production Annual Report, 2004

10 J. Atchison, Review of Progress with Bagasse for Use In Industry (A review of progress in purchasing, handling, storage and preservation of bagasse). J.E. Proc. Intern. Soc. Sugar Cane Technologists 14:1202–1217 (1971)

11 K.E. Gorzell, Finding an Economic and Environmental Balance to the Technology of Producing Building Materials from Agricultural Crop Residue, Paper

Number: 01-16075, 2001 ASAE Annual International Meeting, http://www.meadowoodindustries.com/asae_paper.htm

12 D. Lengel, Ag-Fiber Dot Gone: A Litany of Failure. Panel World July 2001: 8–9, 34–38.

13 D. Glassner, David, James Hettenhaus, Tom Schechinger, Corn Stover Collection Project, Bioenergy '98, Expanding Bioenergy Partnerships, Madison, WI, 1998

14 J. Hettenhaus, T. Schechinger, Corn Stover Harvest: Grower, Custom Operator and Processor Issues and Answers, Oak Ridge National Laboratory Contract 4500008274, 1999.

15 J. Hettenhaus, T. Schechinger, Improved Corn Stover Harvest & Collection Methods, 3rd Annual AgFiber Technology Showcase, Memphis, TN, October 2000

16 E. Lathrop, C. Elbert and B. Treadway, Ind. Eng. Chem. 26:594–598, 1934.

17 H. Hay and Lathrop, E.C. Storage of Crop Fibers and Preservation of their Properties. TAPPI Technical Association Papers, Series XXIV. P 412–418, 1941.

18 J. Salaber and Maza. Ritter Biological Treatment Process for Bagasse Bulk Storage. TAPPI Non-wood Plant Fiber Pulping Progress Report, No 2, October 1971.

19 J. Moebius, The Storage and Preservation of Bagasse in Bulk Form, Without Baling. Pulp and Paper Development in Africa and Near East, United Nations, N.Y. Volume II, 1966.

20 J. Bruin, Gonin, C., McMaster, L., and Morgan, R., Wet Bulk Storage of Bagasse. Proc. Intern, Soc. of Sugar Cane Tech. (ISSCT) XV Congress: 1793–1820, 1974.

21 L. Mann, Tolbert, V. and Cushman, J. (2002) Potential environmental effects of corn (*Zea mays* L.) stover removal with emphasis on soil organic matter and erosion. Agriculture, Ecosystems and Environment 89:149–166.

22 M. Stumborg, L. Townley-Smith, and E. Coxworth (1995) Crop residue export-issues and concerns. Innovations in Straw Utilization Symp, Oct 23–25. 1995, Winnipeg, Manitoba. Agriculture

and Agri-Food Canada Research, Swift Current, Sask.

23 W. Wilhelm, and Cushman, J. (2003) Implications of Using Corn Stalks as A Biofuel Source: A Joint ARS and Doe Project [abstract]. Eos. Trans. Agu. 84(46), Fall Meet. SUPPL., Abstract B51b-05.

24 J. Doran, W. Wilhelm and J. Power, Crop residue removal and soil productivity with no-till corn, sorghum and soybean, Soil Sci. Soc. of Am. J., 48, 3, 1984.

25 D. Linden, C. Clapp and R. Dowdy, Long term corn grain and stover yields as a function of tillage and residue removal in east central Minnesota. Soil Till. Res. 56, 167–174, 2000.

26 V. Beri, Sidhu, B. S., Bahl, G. S. and Bhat, A. K. (1995) Nitrogen and phosphorus transformations as affected by crop residue management practices and their influence on crop yield. Soil Use and Management 11: 51–54.

27 P. Unger, Ed., Managing Agricultural Residues, 1994. CRC Press

28 K. Paustian, J. Brenner, K. Killian, J. Cipra, S. Williams, E. T. Elliott, M. D. Eve, T. Kautza, and G. Bluhm (2002) State level analyses of C sequestration in agricultural soils. Pp. 193–204 in: J. M. Kimble, R. Lal, and R. F. Follett (eds.), Agriculture Practices and Policies for Carbon Sequestration in Soil. Lewis Pub, CRC Press, Boca Raton, Fl.

29 Soil quality web site: http://csltest.ait.iastate.edu/SoilQualityWebsite/home.htm

30 Iowa Farm Custom Rate Survey, 2004, http://www.extension.iastate.edu/Publications/FM1698.pdf

31 Agricultural carbon sequestration, Chicago Climate Exchange, 2004, http://www.chicagoclimatex.com

32 National Commission on Energy Policy, "Ending the Energy Stalemate: A Bipartisan Strategy to Meet America's Energy Challenges," 2004, http://www.energycommission.org

33 CAST 1992. Preparing US Agriculture for global climate change. Council for Agricultural Science and Technology, Task Force Report 199.

34 J. Hettenhaus, R. Wooley, J. Ashworth, Sugar Platform Colloques National Renewable Energy Laboratory, NREL/ACO-1-31051-01, January 2002.

35 Roadmap for Agriculture Biomass Feedstock Supply in the United States, November, 2003, Document Number: DOE/NE-ID-11129 http://devafdc.nrel.gov/pdfs/8245.pdf

36 J. Atchison, J. Hettenhaus, Innovative Methods for Corn Stover Collecting, Handling, Storing and Transporting, National Renewable Energy Laboratory Subcontract No. ACO-1-31042-01, March 2003, www.afdc.doe.gov/pdfs/7241.pdf

37 Levelton Engineering Ltd. and (S&T)² Consultants Inc., Assessment of Net Emissions of Greenhouse Gases From Ethanol-Blended Gasoline in Canada: Lignocellulosic Feedstocks, 2000.

38 Harris Group Inc., Process Design and Cost Estimate of Critical Equipment in the Biomass to Ethanol Process, Report No. 99-10600/13, Baled Feedstock Handling System, Revision 1w, Subcontract No. aco-9-29067-0, October 11, 2000

39 B. Hames, S. Thomas, A. Slitter, C. Roth and D. Templeton, Rapid Biomass Analysis: New Tools for Compositional Analysis of Corn Stover Feedstocks and Process from Ethanol Production, 24th Biotech Symp for Fuels and Chemicals, 2002.

40 W. Gale, C. Gambardella, and T. Bailey (2000) Surface residue- and root-derived carbon in stable and unstable aggregates. Soil Sci Soc Am J 64(1):196–201.

41 D. Reicosky, Kemper, W. D., Langdale, G. W., Douglas, C. L., Jr. and Rasmussen, P. E. (1995) Soil organic matter changes resulting from tillage and biomass production. J. Soil and Water Conservation May–June: 253–261.

42 R. Lal, J. Kimble, R. Follett and C. Cole, The potential of US Cropland to Sequester Carbon and Mitigate the Greenhouse Effect, 1998, Sleeping Bear Press.

43 R. Nelson (2002) Resource assessment and removal analysis for corn stover and wheat straw in the Eastern and Midwestern United States – rainfall and wind-induced soil erosion methodology. Biomass and Bioenergy 22: 349–363.

44 Conservation Technology Information Center, Purdue University, 2004, www.ctic.purdue.edu

45 Managing Cover Crops Profitably, 2nd ed., 1998, Sustainable Agriculture Network. II. Series, USDA. www.sare.org/publications/covercrops/covercrops.pdf

46 S. Sokhansanj and A. Turhollow, Biomass Densification – Operations and Costs, BioEnergy 2002 Proceedings, University of ID, Moscow, ID

47 PAMI, Prairie Agriculture Machinery Institute, Modeling and Comparing Whole Crop Harvest Systems, Research Up-Date 739, 1998, http://www.pami.ca/PDFs/Pami739.pdf

48 R. Quick, and T. J. Tuetken (2001) Harvest, handling, and densification for commercial processing of biomass feedstock. DOE/EE/10595-4. Iowa State Univ

49 A. Turhollow, M. Downing, J. Butler, The cost of silage harvest and transport systems for herbaceous crops, Proc., BIOENERGY '96, September 15–20, 1996, http://bioenergy.ornl.gov/papers/bioen96/turhllw.html

50 K. Shinners, P. Savoie, Single pass Whole-Plant Corn Harvesting for Biomass, 25th Symp. Fuels and Chem, 2003

51 G. Schnitkey, D. Latz and J. Siemens, Illinois Farm Business Management Custom Rate Guide–Machinery Cost Estimates, 2003, http://www.ace.uiuc.edu/fbfm/farmmgmt.htm

52 J. Moebius, The Storage and Preservation of Bagasse in Bulk Form, Without Baling. Pulp and Paper Development in Africa and the Near East, United Nations, Volume II, 1966.

53 J. Billy, Corn stover in eastern Canada as raw material for production of ethanol, Natural Resources Canada and Georges Lê of "Resources naturelles Québec" 2001.

54 J. Salaber, and Maza. Ritter Biological Treatment Process for Bagasse Bulk Storage. TAPPI Non-wood Plant Fiber Pulping Progress Report, No 2, October 1971.

55 W. Huisman, B. M. Jenkins and M. D. Summers, Cost Evaluation of Bale Storage Systems for Rice Straw, BioEnergy 2002, www.bionergy2002.org

56 A. Kumar, J. Cameron, P. Flynn, Pipeline Transport of Biomass, 25th symposium on Biotechnology for fuels and Chemicals, 2003.

57 Roof, R., Farmrail Systems, Inc., Personal Communications, March 2004.

15

The Corn Wet Milling and Corn Dry Milling Industry – A Base for Biorefinery Technology Developments

Donald L. Johnson

15.1
Introduction

15.1.1
Corn – Wet and Dry Milling – Existing Biorefineries

Corn dry milling has existed for hundreds of years – maize was ground with stones into flour for food consumption by early American populations. Modern corn refining, however, began in the mid 1800s when Thomas Kingsford started up his corn refining plant in Oswego, New York [1].

Corn refining is distinguished from corn milling in that the refining process separates the corn grain into its components, starch, fiber, protein, and oil, and further processes the starch into a substantial number of products. Corn "wet milling" is the aqueous slurry process by which the corn grain is separated into its component parts. Corn "dry milling", in contrast, physically alters moist corn granules into composite products such as flakes, grits, meal, flour, and hominy feed, although some operations do separate germ and recover oil. The dry milling process produces food and industrial products based on flakes, meal, and flour, and also fermentation ethanol.

Specialty products such as white corn flour for food uses and yellow corn flour-based adhesives, produced by what are termed the flour millers, are a small part, less than ten percent, of the industrial market [2] and will not be discussed further here. Those interested in the topic are referred to texts available on the subject [3].

Corn refining has been the fastest growing market for US agriculture over the past 25 years. This is attributed to the burgeoning high-fructose corn sweetener market early in the period, followed by rapid growth in fuel alcohol, and, more recently, by fermentation products. Corn refiners now use over 14% of the annual corn crop [4], exceeding 39 million metric tons (MT) of corn refined each year.

Biorefineries – Industrial Processes and Products. Status Quo and Future Directions. Vol. 1
Edited by Birgit Kamm, Patrick R. Gruber, Michael Kamm
Copyright © 2006 WILEY-VCH Verlag GmbH & Co. KGaA, Weinheim
ISBN: 3-527-31027-4

15.2
The Corn Refinery

15.2.1
Wet Mill Refinery

A corn refinery can be described succinctly in five process steps, but is substantially more complicated in operation. Corn grain that has been received by truck and/or rail is inspected for moisture content and debris, passed through cleaners to remove foreign material and steeped in large tanks. Steeped corn is coarsely ground to loosen and free the low-density germ which is removed by centrifugation from the starch and fiber slurry. A second grind releases starch and gluten from the fibrous hulls, the fiber is further washed to remove residual starch and sent to a feedhouse. The low-density gluten is removed by centrifugation and a battery of cyclone cleaners washes residual protein from the starch. The 99.5+ percent pure "refined" starch is ready for further processing.

Germ, which was removed early in the process, is subjected to further processing to remove the oil, which can be refined or sold as crude corn oil. The spent germ is combined with the fiber from the second grind, dried, and sold as corn gluten feed. The gluten is dried and sold as a 60% protein-feed supplement.

"Wet milling" is so named because the corn is steeped in slightly acidic warm water and is processed as an aqueous slurry until dried or solubilized in downstream processing.

15.2.2
Dry Mill Refinery

A dry mill, or "mash," ethanol plant, is a simpler process. Corn is received and cleaned as in the wet mill, but the clean corn is tempered with steam, ground, and wetted to a free flowing "mash," from which the name is derived. The mash is superheated in a continuous cooker, to which acid and/or enzymes are added to solubilize the starch in the corn meal. Additional water is added to adjust the solids and temperature, and saccharifying enzymes are added. This mash is added to a fermenter, adjusted to appropriate solids and temperature, and yeasts are added to convert the sugars to alcohol. When the fermentation is complete, alcohol is removed by distillation and the residual "still bottoms" are recovered for animal feed. In such a plant, the only two products are ethanol and distillers dried grains and solubles (DDGS). Some plants now separate the germ before "mashing" – the added cost is justified by the value of the oil recovered.

A wet mill corn refinery and a dry mill ethanol plant are compared in a process flow schematic diagram of Fig. 15.1. As might be expected, the capital investment for a mash ethanol plant is significantly lower than that of a corn refinery. The operating profits from the multitude of products normally overshadow the investment cost differences, however; this will be discussed later.

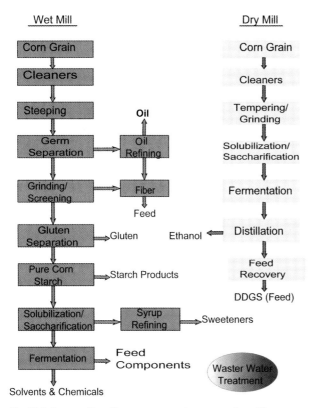

Fig. 15.1 Process flow diagrams comparing wet to dry milling.

15.2.3
Waste Water Treatment

Another common feature of wet and dry mills is, as indicated in Fig. 15.1, the waste water treatment required. Both operations, but especially wet milling, are water-intensive processes. A corn refinery may require two hundred to two hundred fifty gallons per bushel of corn (a bushel is defined as 56 pounds (25.45 kilograms) of corn at 15.5 percent moisture) processed, most of it as process water that is vaporized, condensed, heated, and cooled needing very little treatment before being returned to its source. But five to ten percent contains organic material which must be treated before discharge into the environment. Meeting local, state and federal regulations for liquid wastes may add more than 10% to the total plant investment [5]. The corn milling industry and its equipment suppliers work diligently to minimize water usage.

15.3
The Modern Corn Refinery

15.3.1
Background and Definition

The modern corn refinery is a model for developing future biorefineries. Corn refining has been compared with petroleum refining wherein flexibility of downstream processing is used to maximize profitability [6]. Thus the focus of this chapter is on wet milling, with some reference for comparative purposes to mash ethanol plants.

Corn refining produces several products in large volume. As already mentioned, wet milling refines the corn into four components, starch (carbohydrate), gluten (protein), hull (fiber), and germ (corn oil). Moreover, the carbohydrate fraction, which is nearly 70 percent of the corn composition, is further processed and refined into products such a native starch, modified starch, dextrose, high fructose corn sweetener (HFCS), ethanol, glucose syrup, and special hydrolyzates.

15.3.2
Technologies and Products

In the United States, the largest producer and miller of corn in the world, plant capacities are rated in bushels per day. Refineries in the US range in grind capacity from 55 000 bushels/day (14 000 MT/day) to more than 550 000 bushels/day (14 000 MT/day) [6]. A metric ton of corn grain yields, on average, 684 kg starch, 237 kg corn gluten feed (CGF), 45 kg gluten meal (60% protein) and 34 kg corn oil in a typical wet milling operation. Thus the largest corn refinery produces more than 5 million metric tons of pure carbohydrate per year to be sold as such and further processed into a myriad of refined products.

The wet milling process, as alluded to earlier, is a countercurrent aqueous slurry process. The aqueous stream, called mill water, begins as fresh water entering the final washing step of the pure granular starch stream, flows backward through several recycle loops in intermediate processes, and exits from the freshest corn steeping tank as heavy steep water. The solid phase, beginning as corn kernels, flows from a steep tank forward through the separation processes as components are removed and exits the final washing step as a pure granular starch slurry.

Steeping is accomplished by conveying corn grain into large steep tanks where it is exposed to warm water (circa 122 °F, 50 °C) for 30 to 40 h. A small amount of sulfur dioxide is added to maintain approximately 0.2% concentration to control bacterial growth. The corn kernels soften, loosening the hulls and disrupting gluten–starch bonds as the slightly acidic water diffuses into the swelling kernels. Steeping is currently a semi-continuous countercurrent process. Process water to which sulfur dioxide is added enters the first of a train of steep tanks, each holding as much as 3000 to 5000 bushels (76 to 127 MT) of corn kernels. The steepwater flows continuously through the train while tanks of steeped corn are sequentially removed from the front end and fresh corn tanks added at the back. Flow rates are adjusted to provide the appropriate steeping time. Water exiting the final tank has been exposed to the corn the longest whereas the corn in that tank has been exposed to the steepwater the shortest time. The fully steeped tanks are drained and the kernels are sluiced to the first, or coarse, grind.

Steeping process improvements have been proposed with the objective of shortening steeping time, eliminating sulfur dioxide, and other cost reductions [7] but none has yet been incorporated to any extent.

Steeping yields an additional product, corn-steep liquor (CSL). This nutrient rich product can be concentrated for sale as *condensed fermented corn extractives*, more commonly called concentrated steep liquor. Steep liquor that is not used internally (called thin steep liquor if it has not been concentrated) as a fermentation nutrient or sold to other users as CSL, is combined with corn germ meal (germ from which the oil has been extracted) and hulls, the composite constituting CGF.

Hydrocyclones remove the low-density corn germ from the coarsely ground slurry in the germ separation process. The germ of each kernel contains about 85% of the kernels' oil. Germ is thoroughly washed over bent screens to remove residual starch, then dried and subjected to mechanical and chemical processing to remove the oil. The oil is further processed into either crude or refined corn oil, and the spent germ combined with hulls and steep liquor as described above.

The degermed slurry is subjected to more extensive grinding in attrition mills to free the starch and gluten from the fibrous hull of the kernels. Slurry from the grinding mills flows over concave "bent" screens. The slotted screens enable starch and gluten particles to flow through, but not the fiber, effectively separating the fiber from the starch–gluten slurry. The fiber is rewashed to optimize starch–gluten recovery and combined with spent germ and CSL as already described.

The starch–gluten slurry is centrifuged to remove the gluten (light phase) from the starch water slurry. Gluten, containing 60% protein is dried, and marketed primarily as a premium animal feed ingredient. The starch is subjected to exhaustive countercurrent washing to remove protein to less than 0.5% in the starch, commonly approximately 0.3% range. The last stage, in which the starch is washed to 99.5% purity (some oil and trace minerals also remain), is the only point in the milling process where fresh water is added. This essentially pure carbohydrate stream is ready for further processing into starch products, syrups, or fermentation products.

15.3.3
Refinery Economy

15.3.3.1 Refinery Economy of Scale and Location Considerations
A large corn refinery produces a multitude of products from the pure carbohy-drate stream and strives to minimize the cost per unit of production of the carbohydrate and subsequent products also. Unit production cost consists of the cost of the corn and costs related to plant investment, labor, and conversion. The first two costs decrease as capacity increases whereas conversion cost is usually insensitive to capacity, on a unit production cost basis. Investment-related costs include maintenance, insurance, property tax, and general plant costs, which are a direct function of plant size. Doubling the plant capacity usually increases the investment required by only approximately 50%. Thus, the investment-related cost per unit of production decreases with plant size. Labor cost per unit of production also decreases as production capacity increases. Doubling the capacity may require very little added labor. Unit conversion cost includes charges for utilities such as steam, electricity, and water and are sensitive to volume. That is, doubling the capacity usually doubles the steam, electrical, and water requirements.

As plant capacity increases, the investment per unit production decreases and asymptotes at some minimum. The investment in dollars/annual gallon plotted against annual capacity for a mash alcohol plant, for example, has been shown to level off at about the 70 000 bushel/day grind capacity [8]. The generally accepted size of an "economy of scale" corn refinery is 60 000 to 80 000 bushels/day grind (1525 to 2033 MT/day).

The size and location of a scale plant is also influenced by availability of raw material corn, water, electricity, transportation (rail, water and highway), and labor. To put this in context, a 100 000 bushel/day plant uses more than a square mile of corn crop production per day (based upon national average yield of 142 bushels/acre) [9]. Each days grind requires 28 railcar loads of corn. If the grind were split evenly between two products, corn syrup and ethanol, 25 rail cars of products, including the CGF and the oil would be transported from the plant. Transportation considerations are not trivial.

Most large corn refineries grew from one or two primary products, aside from the attendant co-products, by adding finishing capacity to support a new product with an attendant grind expansion to support the new capacity. For example, a burgeoning HFCS market supported new syrup refining capacity with the attendant grind expansions at existing syrup manufacturers. For HFCS, dramatic growth also spurred green-field plant construction dedicated solely to HFCS production on the scale mentioned above. Even those plants, however, have now been expanded to furnish additional products.

15.4
Carbohydrate Refining

The flexibility in operating a corn refinery is in the downstream processing of the primary product, the carbohydrate. The granular starch slurry can be dried to produce native, or "pearl" corn starch. Alternatively, some or all of the granular starch can be processed using chemical and/or physical methods, into modified starch products. Although important, the over nine billion pounds (4.1 million MT) of corn starch forecasted to be used in the year 2004 [10] is still a distant third to the quantity used for producing corn sweeteners or fuel alcohol.

The greatest portion of the wet milled cornstarch is converted to sweeteners or ethanol. In this process the granular corn starch slurry is solubilized and saccharified using a combination of heat, acid, and enzymes. Large thermal cookers introduce high-pressure steam into the slurry exposing the granules to heat and shear to disrupt the granular structure. Acid and enzymes begin depolymerizing the high-molecular-weight glucose polymer chains. Large vessels, called saccharification tanks, provide long residence time for the continuous flowing starch suspension. Starch-hydrolyzing enzymes are used to saccharify the glucose polymer, converting it to short-chain hydrolyzates. The extent of hydrolysis determines whether it is a corn syrup (20 to 70 dextrose equivalent, DE) or dextrose syrup (94 to 98 DE). (Dextrose equivalent, DE, is a measure of the total reducing sugars in the syrup calculated as dextrose and expressed as a percentage of the total dry substance of the solution. The higher the DE, the greater the extent of hydrolysis.) Corn sweeteners are sold as a wide range of glucose or dextrose syrups depending upon DE and purity. These hydrolyzates are mechanically clarified and refined with carbon and ion exchange to produce the desired syrup.

Converting to 95 or higher DE glucose syrup provides the refiner with three options. It can be refined as dextrose or 95 DE corn syrup, fermented to ethanol, or isomerized to HFCS. Having the high DE glucose stream also provides flexibility in the choice of ethanol fermentation. Batch, semi-continuous, or continuous fermentation are options available with a 95 DE syrup stream. Large refiners producing both HFCS and ethanol provide a common stream which enables production swings, sometimes as much as 50%, from HFCS to ethanol and vice-versa as demand fluctuates. In such circumstances, some of either capacity is idle at times. That "idle capacity" investment is a small part of the overall plant investment, however, and considered a small price to pay for the flexibility.

HFCS requires a 95 DE glucose or higher feed to the isomerization reactors, the higher the better (while avoiding isomaltose reversion, which is discussed later). Fixed isomerizing enzymes convert some of the glucose to fructose, a very sweet carbohydrate monomer. (Sucrose is a dimer of a molecule of glucose and a molecule of fructose). A 42% fructose stream issues from the isomerizing reactors, the balance being glucose and any higher sugars which were present in the feed stream. The product is refined with carbon and ion exchange and concentrated for shipment. Large chromatographic columns are also used in an enriching process in which the components fructose, glucose, and higher sugars are separated. An 85 to 90% fructose product results, which is blended with 42% fructose syrup to produce a range of fructose compositions. The preponderance of product is 55% fructose syrup, an extensively used syrup in the huge soft drink industry.

Corn refiners produce large volumes of glucose syrups. This covers a broad range of products ranging from 20 DE to 70 DE, as already mentioned. Such products are widely used in the baking, canning, and confectionary industries.

If a hydrolysate is to be converted to ethanol, some refiners will provide a somewhat lower DE stream to the fermenter to avoid isomaltose, a non-fermentable reversion sugar of glucose which occurs as a result of an equilibrium reaction at high DE. The higher sugars (oligomers) are hydrolyzed, by enzymes added to the fermenter, to hydrolyzates that are used by the glucose-fermenting organism. The fermenting organism consumes the glucose and other fermentable sugars, reversion conditions are avoided in the saccharification process, and overall yields are improved.

Having appropriate converter capacity also enables the option to produce other fermentation products. Some vitamins and amino acids may require a highly pure dextrose whereas a simultaneous saccharification–fermentation process can readily utilize a low-DE syrup. The range of choices is broad and, as new industrial organisms are introduced, even more options will become available.

15.5
Outlook and Perspectives

The modern corn refinery is a model for the application of biotechnology to the production of fuels, chemicals, and materials from abundantly available natural resources in a sustainable, environmentally acceptable manner. New commodity chemicals and materials, capable of replacing non-renewable petroleum-derived products are being developed and manufactured now from corn-derived glucose in such refineries. Other biomass sources of glucose that are equally or more abundantly available and potentially less expensive than corn can readily be incorporated into such a process environment as the technology for such utilization is developed.

References

1 B.W. Peckham 2000, The First Hundred Years of Corn Refining in the United States, in Corn Annual 2000, Corn Refiners Association, Washington, DC.

2 United States Department of Agriculture 2003, Economic Research Service, Feed Outlook, January 2003

3 See for example, P. White and L.A. Johnson (eds.) 2004, Corn: Chemistry and Technology, 2nd edn, American Association of Cereal Chemists, Eagan Press.

4 Corn Refiners Association 2003, Corn Annual 2003, Washington, DC.

5 P.W. Madson, and J.E. Murtagh 1991, Fuel Ethanol in USA: Review of Reasons

for 75% Failure Rate of Plants Built, *International Symposium on Alcohol Fuels,* Firenze, 1991, available from Katzen International, Cincinnati, Ohio.

6 L. R. Lynd **2002**, Principal Investigator, Strategic Biorefinery Analysis, NREL Subcontract ADZ-2-31086-01.

7 J. Randall et al. **1978**, USP 4,106,487.

8 R. Katzen et al. **1994**, *Ethanol from Corn – State of the Art Technology and Econom-*ics, National Corn Growers Association Corn Utilization Conference V, June 1994, unpublished.

9 US Department of Agriculture, NASS, Agricultural statistics board.

10 US Department of Agriculture, Economic Research Service.

Part IV
Biomass Conversion: Processes and Technologies

Biorefineries – Industrial Processes and Products. Status Quo and Future Directions. Vol. 1
Edited by Birgit Kamm, Patrick R. Gruber, Michael Kamm
Copyright © 2006 WILEY-VCH Verlag GmbH & Co. KGaA, Weinheim
ISBN: 3-527-31027-4

16
Enzymes for Biorefineries

Sarah A. Teter, Feng Xu, Glenn E. Nedwin, and Joel R. Cherry

16.1
Introduction

The total amount of carbon and nitrogen biologically processed by photosynthesis into polymeric organic material is referred to as biomass. Plants are the main source of biomass and it is estimated that the total amount of biomass worldwide is approximately 10^{12} tons. Biomass is a renewable source of carbon building blocks, and there is great potential for converting this resource into a diverse array of biobased products.

Just over a hundred years ago, 90% of our energy needs were supplied by biomass, largely by combustion of wood. Most non-fuel industrial products, including dyes, inks, paints, medicines, chemicals, fibers, and plastics, were made from trees, vegetables, and crops. By the 1970s, 70% of US energy and 95% of industrial products were derived from petroleum rather than from renewable sources. The finite petroleum resources, a host of environmental issues, coupled with a growing interest in reducing the US dependence on foreign energy and industrial feedstock sources, have fueled research and development into alternative energy sources and the economic utilization of biomass as a source of biobased products [1].

The conversion of agricultural commodities such as corn into fuel-grade ethanol is one successful alternative energy initiative. Gasoline containing 10% ethanol was introduced as a fuel for automobiles. Today, ethanol in gasoline continues as an additive replacement for the oxygenate methyl tertiary butyl ether (MBTE). Fuel ethanol production from sugar/starch biomaterials, for example corn and sugar cane, has become an economically viable industry. In North America, approximately 11 billion liters of ethanol are currently produced annually, with a projected growth rate of ~20% for the foreseeable future.

Comparing with sugar and starch based agricultural products, biomass has a much larger potential to become the renewable energy source of the future. Biomass includes agro/forest byproducts such as corn stover (corn leaves and stalks) and wood pulp and paper residues. It is estimated that in the US alone,

Biorefineries – Industrial Processes and Products. Status Quo and Future Directions. Vol. 1
Edited by Birgit Kamm, Patrick R. Gruber, Michael Kamm
Copyright © 2006 WILEY-VCH Verlag GmbH & Co. KGaA, Weinheim
ISBN: 3-527-31027-4

biomass is capable of yielding ~ 100 billion liters of ethanol annually. In the US corn production generates $\sim 100\,000$ dry metric tons of corn stover [2], an excellent raw biomaterial containing a huge amount of under-utilized, energy-rich lignocellulosics.

The concept of the biorefinery is analogous to the concept of the petroleum refinery in the sense that an abundant feedstock is converted into many different products. Unlike a petroleum refinery, a biorefinery utilizes renewable feedstocks, such as plant-based starch or residual biomass (cellulose, hemicellulose, and lignin) which can be harvested and re-planted year after year. In one scenario, the feedstock is harvested, delivered to the refinery, and pretreated to make the cellulose accessible for enzymatic conversion to fermentable sugars. The resulting sugars are then fermented into primary products such as ethanol, lactic acid, or several other materials for industrial use. Unused residual materials are burned as fuel to generate heat and electricity. Biorefineries exist today, to a small but growing extent, where, for example, corn starch feedstocks are converted to high-fructose syrups, animal feed, oil, and various organic acids (for example citric, gluconic, itaconic and lactic acids).

Like the petroleum refinery, it is expected that the process and products from a biorefinery will evolve to meet society's demand. The first refineries in the 1860s produced kerosene for oil lamps to replace a dwindling supply of whale oil, and the byproducts, naphtha and tar, had few low value uses. With the development of the combustion engine, gasoline and light oil became dominant products and spurred the development of industries utilizing chemical byproducts of fuel production as chemical feedstocks for plastics, synthetic fibers, elastomers, drugs, and synthetic rubber. Although the primary focus of the biorefinery concept today is on fuels and energy production, large-scale implementation will stimulate development of a feedstock industry similar to that seen from the petrochemical refinery.

With recent developments in biotechnology, many petrochemical-derived products can be replaced with industrial materials made from renewable resources. Biotechnology has had a positive impact on the cost-efficiency of enzymatic conversion of biomass to fermentable sugars and has increased the range of products that can be produced by genetic engineering of fermentative organisms. Biotechnological improvements may soon enable us to produce plants with altered properties that make them more amenable to refining.

Biobased products have the potential to dramatically alter our world. The availability of technology enabling the refining of biomass will reduce the release of petroleum-originated greenhouse gases into the atmosphere, will largely decentralize fuel and chemical production, with concomitant improvement of rural economies, and will positively impact US national security by reduction of its dependence on foreign oil imports.

In this chapter we consider the biorefining of agricultural residue materials, primarily focusing on recent advances in enzymatic catalysis in the conversion of biomass to fermentable sugars. We conclude with a short discussion of the prospects for various biorefinery products.

16.2
Biomass as a Substrate

16.2.1
Composition of Biomass

A vast carbon source for biobased products is locked up in plant matter, the most abundant source of biomass on earth. The principal components of biomass are cellulose (30–50%), hemicellulose (20–30%), and lignin (20–30%); with starch, protein, and oils as minor components. The exact composition of each biomass varies depending both on the plant and on the residue collected (Table 16.1). The composition, in turn, determines the ease with which the biomass can be converted to useful products and/or intermediates and affects the functionality of the final product.

The complex polymeric structure of crystalline bundles of cellulose embedded in a covalently linked matrix of hemicellulose and lignin poses a formidable challenge for solubilization and conversion to monomeric sugars. As can be seen in Table 16.1, the relative lignin, cellulose, and hemicellulose content of a variety of potential feedstocks is quite similar, yet even a 5% increase in lignin or hemicellulose content can significantly alter accessibility to enzymatic attack. Thus, the variation in the composition of a given biomass requires some tailoring of the conversion method.

16.2.1.1 Cellulose
Cellulose is abundant in plant cell walls and comprises a linear beta-(1 → 4) anhydroglucopyranose polymer (six-carbon sugars). The molecular weights of different celluloses can range from 200–2000 kDa where the number of glucose

Table 16.1 Composition of representative biomass samples.

Samples	Variety	% Mass		
		Total Lignin	Cellulose	Hemicellulose
Monterey pine	*Pinus radiata*	25.9	41.7	20.5
Hybrid poplar	DN-34	24	40	22
Sugarcane bagasse	*Gramineae saccharum* var. 65-7052	24	43	25
Corn stover	*Zea mays*	18	35	22
Switchgrass	Alamo	18	31	24
Wheat straw	Thunderbird	17	33	23
Barley straw	*Hordeum vulgare* sp.	14	40	19
Rice straw	*Oryza sativa* sp.	10	39	15

Source: http://www.eere.energy.gov/biomass/feedstock_databases.html

residues can exceed 15 000 per polymer molecule. Cellulose has such extensive hydrogen bonding, because of the formation of overlapping, staggered flat sheets, that it is a highly recalcitrant and water-insoluble crystalline material. Within a cellulose chain, each D-glucosyl residue is rotated by approximately 180° relative to its nearest neighbor residue, making cellobiose the repeating unit present in cellulose. Only agents that can attack the glycosidic linkages between the glucose residues or which can disrupt the hydrogen bonding can solubilize cellulose.

16.2.1.2 Hemicellulose

Hemicelluloses are plant cell wall heteropolymeric sugars and sugar acids with a backbone of 1,4-linked β-D-pyranosyls in which O4 is in the equatorial orientation. They are usually shorter than celluloses, typically containing fewer than 200 1,4 linkages, highly branched, and easily hydrolyzed by strong acid or base. Hemicellulose serves as an interface between cellulose and lignin in plant cell walls, and may form covalent and non-covalent linkages with other cell-wall constituents, for example pectin, glucans and proteins. One major hemicellulose is xyloglucan, a beta-$(1 \rightarrow 4)$ linked polymer of xylose with mono-, di-, or triglycosyl side-chains, via O6, composed of a variety of substituents, for example acetyl, arabinosyl, or glucuronosyl units. Other hemicelluloses include xylan, glucuronoxylan, arabinoxylan, mannan, glucomannan, and galactoglucomannan.

16.2.1.3 Lignin

Lignin is a highly complex, amorphous and heterogeneous complex of substituted phenolic compounds, often comprising syringyl, guaiacyl, and p-hydroxyphenol components. It binds to hemicellulose and cellulose. Lignin is highly resistant to enzymatic, chemical, and microbial hydrolysis because of its extensive cross linking. It can, however, be pyrolyzed to form oil for fuel and resins.

16.2.1.4 Starch

Starch is composed of glucose, as a mixture of amylose and amylopectin in varying ratios. Amylose is a linear alpha-$(1 \rightarrow 4)$ D-glucopyranose polymer whereas amylopectin has a similar structure but with additional side branches of more than 20 glucose residues with alpha-$(1 \rightarrow 6)$ linkages. Currently, corn starch is the primary raw material of several major grain-based products, for example ethanol, polylactide, plastics, some packing materials, and adhesives.

16.2.1.5 **Protein**

Proteins are polymers of amino acids. In plants, proteins serve as structural, functional, and regulatory agents. Catalytic proteins, the enzymes, are essential for a variety of plant physiological activity.

16.2.1.6 **Lipids and Other Extracts**

Lipids are esters of moderate to long-chain fatty acids, either saturated or unsaturated. Acidic or basic hydrolysis yields the component fatty acid and alcohol. Triglycerides, esters of fatty acids with glycerol, constitute fats and oils. Esters of fatty acids with monohydric alcohols, often mixed with hydrocarbons, constitute waxes. Phospholipids are important components of cell membranes. Another major plant extract is terpene, made from isoprene (isopentane) units.

16.2.2
Biomass Pretreatment

In a natural setting, lignocellulosic biomass is broken down over a period of years by the accumulated action of physical disruption from the forces of nature (wind, rain, snow, heat, sunlight) and by the action of microbes that chemically and enzymatically degrade it into compounds they can use for their growth. The components of the plant cell wall that give it strength and rigidity, namely the intertwined network of cellulose, hemicellulose, and lignin, also make it resistant to breakdown, whether on a forest floor or in a biorefinery reactor. In contrast with natural decomposition of lignocellulose in nature, breakdown of the feedstock in a biorefinery must occur in a matter of hours or days rather than years. To accomplish this requires coordinated steps of physical disruption, chemical modification, and enzymatic action. The recalcitrant cellulose is relatively resistant to breakdown by microbial hydrolytic enzymes in its natural form, with only approximately 20% of the cellulose present in untreated biomass being hydrolyzed to glucose after treatment with high doses of enzymes. In pretreatment, plant materials are physically disrupted, under the action of stress/tear, temperature, pressure, and/or pH. To convert biomass into fermentable sugars, the purpose of the pretreatment is to disorder or remove cellulose–hemicellulose–lignin interactions and thereby improve access of hydrolytic enzymes to sugar polymers in subsequent steps in the biorefinery.

Physical disruption usually begins with a reduction in the size of the plant material by milling, crushing, and/or chopping. For example, in the processing of sugar cane, the cane is first cut into segments and fed by conveyor into consecutive roller presses that both extract the cane juice (rich in sucrose) and physically crush the cane, producing a fibrous bagasse that has the consistency of sawdust. In corn-stover processing, the stover is initially chopped with knives or ball-milled to increase the exposed surface area and improve wetability.

After physical disruption, pretreatment may continue with a chemical extraction designed to maximize subsequent enzymatic hydrolysis of the cellulose.

This usually means modifying or removing lignin, which not only acts as a block to enzyme action by coating cellulose microfibrils in untreated biomass, but also interferes with enzymatic hydrolysis by directly absorbing some cellulose-active enzymes. The result of pretreatment is a cellulose with both improved solvent accessibility and reduced lignin interference with enzyme action. Numerous methods of biomass pretreatment have been described in the literature and are summarized below.

16.2.2.1 Dilute Acid Pretreatment

This process is perhaps the most thoroughly studied of the pretreatment methods and consists of mixing the biomass with a solution of dilute strong acid (e.g. 5% sulfuric) in a pressurized reactor at high temperature (e.g. 160–200 °C) for 1–10 min then rapidly releasing the pressure. This method effectively hydrolyses most (up to 95%) of the hemicellulose to its constitutive C_5 sugars (xylose, arabinose, etc.) [3]. Little lignin is removed by the process, but it is thought to melt and be "redistributed", enabling improved cellulose hydrolysis. Pretreatment conditions must be adjusted, depending on the source of the biomass, to maximize hemicellulose hydrolysis, while at the same time minimizing the formation of compounds such as furfural and hydroxymethyl furan that are toxic to fermenting yeast and probably also to other organisms of industrial interest (a review on this topic is given elsewhere [4]). In literature reports the solids remaining after pretreatment are often washed before enzyme digestion, but this may not be economically practical in a biorefinery.

16.2.2.2 Ammonia Fiber Explosion

This pretreatment utilizes ammonia mixed with biomass in 1:1 ratio under high pressure (1.4–3 atm) at temperatures of 60–110 °C for 5–15 min, then explosive pressure release. Because of it volatility, ammonia can be recycled with near quantitative recovery. Little (10–20%) lignin is removed, but enzymatic cellulose hydrolysis is reported to proceed to as much as 98% of theoretical yield at relatively high cellulase loadings (15 FPU g^{-1} glucan) [5]. Hemicellulose depolymerization is highly variable and depends on the moisture content of the biomass, but is typically quite low. Enzymatic cellulolysis therefore requires the presence of at least some hemicellulase activity to increase cellulose accessibility during hydrolysis.

16.2.2.3 Hot-wash Pretreatment

This method involves passing hot water through a heated stationary biomass bed and, like dilute acid, has been reported to result in solubilization of more than 90% of the hemicellulose fraction [6]. The hemicellulose is largely converted to pentose oligomers which must be enzymatically converted to monosaccharides before fermentation. The performance of the pretreatment depends on temperature and flow rate, and requires washing for ca. 8–16 min. At high flow rates and temperatures, the lignin content is reduced by as much as 46% and the process produces no significant amounts of compounds inhibitory to fermentation [7, 8]. Although the hydrothermal process does not require the acid-resistant reactor materials of acid pretreatment, this advantage may be offset by increased water use and recovery costs.

16.2.2.4 **Wet Oxidation**

Here molecular oxygen and water are applied to the biomass at high temperature and pressure. In a series of experiments reported by Varga [9], 60 g L^{-1} biomass incubated at 195 °C for 15 min under 12 atm O_2 and containing 2 g L^{-1} Na_2CO_3 solubilized 10% of the cellulose, 60% of the hemicellulose, and 30% of the lignin present in corn stover. Enzymatic hydrolysis of the remaining solids after hydrolysis at 50 °C for 24 h using 25 FPU enzymes per gram of dry biomass achieved an 85% conversion of cellulose to glucose.

Other methods of pretreatment involve the use of sodium hydroxide, lime, organic solvent extraction, or lime steam explosion, but are, in general, less studied than the methods described above.

The critical issues in selecting a pretreatment for lignocellulosic biomass are sugar yield and composition, the cost of the process both in terms of energy and chemical costs, and the capital cost of building the system. The pretreatment system selected has an impact on all the downstream processes in the biorefinery and must be evaluated carefully. As described above, increased enzyme digestibility may be accompanied by an increase in byproducts that inhibit downstream fermentation, whereas less severe conditions may produce a substrate requiring excessive enzyme loadings for cellulose hydrolysis. This interplay between pretreatment, enzymatic digestion, and fermentation is the crux of current research projects to develop an integrated biorefinery.

16.3
Enzymes Involved in Biomass Biodegradation

Biomass degradation is required for the survival of many organisms including bacteria, fungi, plants, protozoa, insects, and herbivores (through symbiotic microbes). Investigation into the action of these enzymes on biomass or its components has been active for over sixty years [10–16]. With the advent of large-scale genome sequencing, the complexity of biomass degradation has become more apparent. Bacteria such as *Clostridium thermocellum*, *Cytophaga hutchinsonii*, *Microbulbifer degradans*, *Rubrobacter xylanophilus*, and *Thermobifida fusca*, and the fungi *Trichoderma reesei* and *Phanerochaete chrysosporium* have all been sequenced to at least draft form, revealing a diverse array of enzymes involved in carbohydrate degradation. Organisms devote much of their resources to degrading plant material, with well over fifty genes targeting polysaccharide degradation even in relatively simple bacteria.

16.3.1
Glucanases or Cellulases

On the basis of sequence homology, cellulases can be grouped in the glycoside hydrolase (GH) family classification system of Coutinho and Henrissat (Carbohydrate-Active Enzymes server at URL: http://afmb.cnrs-mrs.fr/~cazy/CAZY/index.html). Cellulases fall into families GH5–9, 12, 44, 45, 48, 61, and 74 [17]. Cellulases are often modular, comprising a catalytic core, a linker, and one or more cellulose-binding modules (CBM, which can be grouped into ~13 families, part of ~39 families of carbohydrate-binding domains). Such modular organization is found with other enzymes active on other insoluble polysaccharides, for example amylases and chitinases. The CBM can be at the N or C-terminus of the catalytic domain and is attached via a linker domain rich in proline, serine, and threonine. The 3D structure of many catalytic domains has been solved [18]. In general, the active site in exoglucanases is enclosed by two surface loops forming a tunnel, believed to be vital for conferring directionality in enzyme action on linear cellulose microfibrils. In contrast, the active site in endoglucanases has an open groove, enabling it to act in the middle of a cellulose chain. The 3D structure of many CBM has also been solved [19]. In general, a CBM has a flat surface with exposed aromatic side-chains that mediate binding to the hydrophobic cellulose surface.

Cellulase is a general term encompassing a diverse set of enzymes that participate in the hydrolysis of cellulose into glucose. Cellulases include exo-1,4-β-D-glucanases or cellobiohydrolases (CBH, EC 3.2.1.91), endo-1,4-β-D-glucanases (EG, EC 3.2.1.4), and β-glucosidases (BG, EC 3.2.1.21). EG act internally within a cellulose chain at amorphous cellulose regions to cleave glycosidic bonds, thereby fragmenting the cellulose polymer. CBH are believed to "processively" degrade a cellulose chain from either the reducing or non-reducing ends, and can cleave glycosidic bonds within crystalline cellulose regions to release the disaccharide cellobiose. Because EG create new reducing and non-reducing ends within cellulose chains for CBH attack, these two enzyme classes act synergistically in cellulose degradation. At high concentrations cellobiose or other cellooligosaccharides can inhibit CBH activity. Thus BG, which hydrolyses these soluble sugars to glucose, is often required in a "complete", effective cellulolytic system.

In addition to cellulase, phosphorylase can also cleave β-glycosidic bonds, especially those in cellodextrin, by phosphorylating a glucosyl unit [20].

16.3.2
Hemicellulases

Hemicellulases are involved in degrading hemicellulose. Some cellulases, for example GH7 and GH74 EG, have significant xylanase or xyloglucanase side-activity. The structural similarity enables many hemicellulases and cellulases to be grouped into the same GH family [17].

On the basis of the products they form xylanases can be classified as endoxylanases (EC 3.2.1.8) and β-xylosidases (EC 3.2.1.37). On the basis of sequence, endoxylanases belong to the GH10 and GH11 families whereas β-xylosidases belong to GH3. Galacto/glucomannan-active mannanases can also be classified as endomannanases (EC 3.2.1.78) and β-mannosidases (EC 3.2.1.25). Other hydrolases are active on other polysaccharides commonly found in biomass, for example pectinase/polygalacturonase, arabinofuranohydrolase, arabinase, galactanase, glucoronidase, and acetylesterase [21].

16.3.3
Nonhydrolytic Biomass-active Enzymes

In addition to hydrolases, various proteins and enzymes are active on lignocellulosics. Expansin and swollenin are not cellulolytic, but seem able to disrupt the hydrogen bond between cellulose chains, leading to structurally weakened cellulose [10]. Polysaccharide lyases cleave glycosidic bond by β-elimination, resulting in a double bond at the newly formed non-reducing end. Laccase, lignin peroxidase, and Mn peroxidase can oxidize lignin, thus loosening lignin–polysaccharide interactions or relieving lignin inhibition of polysaccharide hydrolases [22, 23].

16.3.4
Synergism of Biomass-degrading Enzymes

The selection pressure on organisms to feed efficiently on biomass has led to the evolution of biological cellulolytic systems integrating highly specialized yet synergistic enzymes. Two distinct, effective systems have developed – the multi-component, secreted, and non-complexed fungal/bacterial (aerobic) cellulases and the multi-component, scaffold-assembled, complexed bacterial (anaerobic) cellulosomes.

One representative fungal cellulolytic system is that of *Trichoderma reesei* (syn. *Hypocrea jecorina*) [24]. One of the most effective cellulose degraders known, *T. reesei* secretes an array of cellulases, including CBH I or Cel7A ($\sim$ 60%), CBH II or Cel6A ($\sim$ 15%), EG I or Cel7B, EG II or Cel5A ($\sim$ 20%), and other minor components (for example as EG III or Cel12A, EG IV or Cel61A, EG V or Cel45A, EG VI or XG74A, BG I or Cel3A, Xyn I or Xyn11A, and swollenin). CBH I and CBH II differ in their affinity for reducing and non-reducing ends. The subtle yet significant difference among the various EG can accommodate the need to degrade a heterogeneous substrate such as cellulose. Commercial *T. reesei* cellulase preparations, for example Novozymes's Celluclast 1.5L and Gencor International's Spezyme, are widely used in a variety of applications.

One representative bacteria cellulosome is that of *Clostridium thermocellum*. This cellulase system is organized around a $\sim$ 200 000 molecular mass scaffolding, a protein equipped with a dockerin, a CBM, and many cohesin domains. The dockerin attaches the assembly to the cell surface, and the cohesins anchor a variety of enzyme molecules (CBH, EG, etc.) by interacting with their dockerin domains [10,

12]. Cellulosomes range from 0.5 to 50 megadaltons, and many cellulosomes can further aggregate into polycellulosomes. The catalytic domains of cellulosomic enzymes are very similar to those of their non-complexed counterparts. Co-localization of enzymes in a cellulosome may improve synergism by bringing necessary components together within the same vicinity, but the organization gives the hydrolases limited mobility in comparison with the non-complexed cellulases. Nevertheless, the cellulolytic activity of the supramolecular cellulosome is comparable with that of the multi-component, non-complexed fungal cellulase system [10].

An effective industrial cellulase preparation should include enzymes that can "multi-task", and the enzyme function should be collaborative and synergistic. Several fungal cellulase preparations are available commercially but no bacterial cellulase preparation has yet been produced industrially. Available cellulase products, developed for detergent, textile, and other industries, are too expensive for a viable biorefinery. The economic considerations of protein production led us to choose Novozymes's Celluclast 1.5L, produced by large scale batch fermentation of *T. reesei*, as a starting point for developing the next generation of biomass-targeting cellulase product. We focused on improving the activity of the *T. reesei* cellulase system while maintaining its already high protein productivity during fermentation. All studies were performed using acid-pretreated corn stover (PCS) as the substrate.

16.4
Cellulase Development for Biomass Conversion

16.4.1
Optimization of the CBH-EG-BG System

16.4.1.1 BG Supplement
A "complete" cellulase system requires BG to hydrolyze cellobiose, a potent inhibitor of CBH and a precursor of fermentable glucose. Balancing the ratio of CBH, EG, and BG is vital for improved cellulose hydrolysis. *T. reesei* secretes at least two enzymes with BG activity at a very low level during normal cellulose-induced growth. We observed that Celluclast hydrolyzed cellulose with improved performance when assayed in a diafiltration–saccharification device which enables continuous removal of small sugars by filtration, compared with a closed vessel. Accumulation of CBH-inhibiting cellobiose in a closed vessel resulted in a slowing down of the overall reaction [25]. We exogenously supplemented Celluclast with an *Aspergillus oryzae* BG (belonging to the GH3 family). Addition of small amounts of BG, present as a few percent of total protein, enabled us to achieve equivalent conversion of cellulose in PCS with half the enzyme dosage of the unsupplemented Cellulase mix (Fig. 16.1). By expressing the *A. oryzae* BG in the *T. reesei* strain used to produce Celluclast 1.5L we were able to eliminate the need to ferment BG separately.

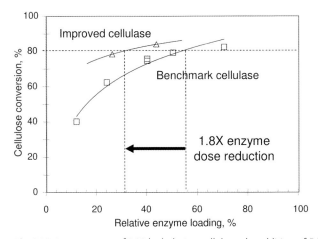

Fig. 16.1 Improvement of PCS-hydrolyzing cellulases by addition of BG.

16.4.1.2 Novel Cellulases with Better Thermal Properties

One focus of our research has been to obtain a collection of CBH, EG, and BG from a taxonomically diverse group of mesophilic, thermotolerant, and thermophilic fungi. Extending the number of cloned and characterized cellulases beyond currently reported enzymes could lead to discovery of enzymes with novel

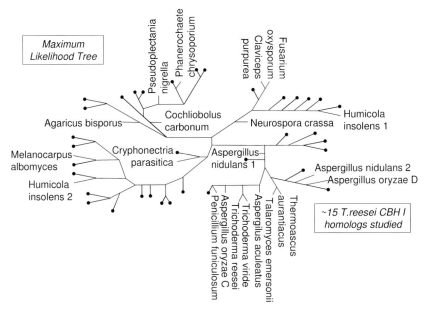

Fig. 16.2 Phylogenetic tree comparing the catalytic core sequences of the novel GH7 CBH I genes to the catalytic core sequences of published genes.

properties. In addition to *T. reesei* we have isolated other cellulolytic fungi that effectively degrade complex lignocellulosic substrates such as PCS, and sought novel CBH I enzymes (from the GH7 family), particularly those from thermophilic filamentous fungi. Thermally stable enzymes could enable cellulose hydrolysis at elevated temperature, which in theory should result in thermal enhancement of the enzymatic rate. We attempted to find a CBH I superior to *T. reesei* CBH I, which has an unfolding temperature T_m of 62.5 °C [26] and is known to be inactivated in hydrolysis reactions above 50 °C [27]. Many genes with a large amount of sequence identity with *T. reesei* CBH I (Cel7A) have been deposited in public databases. We used homology search tools, for example the Smith–Waterman, FASTA, BLAST (gap penalties and scoring matrices), Clustal W (multiple alignment), MEME, and MAST (motif searching) algorithms, to discover numerous GH family 7 genes with wide phylogenetic diversity (Fig. 16.2). They provided a resource for understanding the functional diversity of cellobiohydrolases. Of these genes, 15 were expressed in fungal hosts, purified and characterized. In hydrolyzing various cellulose substrates, a few enzymes from thermophilic fungi had thermal stability/activity superior to that of *T. reesei* CBH I.

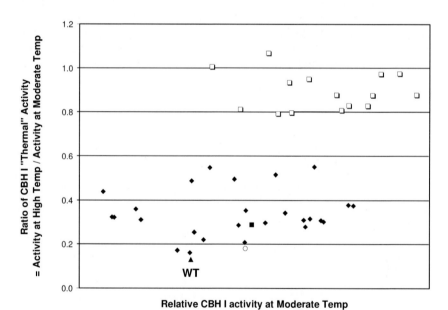

Fig. 16.3 Improved CBH I (Cel7A) variants with enhanced activity at high temperatures. Activity at moderate temperature (at which the wild-type enzyme is stable) is plotted against the ratio of activity at a thermally challenging temperatures (at which the wild-type is unstable) divided by activity at the moderate temperature. The performance of the wild type (wt) is marked as a triangle (▲). The open circle (○) marks the position of a variant obtained by protein design. Closed diamonds (◆) denote variants obtained from primary screens whereas open squares (□) show variants obtained by rounds of shuffling from pools of primary variants.

Because *T. reesei* CBH I has high specific activity on PCS at moderate temperature, we tried to improve its thermal stability, using structure-based design and directed molecular evolution. For structure-based rational design, we compared the coding sequences of thermostable CBH with their less stable counterparts and modeled their structures, informed by the published structures of glycosyl hydrolase domains [28–31]. This comparison revealed specific residues that could be mutated to enhance thermostability, and several of these mutations were created by site-directed mutagenesis. In addition, we generated random mutations in the CBH I gene and identified variants with improved activity at elevated temperature. As a result of both approaches we identified several substitutions in the CBH I gene that led to enhanced performance in hydrolyzing a soluble cellulase substrate at high temperature. DNA shuffling, the process of using recombination between genes with partial sequence identity, was used to find favorable combinations of the identified substitutions and to eliminate detrimental mutations [32] (Fig. 16.3).

We expressed several of our thermally improved CBH I variants in *Trichoderma* host strains that lacked the native CBH I gene. Expression of the improved variants was achieved at levels that approximated those found in the wild-type parent strain, and their expression did not noticeably alter the levels of other proteins in the *T. reesei* secretome. We assayed complete broths containing variant CBH I enzymes for hydrolysis of PCS at temperatures higher than the optimal temperature for *T. reesei* native cellulases. Figure 16.4 shows that the presence of the variant CBH I improved the high-temperature saccharification of

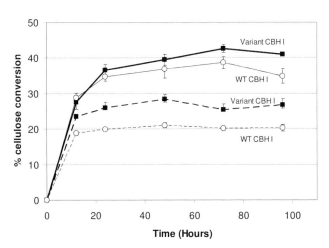

Fig. 16.4 High-temperature hydrolysis by cellulase mix including variant CBH I. Saccharification of pretreated corn stover by two *Trichoderma* broths, one expressing the wild type CBH I ("WT CBH I") and one expressing a CBH I variant ("Variant CBH I"). Solid lines, 55 °C hydrolysis; dotted lines, 60 °C hydrolysis. Cellulases were used at equivalent protein loadings. Cellulose conversion was determined by measurement of reducing sugars.

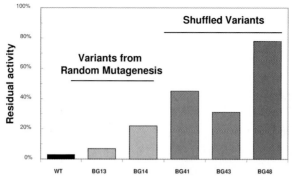

Fig. 16.5 Thermostabilization of *A. oryzae* BG by directed evolution. Residual activity is the ratio of BG activity after heat treatment at 68 °C for 10 min compared with the activity of an untreated sample. Activity was measured using 4-nitrophenyl β-D-glucopyranoside at pH 5.

PCS over the wt strain. The selected variants failed to surpass wt *T. reesei* cellulase mix at its optimum temperature (50 °C), however (data not shown).

In addition to CBH I, we also improved the thermal stability of *A. oryzae* BG by directed molecular evolution. We screened for stabilized variants by measuring enzyme residual activity after brief thermal denaturation at temperatures that partially denature the wt enzyme. Several improved variants had better thermal stability, as measured by assessing residual activity after a ten-minute thermal challenge at 68 °C (Fig. 16.5).

16.4.1.3 Structure–Function Relationship of EG

For efficient cellulose conversion, it is crucial that CBH and EG act synergistically; thus, EG activity and substrate specificity is important for maximizing cellulose hydrolysis. Microbial EG are grouped into many families according to the extent of their sequence identity [17]. *T. reesei* secretes at least six EG, with EG I and EG II making up as much as 15% of the total secreted protein. Although the substrate specificity of several individual representative EG has been thoroughly studied, a systematic, comparative investigation of EG from different GH families has yet to be made [33]. We assayed ~20 EG from GH5, 7, and 45 with a variety of representative substrates to further define their substrate preferences (Fig. 16.6). Cel5 EG had significant mannanase activity, in addition to their cellulase activity. Cel7 EG had significant xyloglucanase activity, in addition to their cellulase activity. In contrast, Cel45 EG were "strict" cellulases, acting almost exclusively on β-1,4 linked glucose polymers. Among the EG, only Cel7 were active on *p*-nitrophenyl-β-D-cellobioside, a commonly used chromogenic surrogate substrate for cellulases. These results suggest that Cel45 have an active site groove that is more defined, or specifically "tuned" to accommodate a β-1,4-D-cellodextrin unit, compared with the active sites found in Cel5 and Cel7.

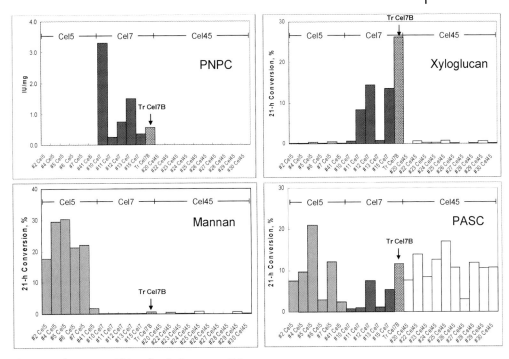

Fig. 16.6 Substrate specificity of endoglucanases. Substrates: PNPC, p-nitrophenyl-β-D-cellobioside; PASC, phosphoric acid-swollen cellulose. *T. reesei* Cel7B is marked with an arrowhead (Tr Cel7B).

Elucidation of this structure–function relationship could assist us in tailor-making cellulase systems specific toward biomass with different cellulose–hemicellulose compositions [34].

16.4.2
Other Proteins Potentially Beneficial for Biomass Conversion

16.4.2.1 Secretome of Cellulolytic Fungi
It is known that the number of cellulase-encoding genes in cellulolytic microbes can far exceed the number (3 to 4) of components in the simplest "complete" cellulase system. The need for a microbe to have an extensive cellulase array might be related to the diversity/heterogeneity of its carbon source, or the requirement of other proteins, beyond the "canonical" composition (reducing-end-preferred CBH I, nonreducing-end-preferred CBH II, EG and BG), for its cellulolytic function.

Different cellulolytic fungi can secrete sets of proteins with significantly different 2D electrophoretic patterns, as exemplified in Fig. 16.7. The explanation for this difference might be twofold. Different fungi use at least one of the four

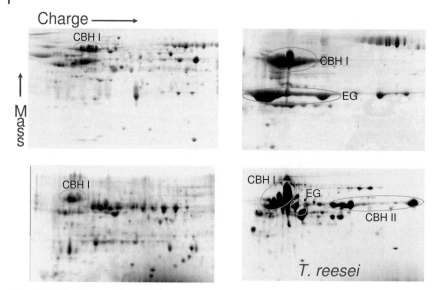

Fig. 16.7 Two-dimensional gels of proteins secreted by *T. reesei* and three other cellulolytic fungi grown on PCS. The "canonical" cellulases are marked.

"canonical" cellulases, but the cellulase(s), although highly similar in terms of amino acid sequence identity, can differ by posttranslational processing (i.e. IEF isoforms). In addition to the major cellulase(s), different fungi can secrete various minor proteins under cellulose-induced growth. The presence of these minor components indicates that other proteins (in addition to the four canonical ones) may play complementary/beneficial roles in cellulosic degradation.

Among the proteins secreted by *T. reesei*, Cel12A, Cel61A, Cel45A, XG74A, Cel3A, Xyn11A, swollenin, and other proteins have been identified in addition to Cel7A, Cel6A, Cel7B, and Cel5A. Microarray cDNA/genomic DNA analysis, Expressed-Signal-Tags (EST), and other molecular biology tools have unveiled many unknown genes whose expression were induced by PCS (Fig. 16.8). Given this evolutionary diversity, we can expect other cellulolytic fungi/bacteria to utilize different sets of proteins. Some organisms may utilize novel component(s) in the enzyme mix; others might be unique with regard to the stoichiometry of the cellulases present.

16.4.2.2 Hydrolases

The two CBH, six EG, and one BG known to be secreted by *T. reesei* belong to eight GH families, representing approximately half of the GH families known to include cellulases. It is possible that cellulases from other GH families could be beneficial to *T. reesei* cellulolytic system, by providing either complementary specificity, stronger synergism, reduced inhibition, enhanced reactivity, or in-

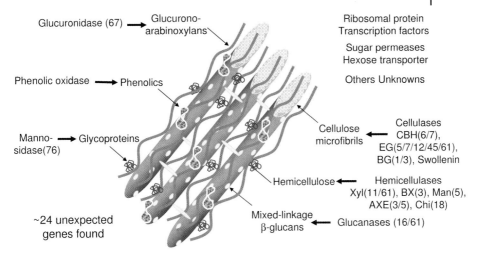

Glucuronidase (67) ⟶ Glucurono-
                        arabinoxylans

Ribosomal protein
Transcription factors

Sugar permeases
Hexose transporter

Phenolic oxidase ⟶ Phenolics

Others Unknowns

Manno- ⟶ Glycoproteins
sidase(76)

Cellulose
microfibrils ⟵

Cellulases
CBH(6/7),
EG(5/7/12/45/61),
BG(1/3), Swollenin

Hemicellulose ⟵

Hemicellulases
Xyl(11/61), BX(3), Man(5),
AXE(3/5), Chi(18)

~24 unexpected
genes found

Mixed-linkage
β-glucans ⟵ Glucanases (16/61)

Fig. 16.8 Schematic of fungal genes induced by growth on PCS. The action of gene products on lignocellulose is depicted.

creased stability. For example, cellulases derived from hyperthermophilic microbes are of particular interest because of their superior thermal profile.

One example of the benefits of pairing the *T. reesei* cellulolytic system with another quite different fungal cellulolytic system is shown in Fig. 16.9. A 1:1 mixture of the two cellulase preparations performed as well as the individual system dosed at *twice* as much as the *T. reesei* cellulolytic system alone, indicating a significant synergism between the two systems. Identification and transfer of those enzymes responsible for this synergism into the *T. reesei* host should create a single organism with significantly improved cellulose-hydrolysis activity.

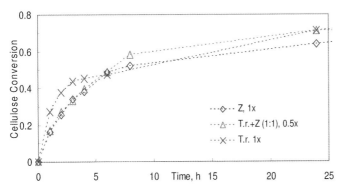

···◇··· Z, 1x
···△··· T.r.+Z (1:1), 0.5x
···✕··· T.r. 1x

Fig. 16.9 Effect of adding fungus Z proteins to *T. reesei* broth in hydrolyzing PCS at 50°C.

Thus, studying non-canonical cellulases is of interest for improving enzymatic PCS hydrolysis.

16.4.2.3 Nonhydrolytic proteins

As shown in Fig. 16.8, several non-hydrolytic proteins seem to be up-regulated under cellulose induction. Some of these can be attributed to cellular processes directly relevant to cellulose utilization, but others apparently cannot. The contributions of these additional components to microbial biomass conversion should be an indispensable part of "cellulolyteomics" – understanding the global network of all cellulosics-active biomolecules. Investigating the mechanism and extent of action of the components on different feedstocks will be an important part of improving biomass conversion. Swollenin and phenolic oxidases are currently attracting attention because of their ability to disrupt cellulose and lignin, respectively; the two reactions are thought to be beneficial to biomass hydrolysis [10].

16.5
Expression of Cellulases

Many individual enzymes acting synergistically form an effective cellulase mix for conversion of lignocellulosics to sugars. Production of cellulase components individually is not economically feasible; instead, all the proteins necessary should be expressed and secreted by a single fungal host. The protein composition must be well balanced to take advantage of the optimum mix for cellulase synergy. At the same time, the overall total protein yield must be high. Considering these factors, it becomes clear that an important aspect of biorefinery research is the technology of protein expression in fungi.

Enhancement of a cellulase production strain can be performed on two different levels; first, classical strain mutagenesis can be used, as has been reported previously for *T. reesei* [35]. Second, genetic engineering can be used to modify levels of endogenous gene expression and to introduce genes for heterologous expression of novel cellulase components.

The use of genetic engineering to introduce and manipulate specific gene expression in *T. reesei* has been indispensable to our cellulase research program. We used several selective genetic markers to follow gene integration into the host and developed a variety of promoter elements to enable variable levels of gene expression. Because we required the ability to introduce several novel genes into the host strain simultaneously, we investigated transformation efficiency, and developed procedures for simultaneous co-transformation of different transgenes. These technological improvements enabled us to investigate, rapidly and efficiently, the effect of introducing different enzymes into the *T. reesei* cellulase mix.

A
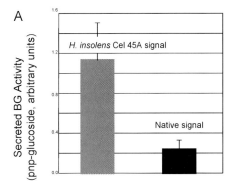

B
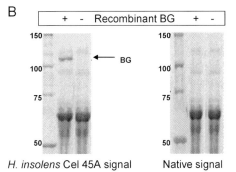

Fig. 16.10 Signal peptide effect on BG secretion in *T. reesei*. *T. reesei* strains were genetically modified to heterologously express *A. oryzae* BG, either behind the native *A. oryzae* BG signal peptide, or behind a signal peptide from the *H. insolens* Cel45A. A. Relative BG activity measured in the secreted fraction, using 4-nitrophenyl β-D-glucopyranoside at pH 5. B. SDS–PAGE of secreted proteins from the two *T. reesei* strains. The positions of molecular weight markers are labeled; the position of *A. oryzae* BG is marked with an arrow. The gels were stained with Coomassie Brilliant Blue.

In addition to controlling gene expression transcriptionally, by using promoters of different strengths, we focused on enhancing individual protein yield by optimizing protein secretion. One example is replacement of the *A. oryzae* BG signal sequence with a signal peptide from *Humicola insolens* Cel45A EG, which improved the BG secretion in *T. reesei* (Fig. 16.10).

The objective of the research discussed here is to produce a single fermentation product with improved capability for converting the cellulose in pretreated corn stover to glucose. The economic impact of these improvements on a corn-stover-based biorefinery that produces fuel ethanol will be discussed below.

16.6
Range of Biobased Products

The goal of the biorefinery is to utilize renewable feedstocks in the production of power, a variety of fuels, and chemicals. Several biobased products are already on the market, including fuel, industrial and potable ethanol, sweeteners (high-fructose syrups and sorbitol), organic acids (citric and lactic acids), MSG, lysine, enzymes, polymers (xanthan gums), food and feed products, and specialty chemicals, with annual multi-billion dollar sales. Biochemicals produced from today's biorefineries find their utility in diverse products such as adhesives, wallboards, resins, paper coatings and additives, textile sizing agents, foam packaging materials, solvents, cosmetics, toiletries, paints, plastics, food, animal feed, and pharmaceuticals.

In deriving products from raw biomaterials, biorefineries employ two fundamental technological platforms – the syngas platform based on thermochemical gasification and the sugar-platform based on biochemical conversion to simple sugars. Biotechnology is currently being applied to the sugar platform, with extensive focus on enzymatic saccharification and whole-cell microbial fermentation of the resulting sugars.

Oxygenated biomass-derived products, for example ethanol and other fermented organic compounds, will be key precursors to many industrial chemicals traditionally dependent on petroleum feedstocks. The tractability of a sugar-platform for biosynthesis of products is apparent in comparison with a petroleum-based industry. Biorefinery-based products have an advantage in that oxygenated intermediates, for example adipic acid or ethylene glycol, can be produced more readily, because of the presence of oxygen in the sugar and starch backbone. Because the raw materials can vary depending on the local source of fermentable sugars, the fermentation of such products is more flexible.

16.6.1
Fuels

In the US, fuels make up approximately 70% of the carbon consumed annually (more than 1.8 billion tons). Biobased ethanol and biodiesel are currently produced at higher cost than gasoline, and these renewable fuels account for less than 2% of total liquid fuel consumption. Developing biobased liquid fuels will require production cost reduction, including use of low-cost carbon sources, for example agricultural/forestry byproducts and urban wastes.

As a direct result of research and development programs worldwide, fuel ethanol production from sugarcane/beet (direct fermentation of material obtained by crushing) and corn/wheat starch (by starch saccharification) has become a viable industry. Yeast-fermentation of simple sugars, particularly sucrose and glucose, has been used economically to produce ethanol, in amounts of more than 20 million tons per year [36]. In Brazil, fermentable sugars are obtained from mechanically processed sugar canes. In the US the sugars come mainly from enzyme-degraded corn and wheat starch. To extend this industry by tapping into inexpensive, readily available biomass materials such as corn stover, wheat straw, and other agro/forestry byproducts as sources for fermentable sugars, intensive research is being conducted to develop enzymes which convert lignocellulosics and other polysaccharides to simple sugars. In addition, research efforts are being focused on obtaining and improving microbes for fermenting diverse sugars [37, 38].

Production of fermentable sugars from cellulose is currently more expensive than their production from amylose (starch). This can partly be explained by the relative recalcitrance of cellulose – amylase hydrolysis is intrinsically faster and the kinetics of cellulase action require relatively higher loadings of enzyme. As a result of significant funding by the US Department of Energy and collaboration between Novozymes and the US National Renewable Energy Laboratory (NREL), however, substantial progress has been made toward reducing enzyme cost for conversion of cellulose to fermentable sugars. After the research

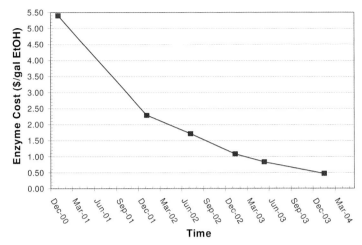

Fig. 16.11 Progress in enzyme cost reduction for corn stover-
based ethanol production. Symbols denote milestones
achieved in reducing enzyme cost for production of ethanol
from pretreated corn stover, as validated by the National Renewable Energy Laboratory (NREL.) Costs are specific to the
corn stover feedstock (PCS) and NREL cost models.

and development advances mentioned above, more than 20-fold cost reduction
has been achieved (Fig. 16.11).

Importantly, the reduction of enzyme cost achieved in the last few years has
had a major affect on the estimated cost of producing fuel ethanol from corn
stover in a biorefinery. In 1999, the total expected cost for producing bioethanol
was dominated by enzyme cost; today enzyme cost is comparable with the estimated costs of biomass feedstock collection or depreciation of capital. Using a
2004 "state of the technology" process cost estimate supplied by NREL, and an
enzyme cost of $0.50 per gallon ethanol produced, ethanol derived from bio-
mass has a total cost of about $2.50 per gallon [39]. Comparing costs for pro-
ducing ethanol from corn starch saccharification (by amylase) and fermentation
to projected costs for lignocellulosic-rich biomass-based ethanol production indicates that the biomass based industry is becoming economically viable.

In addition to fuel ethanol, biomass-derived sugars can be fermented into
combustible "biogas." Mainly methane, the fermentation is accomplished by
anaerobic bacteria, a technology already developed on small to medium-scale.
Fuel ethanol seems to be the future for a biomass-based energy industry, however. Future research and development effort will probably be focused on cellulases with improved reactivity and stability, and on microbes with expanded sugar specificity (e.g. novel yeasts or pathway-engineered microbes capable of fermenting a variety of pentoses, hexoses, or oligomeric sugars).

16.6.2
Fine/Specialty Chemicals

Biomass is abundant in C_6 sugars (hexoses), of which glucose is the most common, and C_5 sugars (pentoses), of which xylose is predominant. Several organic acids are currently produced from these starting sugars via fermentation by microorganisms. As noted in Fig. 16.12, lactic acid and succinic acid fermentation platforms can lead to numerous value-added products. The C_5 sugars can also be fermented into a variety of xylose derivatives including itaconic acid, furfural, furfuryl alcohol, and 2-hydroxymethyltetrahydrofuran (Table 16.2). Among various biomass-derived organic acids being studied, lactic acid and, to a lesser extent, 3-hydroxybutyric acid have attracted the most attention, because of their use in the manufacture of plastics. In addition to biodegradability, reduced CO_2 emission is another benefit of making these biopolymer/plastics [40].

16.6.3
Fuel Cells

A clean, efficient, and easily rechargeable energy source, fuel cells have been actively studied in the past few decades. In fuel cells, chemical energy is converted into electricity by electrochemistry rather than combustion. Biofuel cells, in which enzymes or entire microbial cells serve as electron-transfer catalysts, use

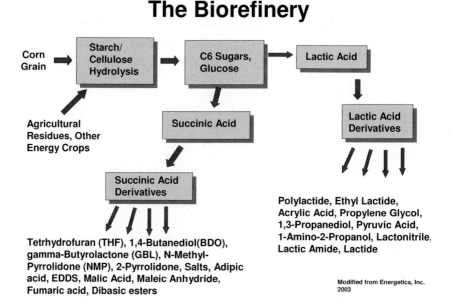

Fig. 16.12 Schematic diagram of biorefinery products based on lactic and succinic acid fermentation platforms.

Table 16.2 Industrial bioproduct opportunities.

Technology platform	Chemical	Applications
Sugar fermentation	Lactic acid (currently biobased)	Acidulant (food, drink), electroplating bath additive, mordant, textile/leather auxiliary
	Polylactide (currently biobased)	Film and thermoformed packaging, fiber, fiberfill
	Ethyl lactate (currently biobased)	Solvent, chemical intermediate
	1,3-Propanediol	Apparel, upholstery, specialty resins, other applications
	Succinic acid	Surfactants/detergents, ion chelators, food, pharmaceuticals, antibiotics, amino acids, vitamins
	Succinic acid derivatives	Surfactants, adhesives, printing inks, magnetic tapes, coating resins, plasticizer/ emulsifiers, deicing compounds, herbicide ingredients, chemical and pharmaceutical intermediates
	Bionolle 4,4 polyester	Thermoplastic polymer applications
	3-Hydroxypropionic acid	Acrylates, acrylic fibers, polymers, resins
	n-Butanol	Solvent, plasticizers, polymers, resins
	Itaconic acid	Aluminum anodizing reagent, methyl acryl

relatively inexpensive, safe, and available "feeds", for example alcohol or sugar, instead of hydrogen gas or its volatile derivatives used in conventional fuel cells [41]. Because of the safety and cost issues of conventional fuel cells, biofuel cells are quickly emerging; in the near future, mini and micro-scale biofuel cells could replace conventional batteries that power a variety of consumer and medical-implant devices. In the more distant future, scaled-up biofuel cells could serve as a major industrial energy source.

Current research on biofuel cells focuses on how to improve performance in terms of speed, output, reliability and durability. Enzyme-mediated electron-transfer between feeds and electrodes is a focus of research and development. For example, alcohol dehydrogenase and sugar oxidase are being studied as facilitators for electron-donation from alcohols or sugars (e.g. glucose) to an anode, and laccase is being studied to facilitate the electron-accepting of O_2 (air) from a cathode. In the future, the focus of biofuel cell research may shift to cheaper, more readily available feedstocks. Because both ethanol and glucose can be generated from biorefineries, we may envisage a next-generation biofuel cell that is powered by biomass. In such a fuel cell, biomass would be enzymatically converted into glucose (e.g. by cellulase), which would then be enzymatically oxidized on an electrode (e.g. by glucose oxidase). The extracted electrons would run through a wire, perform electric work, and then be used to enzymatically reduce O_2 (e.g. by laccase). Biofuel cells may be set up as part of a biorefinery plant that generates electric power from biomass, or be used for wilderness exploration or military operations where fuel transport is logistically costly.

16.7
Biorefineries: Outlook and Perspectives

16.7.1
Potential of Biomass-based Material/Energy Sources

The goal of biorefinery is to utilize renewable feedstocks in the production of power, a variety of fuels, and chemicals. One goal for the next generation of biorefineries will be to more fully integrate facilities that can process a variety of biomass feedstocks into a full range of biochemical products. This integration would enable us to take advantage of the different product streams that might emanate from renewable feedstocks by bioconversion of products (Fig. 16.13).

More than 100 million metric tons of fine, specialty, intermediate, and commodity chemicals are produced annually in the US. Today, only 10% of these

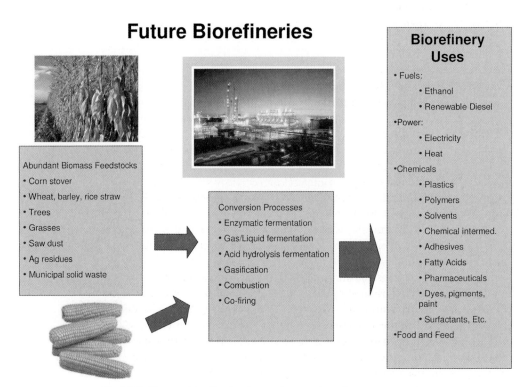

Fig. 16.13 The next biorefineries: Integrating a variety of feedstocks for a multitude of end products.

are biobased. Thus, there is tremendous growth potential for biorefineries, if the economics are competitive, if the environmental impact is favorable, and/or if novel products are created.

16.7.2
Economic Drivers Toward Sustainability

The chemical industry currently consumes approximately 8% of total petroleum and natural gas output to produce approximately 2500 products worth approximately $215 billion [36]. An attempt to replace part of the petrochemical processes with biomass-based biotechnological processes is driven by the need to curb greenhouse gas emission, upgrade agro/forestry industry value production, and reduce reliance on fossil resources.

For biobased production to be economically feasible, the cost of producing the biobased product must compete favorably with the comparable petroleum-derived product. An additional or alternative economic driver for the biorefinery could be synthesis of novel products that provide unique utility, and that are unavailable or uneconomical via petroleum-based chemistry. With regard to improving economy, there are several technologies where cost efficiency should be improved. These include:

• harvesting, collection and pretreatment of the biomass, which serve to unlock the fermentable sugars and increase the carbon conversion to the desired products;
• enzymatic conversion of the polysaccharides in the pretreated biomass stover into glucose and other fermentable sugar monomers; and
• microbial fermentation of the sugars to the desired products.

Efficient enzyme catalysis is one of the primary economic barriers in the challenge to design an overall cost-effective process for converting biomass into fermentable sugars. The research efforts described here, and research efforts in similar work performed at Genencor International, have specifically focused on improving the efficiency of enzymatic hydrolysis, and progress thus far looks quite promising. Further work on metabolic engineering of microbial production strains should continue, as should efforts to better integrate biomass pretreatment, enzyme hydrolysis, and fermentation to avoid complications resulting from isolated efforts.

Several major problems must be solved to enable commercialization of various biorefineries. To satisfy the optimum operating conditions of enzymes and microbes, raw biomass materials collected from diverse regions under diverse climates must be examined to assess the impact of biomass feedstock variability on pretreatment, enzymatic conversion, and fermentation. Optimizing these steps and integrating them into a robust, low cost, efficient, sustainable, and value-generating material–energy cycle is highly challenging, yet offers great social, economic, and environmental promise.

References

1 Finlay, M. Old Efforts at New Uses: A Brief History of Chemurgy and the American Search for Biobased Materials. *J. Ind. Ecology* **7**, 33–46 (2004).

2 Rooney, T. Lignocellulosic Feedstock Resource Assessment. (National Renewable Energy Laboratory, Golden, CO, 1998).

3 Lee, Y. Y., Lyer, P. and Torget, R. W. Dilute-Acid hydrolysis of Lignocellulosic Biomass. *Advances in Biochemical Engineering and Biotechnology* **65**, 93–115 (1999).

4 Zaldivar, J., Nielsen, J. and Olsson, L. Fuel ethanol production from lignocellulose: a challenge for metabolic engineering and process integration. *Appl Microbiol Biotechnol* **56**, 17–34 (2001).

5 Teymouri, F., Laureano-Perez, L., Alizadeh, H. and Dale, B.E. Ammonia fiber explosion treatment of corn stover. *Appl Biochem Biotechnol* **113–116**, 951–63 (2004).

6 Allen, S. G., Kam, L. C., Zemann, A. J. and Antal, M. J. J. Fractionation of Sugar Cane with Hot, Compressed, Liquid Water. *Ind Eng Chem Res* **35**, 2709–2715 (1996).

7 Liu, C. and Wyman, C. E. Impact of fluid velocity on hot water only pretreatment of corn stover in a flowthrough reactor. *Appl Biochem Biotechnol* **113–116**, 977–87 (2004).

8 Nagle, N. J. et al. Efficacy of a hot washing process for pretreated yellow poplar to enhance bioethanol production. *Biotechnol Prog* **18**, 734–8 (2002).

9 Varga, E., Schmidt, A. S., Reczey, K. and Thomsen, A. B. Pretreatment of corn stover using wet oxidation to enhance enzymatic digestibility. *Appl Biochem Biotechnol* **104**, 37–50 (2003).

10 Wilson, D. and Irwin, D. Genetics and properties of cellulases. *Adv Biochem Eng Biotechnol* **65**, 1–21 (1999).

11 Tomme, P., Warren, R. A. and Gilkes, N. R. Cellulose hydrolysis by bacteria and fungi. *Adv Microb Physiol* **37**, 1–81 (1995).

12 Bayer, E. A., Chanzy, H., Lamed, R. and Shoham, Y. Cellulose, cellulases and cellulosomes. *Curr Opin Struct Biol* **8**, 548–57 (1998).

13 Mosier, N. S., Hall, P., Ladisch, C. M. and Ladisch, M. R. Reaction kinetics, molecular action, and mechanisms of cellulolytic proteins. *Adv Biochem Eng Biotechnol* **65**, 23–40 (1999).

14 Maheshwari, R., Bharadwaj, G. and Bhat, M. K. Thermophilic fungi: their physiology and enzymes. *Microbiol Mol Biol Rev* **64**, 461–88 (2000).

15 Schulein, M. Protein engineering of cellulases. *Biochim Biophys Acta* **1543**, 239–252 (2000).

16 Lynd, L. R., Weimer, P. J., van Zyl, W. H. and Pretorius, I. S. Microbial cellulose utilization: fundamentals and biotechnology. *Microbiol Mol Biol Rev* **66**, 506–77 (2002).

17 Bourne, Y. and Henrissat, B. Glycoside hydrolases and glycosyltransferases: families and functional modules. *Curr Opin Struct Biol* **11**, 593–600 (2001).

18 Davies, G. J. Structural studies on cellulases. *Biochem Soc Trans* **26**, 167–73 (1998).

19 Shimon, L. J. et al. Structure of a family IIIa scaffoldin CBD from the cellulosome of *Clostridium cellulolyticum* at 2.2 A resolution. *Acta Crystallogr D Biol Crystallogr* **56 Pt 12**, 1560–8 (2000).

20 Zhang, Y. H. and Lynd, L. R. Kinetics and relative importance of phosphorolytic and hydrolytic cleavage of cellodextrins and cellobiose in cell extracts of *Clostridium thermocellum*. *Appl Environ Microbiol* **70**, 1563–9 (2004).

21 de Vries, R. P. and Visser, J. *Aspergillus* enzymes involved in degradation of plant cell wall polysaccharides. *Microbiol Mol Biol Rev* **65**, 497–522 (2001).

22 Kirk, T. K. and Farrell, R. L. Enzymatic "combustion": the microbial degradation of lignin. *Annu Rev Microbiol* **41**, 465–505 (1987).

23 Gronqvist, S. et al. Lignocellulose processing with oxidative enzymes. in *Applied Enzymology to Lignocellulosics* (eds. Mansfield, S.D. and Saddler, J.N.) 46–65 (Am. Chem. Soc, Washington, DC, 2002).

24 Kubicek, C., Eveleigh, D. E., Esterbauer, E., Steiner, W. and Kubicek-Pranz, E. *Trichoderma reesei Cellulases*, (Royal Society of Chemistry, Cambridge, UK, 1990).

25 Sternberg, D., Vijayakumar, P. and Reese, E. T. beta-Glucosidase: microbial production and effect on enzymatic hydrolysis of cellulose. *Can J Microbiol* **23**, 139–47 (1977).

26 Boer, H. and Koivula, A. The relationship between thermal stability and pH optimum studied with wild-type and mutant *Trichoderma reesei* cellobiohydrolase Cel7A. *Eur J Biochem* **270**, 841–848 (2003).

27 Baker, J. O. et al. Thermal denaturation of *Trichoderma reesei* cellulases studied by differential scanning calorimetry and tryptophan fluorescence. *Appl Biochem Biotechnol* **34/35**, 217–231 (1992).

28 Kraulis, P. J. et al. Determination of the three-dimensional solution structure of the C-terminal domain of cellobiohydrolase I from *Trichoderma reesei*. A study using nuclear magnetic resonance and hybrid distance geometry-dynamical simulated annealing. *Biochemistry* **28**, 7241–7257 (1989).

29 Divne, C., Stahlberg, J., Teeri, T. T. and Jones, T. A. High-resolution crystal structures reveal how a cellulose chain is bound in the 50 A long tunnel of cellobiohydrolase I from *Trichoderma reesei*. *J Mol Biol* **275**, 309–25 (1998).

30 Mattinen, M. L. et al. Three-dimensional structures of three engineered cellulose-binding domains of cellobiohydrolase I from *Trichoderma reesei*. *Protein Sci* **6**, 294–303 (1997).

31 Mattinen, M. L., Linder, M., Drakenberg, T. and Annila, A. Solution structure of the cellulose-binding domain of endoglucanase I from *Trichoderma reesei* and its interaction with cello-oligosaccharides. *Eur J Biochem* **256**, 279–86 (1998).

32 Stemmer, W. P. Rapid evolution of a protein in vitro by DNA shuffling. *Nature* **370**, 389–91 (1994).

33 Lawoko, M., Nutt, A., Henriksson, H., Gellerstedt, G. and Henriksson, G. Hemicellulase activity of aerobic fungal cellulases. *Holzforschung* **54**, 497–500 (2000).

34 Vlasenko, E., Xu, F. and Cherry, J. R. Thermostability, substrate specificity and hydrolysis of cellulose by endoglucanases from families 5,7, and 45 of glycoside hydrolases. in *25th Symposium on Biotechnology for Fuels and Chemicals* (Breckenridge, CO, 2003).

35 Eveleigh, D. E. and Montenecourt, B. S. Increasing yields of extracellular enzymes. *Adv Appl Microbiol* **25**, 57–74 (1979).

36 Danner, H. and Braun, R. Biotechnology for the production of commodity chemicals from biomass. *Chem Soc Rev* **28**, 395–405 (1999).

37 van Wyk, J. P. H. Biotechnology and the utilization of biowaste as a resource for bioproduct development. *Trends in Biotechnology* **19**, 172–177 (2001).

38 Himmel, M. et al. Advanced bioethanol production technologies: A perspective. in *Fuels and Chemicals from Biomass*, Vol. 666 (eds. Saha, B. C. and Woodward, J.) 2–45 (American Chemical Society, Washington, DC, 1997).

39 Ibsen, K. Personal Communication. (National Renewable Energy Laboratory, Golden, CO, 2004).

40 Ohara, H. Biorefinery. *Appl Biochem Biotechnol* **62**, 474–477 (2003).

41 Wong, T. S. and Schwaneberg, U. Protein engineering in bioelectrocatalysis. *Current Opinion in Biotechnology* **14**, 590–596 (2003).

17
Biocatalytic and Catalytic Routes for the Production of Bulk and Fine Chemicals from Renewable Resources

Thomas Willke, Ulf Prüße, and Klaus-Dieter Vorlop

17.1
Introduction

17.1.1
Renewable Resources

The most important sources of renewable resources for industry are oil plants, starch plants, sugar plants, energy plants, and wood, but also waste and residues from agriculture and industry. The corresponding substrates for conversion processes are manifold and belong to such heterogeneous substance classes as oils, fats, glycerol, lignocellulose, cellulose, starch, inulin, sugar, complex biomass, etc. Fats and oils are already being used as feedstock in industry at a level of 15 million t a^{-1}. The corresponding products are mainly applied in plastics, paints, lacquers, biotensides, and energy (as biodiesel). The potential of carbohydrates (starch, sugar, cellulose) is far from being fully exploited. In the year 2002/2003, approximately 143 million tons of sugar were produced worldwide (Germany 4 million tons). Of these, only 70 000 t (1.7%) were industrially employed as renewable resources in the pharmaceutical and chemical sector in Germany [1].

Because of the substantial quantities of (ligno)cellulose available, utilization of the material of biomass (wood, straw, waste, and residues) has huge potential. Countries with large amounts of wood, for example Canada, the USA, Scandinavia, or Austria, invest much effort to utilize this potential. There is much need for research. If it were possible to establish highly efficient enzymatic pulping processes, numerous bulk products (ethanol, butanol, lactic acid, etc.) could be produced at competitive prices.

Biorefineries – Industrial Processes and Products. Status Quo and Future Directions. Vol. 1
Edited by Birgit Kamm, Patrick R. Gruber, Michael Kamm
Copyright © 2006 WILEY-VCH Verlag GmbH & Co. KGaA, Weinheim
ISBN: 3-527-31027-4

17.1.2
Products

In 2001 the organic chemicals produced worldwide were estimated to be worth almost 1,900 billion Euros. Asia leads, with 586 billion Euros, followed by the European Union (519 billion Euros) and North America (508 billion Euros). The German chemical industry, with approximately 25% of the total European amount, recorded sales in 2002 of 133 billion Euros.

In respect of price and amount, the products can be roughly classified into two sectors: (1) bulk chemicals or commodities (>1 million t a^{-1}, $<$ US\$2–4 kg^{-1}), and (2) fine and specialty chemicals (<1 million t a^{-1}, $>$ US\$2–4 kg^{-1}). Worldwide the sales of fine and specialty chemicals is approximately 250 billion US\$ (Europe 120 billion US\$), which, for Europe, is approximately 20% of all the chemical products sold.

17.1.2.1 Bulk Chemicals and Intermediates
In bulk chemical synthesis the use of renewable resources as feedstock is rather limited. Relevant future applications include biobased synthesis gas, and products thereof, and a few selected products, for example ethanol. The potential use of renewable resources for the production of intermediates, for example, monomers or plasticizers for polymers, is mainly a question of the price of crude oil. At a crude oil price (2004) of approximately 50 US\$ per barrel ($0.25 \, € \, L^{-1}$), biotechnological processes can hardly compete. With rising crude oil prices, chemical and biotechnological processes based on renewables become increasingly competitive with petrochemical-derived products, especially for product prices >2 US\$ kg^{-1}.

17.1.2.2 Fine Chemicals and Specialties
For fine chemicals the price of the product is not so critical – product functionality and purity, and quality assurance, are much more important. Extremely high prices are charged for pharmaceuticals, followed by cosmetics and food ingredients and some intermediates for industry. If such high prices are accepted by the market, sustainability forces the chemical industry to use economical and environmentally friendly processes. Thus largest chances of broader application of renewable resources, either by biotechnological or chemical processes, are in fine chemicals. Often, biotechnology is the only way to obtain the required product.

17.2
Historical Outline

Until 1930 many important bulk products, for example fuels (ethanol, butanol), organic acids (acetic acid, citric acid, lactic acid), and other basic chemicals, were mainly produced from renewable resources. Process engineering was limited to fermentation by use of fungi or bacteria. In the past some basic chemicals (for example butanol and acetone) were produced exclusively by fermentation. With the development of petroleum chemistry, however, they were replaced by chemical–technical products. In the production of other chemicals (ethanol, citric acid, lactic acid, and acetic acid), biotechnological techniques have always been predominant, because the chemical–technical alternatives are not economical.

There are several prognoses of the amount and range of worldwide petroleum reserves. Most of the experts predict that maximum production will be achieved in the next few decades [2] (Fig. 17.1). Countries with high energy demands and limited resources, for example the USA, have already realized this and are investing much effort in appropriate research [3]. In the USA, for example, substitution of fossil fuel with renewable resources in the production of liquid fuels and organic chemicals is envisaged to be 50% and 90%, respectively, by 2090 [4]. More realistic prognoses expect an increase to 25% in the next 30 years [5]. Shell Oil, for example, intends to provide 30% of the world's chemical and energy needs by use of biomass by 2050, corresponding to nearly US$ 150 billion [6]. DuPont, one of the largest manufacturers of plastics, intends to produce 25% of its products from renewable resources by the year 2010 [7]. Figure 17.2 summarizes several prognoses for the USA.

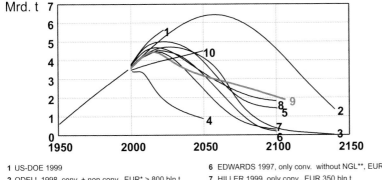

1 US-DOE 1999
2 ODELL 1998, conv. + non conv., EUR* > 800 bln t
3 ODELL 1998, only conv., EUR about 450 bln t
4 CAMPBELL 1997, only conv. EUR about 250 bln t
5 EDWARDS 1997, conv. + non-conv., EUR > 500 bln t

6 EDWARDS 1997, only conv. without NGL**, EUR 385 bln t
7 HILLER 1999, only conv., EUR 350 bln t
8 HILLER 1999, conv. + non-conv., EUR 580 bln t
9 Shell 1995, conv + non-conv., EUR about 600 bln t
10 WEC 1999, conv. + non-conv.

*EUR = estimated ultimate recovery
**NGL = natural gas liquids

Fig. 17.1 Prognoses of crude oil production and estimated ultimate recovery (EUR) [2].

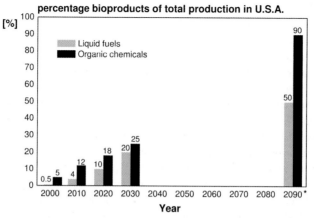

Fig. 17.2 Biotechnologically produced liquid fuels and organic chemicals in the USA as share of total production [3] (estimated data for 2090).

17.3
Processes

Large-scale chemical processes are usually very sophisticated, because environmentally friendly catalytic conversions are used almost exclusively. Although they are usually performed at high temperatures and pressures, and although substrates and products are often detrimental to health or are environmentally significant, they can be regarded as clean processes. Nevertheless, chemical processes with low annual production volumes and/or multi-step synthetic path-

Table 17.1 Typical problems of biotechnological processes and possible solutions.

Problem	Solution
Appropriate biocatalyst not available	Cell screening Strain optimization, mutation/selection Metabolic pathway design (MPD)
Productivity too low	High-cell density fermentation Cell recycle Immobilization
Substrates too expensive	Cell screening, substrate screening
Cheap substrates often not suitable	Genetic engineering, MPD
Unwanted by-products	Strain optimization, mutation/selection
Metabolic pathways not optimum	
Low product concentration (production inhibition)	
Product recovery	In situ processes
Process control	On-line analysis

ways, especially in the fine and specialty segment, are less efficient and less environmental friendly. In this segment more classic organic chemistry is used than catalytic processes, resulting in significant waste generation, emissions, and energy consumption.

Biotechnological processes usually occur under mild conditions. Biocatalysts, substrates, intermediates, and by-products, and the product itself, are biodegradable. Water is usually used as a solvent. There are also frequent disadvantages, however, including low product concentration, low productivity and, hence, high recovery costs. Table 17.1 lists some problems and possible solutions. Some products are only accessible chemically, whereas biotechnology is more appropriate for others (chiral substances, some vitamins and amino acids, highly selective transformations with polyfunctional substrates, such as sugars). Numerous syntheses are conducted exclusively using enzymes (lipases, amylases, proteases, and, also, increasing in the future, cellulases). To establish a large-scale process based on a biochemical reaction it is preferable to have means available to hold back the catalyst (i.e. enzyme) in the bioreaction vessel. By immobilizing catalysts, for example growing, resting, or dead cells or enzymes, it is possible to retard them.

17.3.1
Immobilization

Different types of immobilization procedure have been developed for this purpose, as is shown in Fig. 17.3 [8]. Besides the advantage of easy retention, immobilized catalysts are also often more stable with regard to, for example, pH and temperature. When entrapped the catalysts are, moreover, protected against other bacteria and thus processes can run under non-sterile conditions, because potential contamination is washed out while the favored catalyst is specifically protected.

Encapsulation of catalysts also has disadvantages, however: during the immobilization process the catalyst may be inactivated by physicochemical or physiological effects. Even if this does not happen, the overall activity of the immobilized system could be lower than that of the free catalyst, because of diffusion

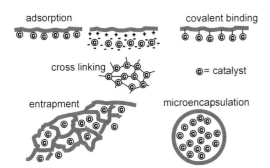

Fig. 17.3 Different ways of immobilizing biocatalysts [8].

limitations. To minimize this effect the particles should be small and applicable for the later application.

Examples of processes developed, investigated, and optimized at the Institute of Technology and Biosystems Engineering are discussed in the sections below.

17.3.2
Biocatalytic Routes from Renewable Resources to Solvents or Fuels

17.3.2.1 Ethanol Production with Bacteria or Yeasts?

Introduction Ethanol can be used as a liquid energy carrier, fuel additive, and feedstock in the chemical industry. Because of the costs – except for use in foods or stimulants – biotechnological production in Europe has not yet been profitable. In May 2003 an EU directive on the use of biofuels set a minimum level of 5.75% bio-fuels (including bioethanol) for all transport fuels sold by 2010 [9]. Thus ethanol will be more highly in demand in the future. The biotechnological production of ethanol – at the beginning of the 20th century mainly for fuel – is currently experiencing a renaissance.

In the year 2001, worldwide annual ethanol production amounted to more than 30 billion liters. The leading role played by Brazil, where bioethanol from sugar cane has been used for more than 25 years, has currently been taken over by the USA, which will probably continue to occupy first place. In the USA, mainly corn or wheat starch is used. In the EU, with a total of approximately 2 billion liters, France (approx. 0.8 billion liters) is the largest producer; Germany produces only approximately 0.3 billion liters [10].

The Process Ethanol is produced by fermentation with yeasts or bacteria (Fig. 17.4). The classic route by use of yeasts has been known for thousands of years and is one of the oldest biotechnological processes used by mankind. Substrates are sugar-based feedstocks (sucrose, glucose, molasses) and also starch hydrolyzates. A study recently promoted by the German Research Foundation (DFG) determined costs based on grain starch for the German market. According to this study, substrate costs account for up to 50% of total production costs [11].

To find cheaper sources of renewable raw materials, various routes are being followed:

- A search for organisms which, in addition to glucose, can utilize other sugars, for example pentoses (xylose, arabinose). Such sugars are the products of hydrolysis of hemicellulose, the basic constituent of wood, straw, and a variety of other plant residues [12–14].
- Screening for enzymes which split the raw materials into usable sugars as efficiently as possible, either directly or in coupled processes [15].
- Alteration of known or new organisms by genetic engineering (genetically modified microorganism, GMO) to enlarge their substrate spectrum [16, 17]. In the USA a new technique is currently being implemented on a pilot scale

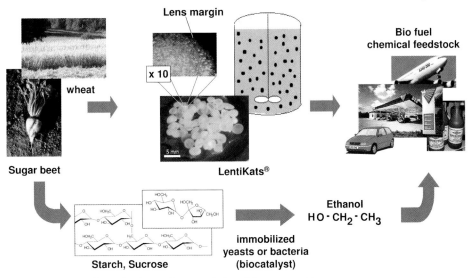

Fig. 17.4 Process scheme for the production of ethanol from renewable resources.

[18]. The process uses genetically modified *Zymomonas mobilis*, which was given the ability to use pentoses (xylose) in addition to hexoses (glucose, fructose). This enables inexpensive substances which could not previously be used, for example, rice straw, to be transformed into ethanol with high yields [19].

Reduction of the process costs can be achieved by several methods:

- Screening or genetic engineering of microorganisms with the goal of increasing productivity, ethanol tolerance (and hence achievable final product concentration), and yield. For example, use of the bacterium *Zymomonas mobilis* instead of conventional yeasts (*Saccharomyces spp.*) also results in increased product yields, besides the fivefold higher productivity. In addition, immobilization boosts volumetric productivity and, again, product yield. Furthermore, product tolerance, and with it the final ethanol concentration, is enhanced. Essential data for the process are listed in Table 17.2.

Table 17.2 Ethanol production with yeast or bacteria.

Biocatalyst	Productivity in kg ethanol m^{-3} h^{-1}	
	Suspended cells	Immobilized cells
Yeast *Saccharomyces cerevisiae*	0.5–2	10–30
Bacterium *Zymomonas mobilis*	4–5	50–80

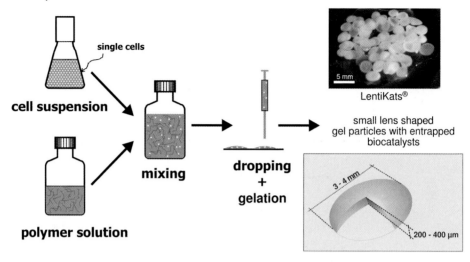

Fig. 17.5 Cell-Immobilization procedure for the production of lens-shaped particles (LentiKats).

- Development of new fermentation methods which, in particular, include the use of immobilized (entrapped) cells, so that the process can be run under non sterile conditions or the biocatalyst can be easily recycled. The latter is particularly important for high-performance strains or genetically engineered microorganisms.

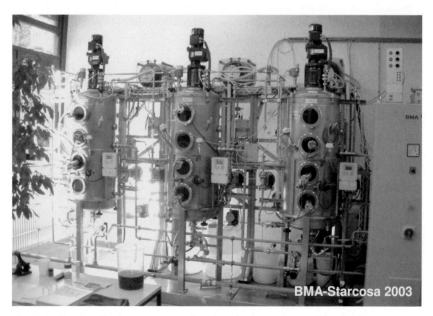

Fig. 17.6 Pilot plant for the continuous ethanol production with immobilized cells.

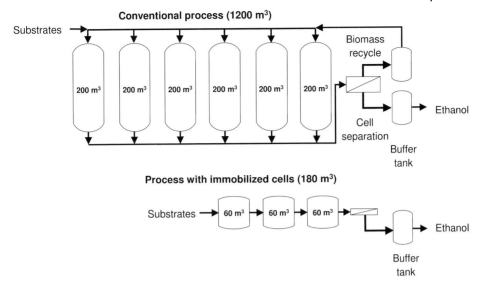

Fig. 17.7 Process design of an ethanol production plant.
Effect of type of biocatalyst on plant size. Source:
BMA–Starcosa 2001, Brunswick, Germany, capacity 60 000 L
ethanol day^{-1}.

For example, new immobilization technology based on lens-shaped particles
(Fig. 17.5) [20] was adapted for production of ethanol from molasses in cooperation with the company BMA–Starcosa (Braunschweig, Germany). Continuous
and stable ethanol production from untreated molasses was achieved over several
months, even under nonsterile conditions. A pilot plant (Fig. 17.6) has been run-
ning at BMA–Starcosa, under the described conditions, since 2003. Figure 17.7
shows clearly the extent to which plant size, and consequently investment costs,
can be reduced solely by introduction of immobilized cell systems for the biotechnological ethanol production. In combination with the above-mentioned improvements ethanol could be produced economically in the future.

17.3.3
Biocatalytic Route from Glycerol to 1,3-Propanediol

17.3.3.1 Introduction
One of the applications of 1,3-propanediol (PD) is its use as a diol component
in the plastic polytrimethyleneterephthalate (PTT), a new polymer with properties comparable with those of Nylon. It is preferably used for carpets (Corterra
by Shell) or special textile fibers (Sorona by DuPont). Further applications are
appearing in polyester resins, mainly in the paint industry.

17.3.3.2 **The Process**

PD can be produced biotechnologically from glycerol with the aid of bacteria (Fig. 17.8). Glycerol is mainly a by-product of fat splitting and biodiesel production. Further growth of the biodiesel market would result in a fall in the price of glycerol. One of the largest biodiesel producers in Germany (Nevest, Schwarzheide) filed for insolvency in December 2003, partly because of the decline in the price of glycerol from 1000 €/t to nearly half [21]. Some companies even pay to dispose of their glycerol. Glycerol–water from RME production, in particular, would be an interesting raw material if it could be used in fermentation without further pretreatment. Another method would be the utilization of glucose instead of glycerol, which would provide independence from the fluctuating glycerol market. Because no microorganisms are known which directly convert glucose into 1,3-propanediol, however, this technique requires mixed cultures or microorganisms designed by genetic engineering. Both possibilities have been examined. The gene-technological variant is favored by DuPont in cooperation with Genencor and is on the verge of technical implementation [22].

Under some conditions, however, the classic technique based on glycerol can be quite interesting technically and economically. A concerted, extensive search for new microorganisms (screening) and improved process design (fed-batch with pH-controlled substrate dosage) enabled product concentrations, which were relatively low at a maximum of 70 to 80 g L^{-1} as a result of product inhibition (Fig. 17.9), to be increased to more than 100 g L^{-1} (Fig. 17.10). Another advantage of the new technique and the new isolated strains is the use of low-priced crude glycerol or glycerol–water (Fig. 17.11). This is a factor which should not be underestimated and has a direct effect on product costs

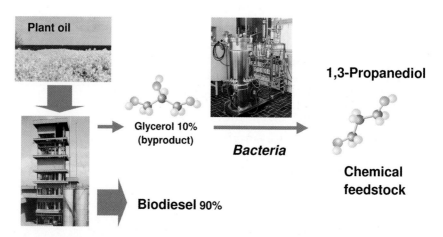

Fig. 17.8 Process scheme for 1,3-propanediol production from plant oil via glycerol or glycerol–water as a byproduct of biodiesel production.

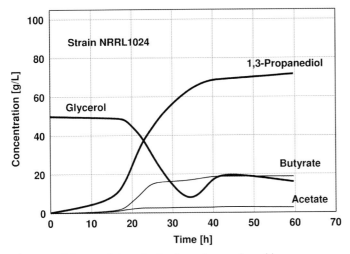

Fig. 17.9 1,3-Propanediol production from pharma glycerol by use of a commercially available strain (pH-controlled fed batch, mineral medium with YE, 32 °C, pH 7.2).

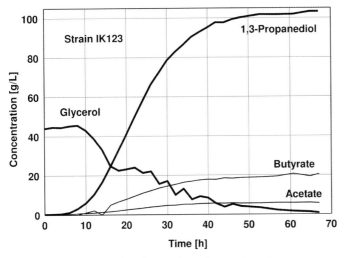

Fig. 17.10 1,3-Propanediol production from pharma glycerol with a new strain from screening (35 °C, pH 7.0, other conditions as for Fig. 17.9).

(Fig. 17.12). Further on, use of immobilized cells (LentiKats; Section 17.3.2.1, above) rather than freely suspended cells, enables productivity to be increase from approximately 2 to 30 g_{PD} L^{-1} h^{-1}.

Comparison of current (chemical) techniques with the new biotechnical techniques based on different substrates and glycerol qualities (= raw glycerol costs)

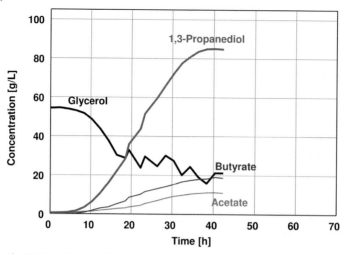

Fig. 17.11 1,3-Propanediol production from raw glycerol–water with a new strain from screening (conditions as for Fig. 17.10).

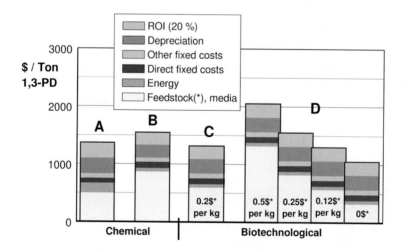

A: Shell from ethylene oxide, 60,000 t/a
B: Degussa from acroleine, 45,000 t/a
C: DuPont from glucose, 25,000 t/a
D: ? from glycerol, 25,000 t/a

Fig. 17.12 Cost comparison of industrial 1,3-propanediol production, effect of substrate costs, (*) glucose or glycerol, respectively (Data from PERP 1998, substituted).

shows that biotechnology might be competitive with chemical techniques if crude glycerol is used (PERP 1998).

17.3.4
Biocatalytic Route from Inulin to Difructose Anhydride

17.3.4.1 Introduction
Inulin is a linear β-2,1-linked polyfructane terminated with a glucose residue. Large amounts of inulin are contained in the roots and tubers of crops like dahlia, chicory, and Jerusalem artichoke. Inulins have a very limited market thus far, mainly because of the high cost of expensive separation and purification steps. For 1.5 to $2 \in kg^{-1}$ it is approximately four times as costly as competing glucose, starch, or sucrose. This also explains why short oligofructoses are synthesized enzymatically from sucrose for probiotic products rather than by partial hydrolysis of inulins. Future use of inulin-derived products is thus either in high-value markets, for example the functional food segment, or by converting inulin into intermediates which can be separated and purified at lower cost. One promising compound derived from inulin for this purpose is difructose anhydride (DFA III, Fig. 17.13).

DFA III can be the basis for plastics and tensides. It can be crystallized as easily as sucrose after an ion-exchange step and hence can be produced at a price well below that of inulin. So far DFA III has not been introduced to the market, because no efficient enzyme and biotechnical process was available for the necessary bioconversion of inulin.

To produce DFA III on a technical and industrial scale, large amounts of enzyme are needed. The following sections introduce a strategy showing how this problem can be solved [23, 24].

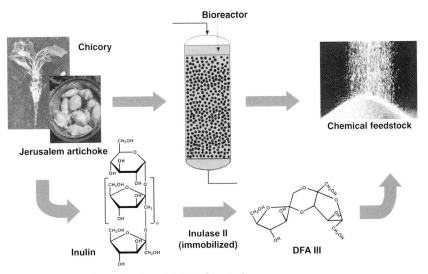

Fig. 17.13 Process for production of DFA III from inulin.

17.3.4.2 Enzyme Screening

From 65 tested samples from extremophile locations, approximately 400 bacterial strains were obtained and investigated further. Four strains were found to produce DFA III and one strain (Buo141) identified as an *Arthrobacter* sp. expressed an enzyme, stable for weeks at elevated temperatures of 60 °C whereas the activity of the other strains declined within a few hours (Fig. 17.14). The new strain grows aerobically at ambient temperatures and secreted inulase II extracellulary but only with low activity, too low for economical industrial process. To overcome these limits, genetic engineering was used.

17.3.4.3 Genetic Engineering

To increase production of the enzyme the gene encoding for the inulase II (*ift* gene) should be transferred to and expressed in an *E. coli* host. To gain access to the bacterial gene suitable primers for a polymerase chain reaction (PCR) were needed. For primer design, only two highly divergent sequences of inulase proteins were known.

A special primer design based on phylogenetic analysis substantially accelerated isolation of the *ift* gene. The complete *ift* gene was obtained by screening the genomic library with this probe. As a result a plasmid was constructed which expressed an enzyme of 477 amino acids when transferred to *E. coli*. A cell-free extract of such a culture had an activity of 3000 U L^{-1}, whereas most of this activity was detected intracellularly. In *Arthrobacter* the inulase II enzyme is expressed as an extracellular enzyme. Transport through the cell membrane is accomplished by means of a specific signal-transfer peptide which is part of the *ift* gene. Because of phylogenetic differences between the species *Arthrobacter* and *Escherichia* the transfer-peptide does not work in *E. coli*. In *E. coli* the enzyme remains intracellular, as was shown by analysis of the activity of disrupted cells and the supernatant of cultivations. Exact removal of the complete transfer-peptide resulted in a one-hundredfold increase in activity. A further increase in

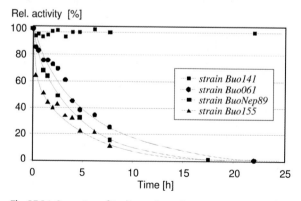

Fig. 17.14 Screening of inulinase II producers: comparison of long-term stability.

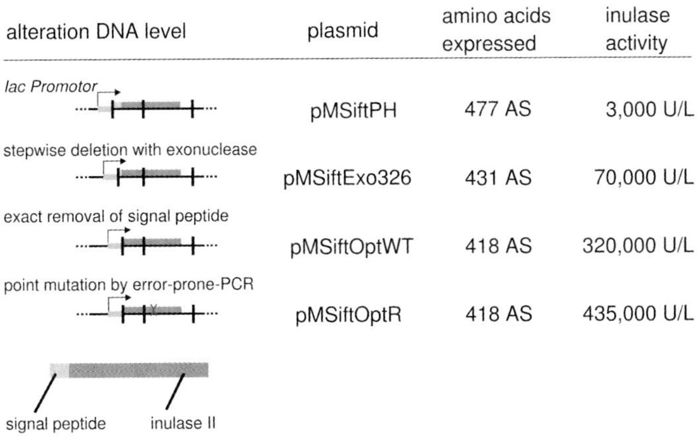

alteration DNA level	plasmid	amino acids expressed	inulase activity
lac Promotor	pMSiftPH	477 AS	3,000 U/L
stepwise deletion with exonuclease	pMSiftExo326	431 AS	70,000 U/L
exact removal of signal peptide	pMSiftOptWT	418 AS	320,000 U/L
point mutation by error-prone-PCR	pMSiftOptR	418 AS	435,000 U/L

signal peptide   inulase II

Fig. 17.15 Increase of inulinase II activity by genetic engineering.

activity of approx. 35% was possible because of a point-mutation induced by error-prone PCR. In position 221 of the enzyme a glycine was exchanged with arginine. (Fig. 17.15). To obtain sufficient large quantities of the enzyme the genetically modified organism was fermented.

17.3.4.4 Fermentation of the Recombinant *E. coli*

The recombinant *E. coli* pMSiftOptR was fermented using an inexpensive technical medium. During the fermentation inulase activity was monitored. A final biomass concentration of $11\,\mathrm{g\,L^{-1}}$ (dry weight) and an overall activity of $1\,760\,000\,\mathrm{U\,L^{-1}}$ was measured (Fig. 17.16). Because high-density fermentations of *E. coli* are known to reach biomass concentrations of approximately $100\,\mathrm{g\,L^{-1}}$ it seems possible that after optimizing the fermentation step activity of at least $15 \times 10^{6}\,\mathrm{U\,L^{-1}}$ is possible.

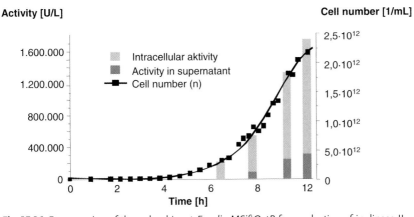

Fig. 17.16 Fermentation of the redombinant *E. coli pMSiftOptR* for production of inulinase II.

17.3.4.5 Enzyme Immobilization and Scale-up

For immobilization of inulinase II, the molecular weight of the enzyme must be increased, otherwise the enzyme will be lost by diffusion out of the particle. Inulase II was therefore flocculated from a cell-free extract by co-crosslinking with glutardialdehyde and chitosan (Fig. 17.17). Fortunately, the enzyme is not damaged by glutardialdehyde. The crosslinked enzyme was then immobilized in alginate beads of different diameter in the range 500 to 800 μm and analyzed to compare their activity with regard to bead diameter (Fig. 17.18.) Although beads 500 μm in diameter had 54% activity compared with the value when the same beads were dissolved, beads of 600 μm had only 42% of the activity. For 850-μm beads only one third of the original activity was observed. This shows once again the benefits of using sufficiently small particles when working with encapsulated systems.

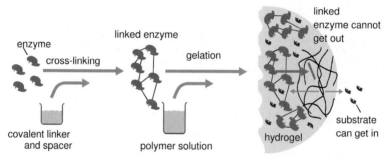

Fig. 17.17 Enzyme-immobilization: cross-linking of inulase II for molecular-weight enhancement to prevent enzyme loss by diffusion.

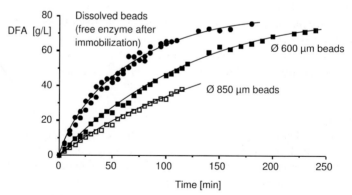

Fig. 17.18 Effect of bead diameter on the activity of encapsulated inulase II. Dissolved beads means that the formerly immobilized enzyme is released to prevent diffusion limitation.

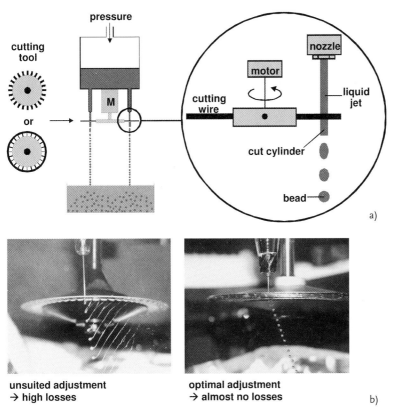

Fig. 17.19 Principle of JetCutting, and high-speed-motion picture of the cutting process showing the effect of correct adjustment.

To accomplish the task of producing the desired small droplets from the very viscous alginate–enzyme solution, a novel JetCutter technology was used. In comparison with other techniques, for example blow-off devices, vibrating nozzles or electrostatic forces, the JetCutter uses mechanical cutting of a continuous jet of liquid to produce small droplets; this is shown in Fig. 17.19 [25].

17.3.4.6 Summary

Complete process development has been shown, starting from screening for an enzyme with the desired properties – an inulase II converting inulin to DFA III at elevated temperatures (60 °C). After screening and successful optimization of the enzyme by genetic engineering and construction of a genetically modified organism which expresses the enzyme in very high numbers, this strain was fermented to furnish large amounts of enzyme for immobilization. After immobilization by entrapment of the enzyme in hydrogel particles, an industrially applicable enzyme formulation with an activity of 196 U g^{-1} (wet matter) is obtained.

17.3.5
Chemical Route from Sugars to Sugar Acids

17.3.5.1 Introduction
The increasing use of low-molecular-mass carbohydrates (sugars) for production of chemical building blocks is of great interest both economically and ecologically. Besides the biotechnological routes presented above, chemical catalysis has great potential for functionalization of sugars to furnish fine chemicals or building blocks for the chemical industry. Sugar oxidation in the presence of supported noble metal catalysts has always been an attractive subject. The products are biodegradable compounds and have many potential applications. Gluconic acid, for example, is of great industrial interest. Annual production amounts to nearly 80 000 t; this is used as a noncorrosive and biologically degradable complexing agent in industry, and in numerous applications in food, pharmaceuticals, and cosmetics. Lactobionic acid and maltobionic acids – the oxidation products of the corresponding sugar monomers lactose and maltose, respectively – can be used in the detergent and pharmaceutical and food industries.

Gluconic acid is mainly produced biotechnologically, because chemical catalysts are inadequate. With gold catalysts, this could be changed in the future (Fig. 17.20).

Table 17.3 gives an overview of some important milestones in chemical catalytic glucose oxidation. The work of Prati and Rossi describes an charcoal-supported gold catalyst for glucose oxidation, which exceeds the previous Pt- and

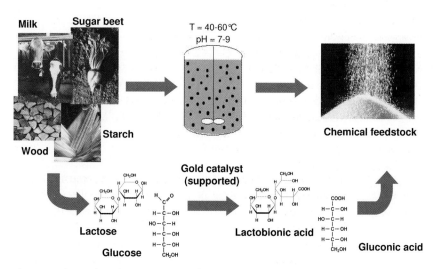

Fig. 17.20 Chemical catalytic conversion of carbohydrates from renewable resources.

Table 17.3 Milestones in the chemical catalytic oxidation of carbohydrates.

Topic	Description	Working group
Beginnings	"Mannitol acid" with platinum-Mohr Oxidation of carbohydrates on platinum interpreted as oxidative dehydration	Group-Besanz (1861) Wieland (1912)
Systematic	Reactivity sequence of the moieties in carbo-hydrates on platinum	Heyns and Paulsen (1950s/60s)
Bimetal catalysts	Doping of platinum and palladium catalysts with bismuth or lead (problem: long-term stability, Bi/Pb leaching)	Kuster/Bekkum (1980s)
Gold catalysts	Au/C for oxidation of glucose to gluconic acid highly active and selective (problem: long-term stability)	Prati and Rossi (2001)
	Enhancement of long-term stability by new preparations on TiO_2	Mirescu and Prüße (2003)

Pd-based catalysts in activity and selectivity, which is nearly 100% to gluconic acid [26]. Nevertheless long-term stability is still far too low for industrial appli-cation. A breakthrough could be achieved by the use of titania- or alumina-sup-ported gold catalysts, which combine high activity and selectivity with long-term stability, which seems sufficient for industrial applications.

17.3.5.2 Gold Catalysts

For glucose oxidation a comparative study of catalysts used industrially for the same reaction shows the high selectivity of the new gold catalysts (Fig. 17.21). This gold catalyst is highly active over a wide range of pH, temperature, and glucose concentrations. Except for formation of small amounts of fructose by isomerization at temperatures above 70 °C and pH > 10, selectivity to glucose al-ways exceeds 99.5%. These results confirm the outstanding properties of the gold catalysts in this reaction.

Whereas the charcoal-supported catalysts of Prati and Rossi lose 50% activity after four replicate batches, the TiO_2-supported catalysts remain stable. After 17 replicate batches no activity loss was observed. The mean activity was 425 $mmol_{glucose}\,g_{metal}^{-1}\,min^{-1}$, corresponding to an overall productivity of 5 $kg_{gluconic\ acid}\,g_{gold}^{-1}\,h^{-1}$.

In addition to glucose, several other carbohydrates were tested with both TiO_2 and Al_2O_3-supported gold catalysts. Fast and complete reaction occurs with pen-toses (arabinose, ribose, xylose, and lyxose), hexoses (mannose, rhamnose, galac-tose, and n-acetylglucosamine), and some di- and oligosaccharides (lactose, cello-biose, melibiose, maltose, maltotriose, maltotetrose) each with a selectivity of vir-tually 100% (Fig. 17.22, Table 17.4). No reaction occurred with ketoses or blocked aldoses (fructose, isomaltulose, methylglucose, sorbose, sucrose, and trehalose).

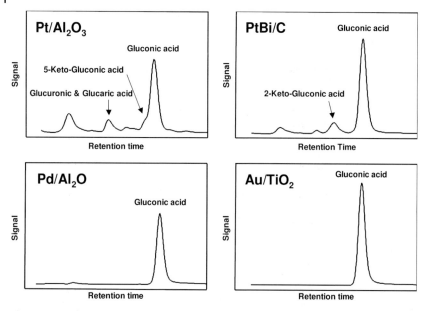

Fig. 17.21 Catalytic oxidation of glucose: screening of catalysts and selectivity proven by HPLC.

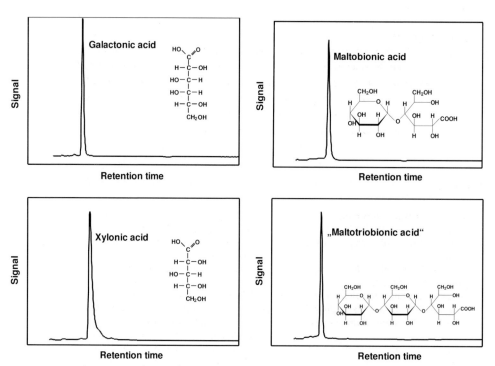

Fig. 17.22 Catalytic oxidation of other carbohydrates: galactose, xylose, maltobiose and maltotriose with Au/TiO₂ catalyst.

Table 17.4 Catalytic oxidation of carbohydrates (conditions: cat: 0.6% Au/Al_2O_3, 40 °C, pH 9, 100 mmol substrate, conversion >99%).

Type	Substrate	Activity (mmol min^{-1} g$_{Me}^{-1}$)	Activity (kg$_{product^*}$ h^{-1} g$_{Me}^{-1}$)$^{a)}$	Selectivity (%)
Pentose (C$_5$)	Arabinose	334	4.1	>99.9
	Lyxose	145	1.8	>99.9
	Ribose	234	2.8	>99.9
	Xylose	251	3.1	>99.9
Hexoses (C$_6$)	Galactose	338	4.8	>99.9
	Glucose	165	2.3	>99.9
	N-Acetylglucose	295	4.8	>99.9
	Mannose	172	2.4	>99.9
	Rhamnose	180	2.3	>99.9
Disaccharides (C$_{12}$)	Cellobiose	282	6.7	>99.9
	Lactose	84	1.9	>99.9
	Maltose	177	4.0	>99.9
	Melibiose	54	1.3	>99.9

a) Potassium salt of acid

17.3.5.3 Summary

The newly developed Au/TiO_2 catalysts have outstanding properties, including pronounced substrate selectivity and extremely high product selectivity. Combination of these with very high activity and excellent long-term stability results in catalysts that meet all the requirements demanded from a "Synzyme" (synthetic enzyme). In the future, gold catalysts may be an alternative to the biotechnological process for industrial production of gluconic acid.

References

1 WVZ, Wirtschaftliche Vereinigung Zucker, Informationen zum Zuckermarkt Stand 12/2003. **2003**, http://www.zucker-wirtschaft.de

2 K. Hiller and P. Kehrer, *Erdöl Erdgas Kohle,* **2000**, 116, 9, 427.

3 BRDTAC, Roadmap for Biomass Technologies in the United States. **2002**, Biomass R&D Technical Advisory Committee.

4 NRC, Biobased industrial products: priorities for research and commercialization. In: National Research Council (ed.), **2000**, Washington, DC.

5 BRDTAC, Vision for Bioenergy and Bio-based Products in the United States. **2002**, Biomass R&D Technical Advisory Committee.

6 OECD, Biotechnology for clean industrial products and processes, p. 30. **1998**, OECD Publications, Paris Cedex.

7 Dupont, Press release: Genencor International and Dupont expand R&D collaboration to make key biobased polymer. **2001**, http://www1.dupont.com/NASApp/dupontglobal/corp/index.jsp?-page=/content/US/en_US/news/product/2001/pn03_12_01.ht ml

8 J. Klein and K. D. Vorlop, Immobilization techniques: Cells. In: M. Moo-Young
(ed), Comprehensive Biotechnology,
1985, 203–224. Pergamon Press, Oxford.

9 EU, Directive 2003/30/EC of the European Parliament and of the Council of 8
May 2003 on the promotion of the use
of biofuels or other renewable fuels for
transport. *Official Journal of the European
Union*, **2003**, 46, L123, 42–47.

10 C. Berg, World ethanol production 2001.
2001.

11 A. Rosenberger, H. P. Kaul, T. Senn, W.
Aufhammer, Costs of bioethanol production from winter cereals: the effect of
growing conditions and crop production
intensity levels. *Industrial Crops and
Products*, **2002**, 15, 2, 91–102.

12 J. Zaldivar, J. Nielsen, L. Olsson, Fuel
ethanol production from lignocellulose:
a challenge for metabolic engineering
and process integration. *Applied Microbiology and Biotechnology*, **2001**, 56, 1–2,
17–34.

13 Q. A. Nguyen, J. H. Dickow, B. W. Duff,
J. D. Farmer, D. A. Glassner, K. N. Ibsen,
M. F. Ruth, D. J. Schell, I. B. Thompson,
M. P. Tucker, NREL/DOE ethanol pilot-
plant: Current status and capabilities.
Bioresource Technology, **1996**, 58, 2, 189–
196.

14 H. G. Lawford and J. D. Rousseau, Cellulosic fuel ethanol – Alternative fermentation process designs with wild-type and
recombinant zymomonas mobilis.
Applied Biochemistry and Biotechnology,
2003, 105, 457–469.

15 Iogen, EcoEthanol. **2003**,
http://www.iogen.ca/

16 L. O. Ingram, P. F. Gomez, X. Lai, M.
Moniruzzaman, B. E. Wood, L. P. Yoma-
no, S. W. York, Metabolic engineering of
bacteria for ethanol production. *Biotechnology and Bioengineering*, **2002**, 58, 2–3,
204-214.

17 J. Zaldivar, A. Borges, B. Johansson,
H. P. Smits, S. G. Villas-Boas, J. Nielsen,
L. Olsson, Fermentation performance
and intracellular metabolite patterns in
laboratory and industrial xylose-ferment-
ing *Saccharomyces cerevisiae*. *Applied
Microbiology and Biotechnology*, **2002**, 59,
4–5, 436–442.

18 US-Department of Energy: The DOE
ethanol pilot plant – a tool for commercialization. **2000**. http://www.ott.doe.gov/
biofuels/pdfs/28397.pdf

19 D. de Jesus and N. P. Nghiem, Student
Abstracts: Chemistry at ORNL – Abstract
Ethanol Production from Rice-Straw Hy-
drolyzate Using *Zymomonas mobilis* in a
Continuous Fluidized-Bed Reactor
(FBR). **2002**, http://www.scied.science.
doe.gov/scied/abstracts2000/
ornlchem.htm

20 P. Wittlich, E. Capan, M. Schlieker, K.-D.
Vorlop, U. Jahnz, Entrapment in Lenti-
Kats. In: V. A. Nedovic and R. Willaert
(ed.), Fundamentals of Cell Immobilisation Biotechnology, **2004**, 53–63. *Focus
on Biotechnology*. Hofman, M. and Anné,
Jozef. Kluwer Academic Publishers, Dordrecht.

21 VDI, Ökosprit mit Makel. *VDI-Nachrich-
ten*, **2004**, 9, 11.

22 S. K. Ritter, Green Reward – Presidential
honors recognize innovative syntheses,
process improvements, and new products that promote pollution prevention.
*Chemical and Engineering News, Science
and Technology*, **2003**, 81, 26, 30–35.

23 U. Jahnz, M. Schubert, H. Baars-Hibbe,
K. D. Vorlop, Process for producing the
potential food ingredient DFA III from
inulin: screening, genetic engineering,
fermentation and immobilisaton of inulase II. *International Journal of Pharma-
ceutics*, **2003**, 256, 199–206.

24 U. Jahnz, M. Schubert, K. D. Vorlop,
Effective development of a biotechnical
process: Screening, genetic engineering,
and immobilization for the enzymatic
conversion of inulin to DFA III on industrial scale. *Landbauforschung Völken-
rode*, **2001**, 51, 3, 131–136.

25 U. Prüße and K. D. Vorlop, The Jetcutter
technology. In: V. A. Nedovic and R.
Willaert (eds.), Fundamentals of Cell
Immobilisation Biotechnology, **2004**,
295–309. *Focus on Biotechnology*. Hofman, M. and Anné, J., Kluwer Academic
Publishers, Dordrecht.

26 S. Biella, L. Prati, M. Rossi, Selective oxidation of D-glucose on gold catalyst.
Journal of Catalysis, **2002**, 206, 2,
242–247.

Subject Index

Numbers in front of the page numbers refer to Volume 1 and 2: e.g., 2: 282 refers to page 282 in volume 2

Biorefineries – Industrial Processes and Products. Status Quo and Future Directions. Vol. 1
Edited by Birgit Kamm, Patrick R. Gruber, Michael Kamm
Copyright © 2006 WILEY-VCH Verlag GmbH & Co. KGaA, Weinheim
ISBN: 3-527-31027-4

paper industries, starch usage   2: 83
paper mill waste   1: 134
parasorbic acid, glucose product family
    1: 21
partial glycerides   2: 270
particle size, feedstock materials   1: 144
paste reactions, starch modifications   2: 77
pasture lands   1: 52
patents
– protein-based polymers   2: 245–249
– reexamination request   2: 245–249
Payen, A.   1: 6
PC   1: 30, 269, 271
– downstream processing   1: 281
PCB, lignin containing   2: 194
PCR technique   2: 225
PCS-hydrolyzing cellulases, improve-
    ments   1: 367
PD   1: 393–397
PDLA   2: 395
PDO   1: 11
peanut   2: 281
pearl corn starch, carbohydrate refining
    1: 351
pearling   1: 173–176
– oat grain   1: 183
pectin substances   1: 265
Penicillium   1: 202
pentaerythritol esters   2: 308
2,3-pentane dione, glucose product
    family   1: 21
"pentanes-plus"   1: 151
pentosan change, wet storage   1: 336
pentosans, conversion   2: 28
pentose fermentation   1: 206
pentose sugars   1: 78
pentoses   1: 91
– conversion   2: 28
peptide sequences, repeating   2: 217
Peptostreptococcus productus   1: 235
perfluoroalkyl iodides, addition   2: 263–264
perfluoroalkylated products, synthesis
    2: 263
performic acid procedure   2: 254
pericarp   1: 183
– wheat   1: 167
pericyclic reactions   2: 260–261
pesticides, lignin-based dispersants   2: 193
PET   2: 133
petrochemical industry   1: 86
– transformation steps   1: 88
petrochemical technology   2: 373
petroleum

– dependence   1: 115
– structural shift   1: 116
petroleum-based pathways, polyamides
    2: 45
petroleum chemistry, comparison with bio-
    mass   1: 118–122
petroleum costs   1: 48–50
petroleum dependence, reduction   1: 71
petroleum feedstocks   1: 45
petroleum refineries   1: 16
petroleum refining industry, develop-
    ment   1: 41
petroleum reserves, prognoses   1: 387
petroporphyrin formation   2: 332
petroporphyrins   2: 331–332
PF   2: 181
PF resins, markets   2: 183
pH adjustment   1: 79
PHA   1: 182, 214, 236, 239, 2: 44
– accumulation   1: 236
pharmaceuticals   1: 13, 2: 14–15
– intermediate   2: 40
– preparation   2: 26
– purification target level   2: 230
– starch usage   2: 88–89
phase III-biorefineries   1: 19–20
phase separated product, gross visualiza-
    tion   2: 229
phase separation, purification   2: 228
phase transition, Gibbs free energy   2: 234
PHB   1: 209, 238
– chemical structure   1: 214
– copolyesters   1: 215
– intracellular reserve material   2: 423
– lifetime of products   1: 214
– synthesis   1: 237–238
– yield determination   1: 238
PHB-PHV copolymer, brittleness   2: 426
phenol–formaldehyde resin   2: 181
phenol–formaldehyde resin markets,
    lignin   2: 187
phenolic acids   1: 178
phenolic–carbohydrate complexes, *Lolium
    perenne*   1: 264
phenolic molding compound market
    2: 184
phenolic resins   2: 16, 181, 185
– biorefinery lignin   2: 181–183
phenomenological axioms, engineering pro-
    tein-based polymers   2: 232–234
phenyl-propanoid units, crosslinked   2: 181
phenylpropane units   2: 157, 159
– bonding   2: 153–156